Essential Exercises for the Childbearing Year

Other Books by Elizabeth Noble

Having Twins: A Guide to Health and Comfort Before and After Your Baby is Born (2nd ed. 1991)

Childbirth with Insight

Marie Osmond's Exercises for Mothers-to-Be

Marie Osmond's Exercises for Mothers and Babies

Having Your Baby by Donor Insemination

Primal Connections: How Our Experiences from Conception to Birth Influence our Emotions, Behavior, and Health

The Joy of Being a Boy, with Leo Sorger, M.D.

Essential Exercises for the Childbearing Year

A Guide to Health and Comfort Before and After Your Baby is Born

Elizabeth Noble, P.T.

Foreword by Raul Artal, M.D.
Chairman and Professor of Obstetrics and Gynecology,
State University of New York, Syracuse

Editorial Consulting and
Afterword by Louis Keith, M.D.
Professor of Obstetrics and Gynecology,
Northwestern University Medical School, Chicago

Fourth edition

New Life Images

To Leo—my partner in love, life, and work.

Library of Congress Cataloging-in-Publication Data

Noble, Elizabeth, date 1995. Essential exercises for the childbearing year: a guide to health and comfort before and after your baby is born/ Elizabeth Noble: foreword by Raul Artal. 4th edition.
288p.
Includes bibliographical references and index.
ISBN 0-9641183-1-9
1. Pregnant women—Health and hygiene. 2. Exercise for women.
3. Prenatal care. 4. Postnatal care. 1. Title. RG558.7. N62 1995
618.2'4—dc19
95-070933
CIP
Printed in the United States of America

CRS 14 13 12 11 10 9 8 7 6 5 4 3 2

Typesetting and layout by Amy Rothstein, Waltham, Massachusetts

Contents

Acknowledgments

My thanks to Raul Artal for many years of friendship, for his continuing interest in linking physical therapy and obstetrics, and for inviting me to address obstetricians attending a course at the Annual Congress of the American College of Obstetricians and Gynecologists (ACOG). Dr. Artal spearheaded the Guidelines for Exercise first issued by ACOG in 1985 and again in 1994. The foremost pioneer in the realm of pregnancy and exercise, his foreword to this fourth edition of *Essential Exercises* is an endorsement I deeply appreciate.

I also thank Louis Keith for his excellent editing of this manuscript. He brings to this edition not only his thirty years of clinical knowledge as an obstetrician, but a remarkable command of English grammar and expression. His thoroughness is truly impressive. Time and again, his turn of phrase dramatically clarified a point. I was fortunate to benefit from his dual expertise on an earlier occasion, in 1988, when he kindly wrote the foreword to the second edition of *Having Twins.*

My husband, Leo Sorger, also scrutinized the manuscript, sharing his obstetrical expertise and proof-reading skills. My seven-year old son Carsten, who nursed at the keyboard during my prior writing project, now helped by walking on my back after long sessions at the computer!

The thousands of childbearing women who have joined my classes or consulted me over the years have taught me more than any text. I am grateful for these experiences and trust that the continued life of *Essential Exercises* stands as my commitment to their health and well-being.

Most of the art work in each addition has been done by Maya M. Jacob with some occasional alterations. We have watched the featured pregnant woman mature over twenty years!

Mike Andolina, computer consultant, brought good humor to some frustrating situations in the creation of the jacket. Amy Rothstein helped to pull it all together for this author when becoming a publisher as well grew overwhelming.

My family—Leo, Julia, and Carsten—provide the personal inspiration and support that every writer needs during the gestation and birth of a book. My love and thanks to them, as always.

Foreword

In my twenty-five years of practicing obstetrics, I have witnessed two revolutions in pregnancy and childbirth. One revolution centers on today's advanced medical technology and our increased scientific understanding of reproduction. The second revolution rests with today's woman and the way that she and her partner approach pregnancy, childbirth and parenthood. The days are now gone when it was the doctor who "called the shots" throughout the pregnancy, even dictating when and how a baby would be born. Even though I was an obstetrician, I was not allowed to be present for the birth of my first child!

Today, the woman, and usually, her partner, make the decisions with the guidance of her health care provider who can provide medical intervention if it's needed. Therefore, today's woman needs to be fully informed. Typically, she combines a career with pregnancy and parenthood, and is also more physically active than women of her mother's generation. Pregnancies are often carefully planned, with a renewed focus on health, diet, medication and exercise even before conception. Pregnancy is a time for the entire family to take stock of health habits and to alter those that are detrimental. Elite athletes are concerned to maintain their competitive status, but they also want to know about nutrition, possible occupational hazards, and numerous other aspects of pregnancy and childbirth. Women who are at high risk for pregnancy loss are even more concerned about the effects of lifestyle on their pregnancies.

Throughout history, women have been given all sorts of advice on physical activity during pregnancy, and how best to deal with pregnancy and childbirth. These advisers have ranged from physicians and midwives to some of our greatest philosophers and statesmen. Early observers correlated an uneventful pregnancy and easy labor with physical activity. In the third century B.C., for example, Aristotle attributed difficult childbirth to a sedentary lifestyle. In Exodus, Chapter 1, Verse 19, the Biblical writers observed that the Hebrew slave women had an easier time giving birth than their Egyptian mistresses: ". . . the Hebrew women are not as the Egyptian women; for they are lively, and are delivered ere the midwives come in unto them."

By the eighteenth century, physicians generally supported the notion that physical activity during pregnancy was beneficial. In 1788 James Lucas, a surgeon at the Leeds General Infirmary in England, presented a paper to the Medical Society of London in which he advocated exercise during pregnancy on the premise that exercise would result in a smaller baby that would pass more easily through the birth canal.

Still, there were dissenters, and many physicians felt that pregnancy should be a time of rest and confinement. During the Victorian era an even more confining and paternalistic view toward women and what was fitting and healthy prevailed. To the Victorian lady, the confinement of pregnancy was just that. It was considered unseemly for a pregnant woman to engage in social activities or to even be seen outside her family setting.

However, by 1913 a handbook for pregnant women advised: "Walking is the best kind of exercise. Most women who are pregnant find that a two- to three-mile walk daily is all they enjoy, and very few are inclined to indulge in six miles, which is generally accepted as the upper limit. Very few outdoor sports can be unconditionally recommended to the prospective mother. Because athletic exercise is either too violent or else jolts the body a great deal, it is especially dangerous in the early months of pregnancy. All kinds of violent exertion should be avoided—a rule which at once excludes sweeping, scrubbing, laundry work, lifting anything that is heavy, and going up and down stairs hurriedly or frequently. The use of a sewing machine is also emphatically forbidden." Fortunately, by 1949 the US Children's Bureau recommended: "A moderate amount of exercise is good for anyone, and this is particularly true for pregnant woman. Unless you have been ill or unless there is some complication, you can continue your housework, gardening, daily walks, and even swim occasionally."

In 1993, Grantly Dick-Read, a South African obstetrician practicing in London, emphasized knowledge, relaxation and some specific prenatal exercises to reduce the need for pain medication in labor. A Russian named Velvovsky developed a psychoprophylaxis regimen for "painless" childbirth, which was introduced to the West in the 1950s by Dr. Fernand Lamaze and brought to the United States by a one of his patients, Marjorie Karmel. She, together with an Austrian-born physical therapist Elisabeth Bing, developed what has become the Lamaze Method. This preparation focused on mental distraction and breathing techniques to take the mother's mind off the pain of labor contractions. An American physical therapist, Mabel Lum Fitzhugh, published a handbook for use in exercise classes for expectant parents in 1955 and began training teachers of childbirth preparation.

Childbirth preparation classes continued to be offered in late pregnancy and emphasized mental preparation and relaxation techniques for labor, more than exercises in the prenatal and postpartum months. However, a British physiotherapist, Helen Heardman, advocated prenatal and postpartum exercise through her books and had traveled to Yale at the invitation of Dr. Herbert Thoms. Unfortunately, Heardman's career, and the adoption of prenatal and postpartum exercises, were set back several decades when she died in a car accident during that visit.

Heardman's text, *Physiotherapy in Obstetrics and Gynecology* was part of the curriculum studied by Elizabeth Noble in Australia during 1965. After gaining extensive experience as a physical therapist in obstetrics and gynecology, Elizabeth Noble moved to the Boston area. *Essential Exercises for the Childbearing Year*, her first of several books, was the result of the need she saw for pregnant women to begin basic exercises much earlier than the last trimester, when childbirth classes commenced. As Emmanuel Friedman, M.D. wrote in the foreword to the first edition, twenty years ago, one would expect the field of obstetrics and physical therapy to integrate naturally. But that did not begin in the United States until Elizabeth Noble founded and took a leadership role in the Section on Obstetrics and Gynecology (now the Women's Health Section) of the American Physical Therapy Association in 1977.

The first edition of this book was published in 1976, and soon after Elizabeth Noble established the first physical therapy clinic for women's health in the United States. There, she provided both the treatment and prevention of many orthopedic and gynecological problems that typically follow pregnancy in sedentary women. As she lectured around the country, childbirth educators began to offer more information about the abdominal and pelvic floor muscles, and special exercise classes for prenatal and pregnant women could be found in some of the larger cities.

The fitness boom of the 1970s also extended itself to pregnancy. By the 1980s, "go for the burn" became something of a rallying cry, and pregnant women were encouraged to join a rash of aerobic exercise programs and classes. Experts began to question whether the pendulum had again swung too far. Is it really safe for a pregnant woman to "go for the burn"? Did these classes consider the challenges and vulnerabilities of childbearing women? Too often, pregnant women just joined the ranks of the non-pregnant and attempted to keep up the pace—until they dropped out. Injuries affected pregnant women as much as non-pregnant, and the effects of these aerobic classes was counter to the primary intent of engaging in physical activities.

It is now well-established that exercise can have profound benefits for health. Nowadays there are some general guidelines for exercise during pregnancy that have evolved from the research and the experience of physicians and physical therapists. Of course, these are only guidelines—there's no single right way, and what is best for one woman is not necessarily so for another. I strongly support the concept that the woman should have the final say, together with the advice of her own obstetrician, who knows her personal health background. I also believe that pregnancy should not be a state of confinement.

Pregnant women are well-advised to participate in a sound program that incorporates regular, moderate exercise to aid circulation, increase muscle strength, improve posture, and enhance sleep and well-being. *Essential*

Exercises offers such a program, as well as exercises designed for women on bed rest. The author of this book has a profound understanding of the physical aspects of exercise and explains in detail the role of the muscles involved during pregnancy, labor, birth and postpartum. The rationale for each position and movement is provided, along with warnings about errors and misunderstandings. There are valuable tips on posture, relaxation, and also exercises to involve a partner in preparation for labor.

For over thirty years, Elizabeth Noble has seen the benefits of her well-supervised, sensible program for pregnant and postpartum women, and she has shared her extensive experience across the United States and abroad. I personally have invited Elizabeth to teach at the facilities I have directed, and to introduce the physical therapist's view to obstetricians. It is with great respect and admiration for her work that I introduce this book to you. It undoubtedly presents the role of physical therapy during pregnancy and postpartum in the most complete fashion.

Raul Artal, M.D., F.A.C.O.G.
Professor and Chairman
Department of Obstetrics and Gynecology
State University of New York
Syracuse, New York

Introduction

Essential Exercises for the Childbearing Year was my first book, and I now have the pleasure of publishing this expanded and updated fourth edition myself, after gaining experience and insights from several other publications. I can offer my readers the broadest possible revisions, new content, and additional methods of presentation, without the inevitable constraints of a publisher. Perhaps more importantly in this age of changing communication, *Essential Exercises* is also available by individual chapters, as well as electronically.

Twenty years have passed since I wrote the first edition of *Essential Exercises*. The structure and function of the human body hasn't changed, and neither have the basic exercises. However, after two children, thousands of hours of experience with pregnant and postpartum women, and the opportunity to polish my material through many lectures and workshops, simply put, I have changed. I have more to say, and I can say it better. I have been surprised at just how extensively I have rewritten this book, this fourth time around; barely a sentence remains unrevised.

I've been privileged to work in women's health for thirty years. My training as a physiotherapist was in Australia, where prenatal and postpartum exercise, childbirth education and non-surgical treatments for gynecological conditions such as incontinence were and remain mainstream for my profession. On moving to the United States in 1973, I was surprised to discover how poorly recognized women's health issues were in general, and by physical therapists in particular. In those days, fortunate pregnant women could find only a childbirth preparation class during the last trimester—which couldn't possibly help them with the backache or leaky bladder that had happened long before. Moreover, the concept of postpartum exercise in American hospitals was virtually non-existent and absolutely not offered to Cesarean mothers who needed it more. Rather, these mothers were routinely encouraged to stay in bed for seven to ten days in order to "regain their strength." Sadly, a great number of women went through their entire reproductive cycle of many pregnancies with little education and support.

Despite these rather bleak circumstances, I discovered a grassroots network of women willing to share information. *Our Bodies, Ourselves* was first published in 1970 and I joined a group of women who met for self-examination of the cervix, with speculum and mirror, among other activities. I became the medical liaison for *Homebirth Inc.*, to search for doctors willing to provide back-up obstetric assistance if required. Hospital birth in the early Seventies was either the style of huffing/puffing/breath-holding or spinal anesthesia that so numbed women they could only observe the event in a small overhead mirror instead of feeling their birth. Typically they would comment, as they watched the emergence of their babies from their shaved, heavily-draped bodies, "Oh, it's like watching TV!" It was inspiring to meet women from the other camp, who would cross state lines and fight like a tiger for a natural birth or VBAC.[1] Regrettably, those earth mothers were more prevalent in the Seventies than they are in the Nineties.

The Growth of Physical Therapy in Women's Health

In 1977 I founded the section on Obstetrics and Gynecology of the American Physical Therapy Association (APTA), which is now called the Section on Women's Health. (Readers can find referrals to a physical therapist in their area by contacting the APTA. See Resources.) Physical therapists have always been aware that back pain—that ubiquitous complaint in modern sedentary society—invariably started in their women patients during or after a pregnancy. There are wide-ranging opportunities for prevention and education in a host of other common conditions, such as pelvic pain, incontinence, menstrual disorders, osteoporosis, to name just a few.

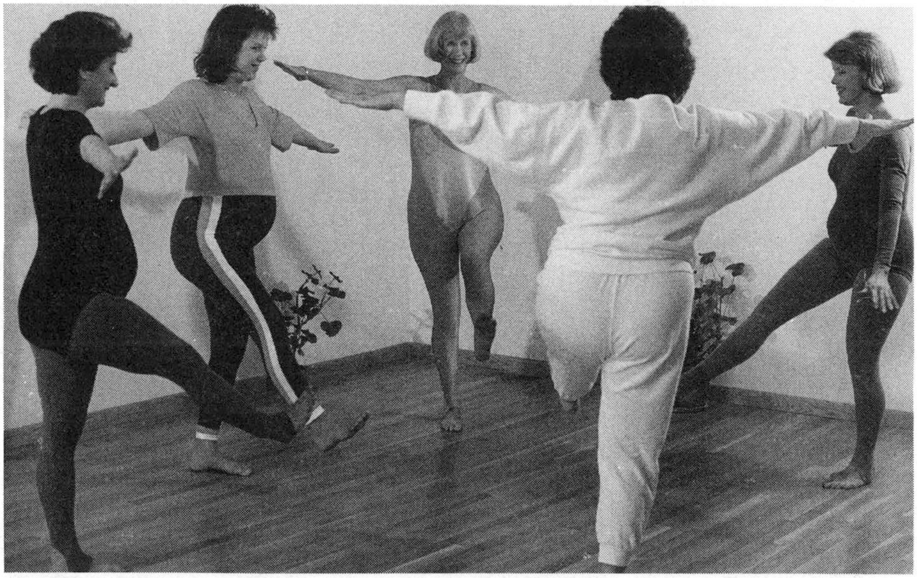

DOUG LONG, LONGSHOTS

Figure 1. Group exercise brings pregnant women together.

I also established a women's health clinic in the Boston area with the vision of providing a comprehensive center where I could pursue such a clinical practice and to offer families support and sharing throughout the entire childbearing year,[2] from conception through to postpartum. Back then, women needed a haven where they were welcome **because** they were pregnant, rather than following a lifestyle **in spite** of being pregnant. Today I think they need it even more. The economic pressures on many women to earn income until the day they deliver, together with the desire to keep their jobs, along with the social conventions that push impossible ideals of motherhood, create highly stressful challenges for increasing numbers of individuals.

When I handed over that practice in 1990, a variety of programs were offered, including ten prenatal and postpartum exercises classes each week. In addition, the Center held *Childbirth Preparation* classes, *Mom and Baby* classes, *Parenting* groups, and occasionally sessions such as *Father and Baby* (the mothers went out to lunch), *Massage for Pregnant Couples, Gender Issues for Expectant and New Parents, Breastfeeding,* and movement and music classes for crawlers, and even toddlers. I also developed the *Pregnancy Playshop*[3]—an experiential weekend for five couples to explore personal issues that might undermine spontaneous birthing.

All the classes and courses that I teach are limited to a small number of participants to facilitate optimal sharing and personalization. For balance, I encourage pregnant women to do safe aerobic exercise recreationally, so that group time can be spent on precise positions and movements done under close supervision. With slow speed and soft music, extensive discussion is possible. The combination of psychosocial support and shared information, together with the library of books, videos and audiotapes turned out to be just as important to the women as the stretching, calisthenics and relaxation. In a 1½ hour prenatal exercise class, I devote at least twenty minutes to an experience such as guided imagery, meditation, communicating with the unborn baby, singing or exchanging a massage of the face, feet or back.

Education for Major Lifestyle Changes

For several years now I have trained others to provide such services. I travel to hospitals and clinics all around the country and help them set up similar programs. Exercise classes that begin in early pregnancy offer the chance for major lifestyle changes. Rarely do a group of healthy people meet at a critical time when they are highly-committed to improving their diet, self-care and relationships with others, including that of their unborn child. It is usually this last concern that provides the most powerful motivation for the women to attend an average of a hundred or more sessions of a prenatal exercise class. A secondary gain is the stronger sense of autonomy and empowerment that develops as these women move and stretch while exchanging information, expectations and fears. Placing childbearing year exercise programs in this broad context of lifestyle change and developing healthy habits is critical in these days of managed care. Most disease and early death in the United States are due to behavioral factors, typically poor nutrition and inadequate exercise. Women consume more health care services than do men, and they also make the most health care decisions for other family members. Ideally, health care targets women during a period of intense focus and commitment—the childbearing year.

After a book of detailed explanations about the childbearing body has been in print for two decades, one might ask if such a book is still needed. The answer is yes, very much so. The aerobics programs that have become popular (and in which the participants often look like they are afflicted with a form of the medieval "St. Vitus' Dance") help prevent cardiovascular disease, but do little for the abdominal muscles, pelvic floor or general body awareness. In the childbearing year, aerobic exercise can actually be a liability if the essential muscles—those of the abdomen and pelvic floor—are weak. The word *essential* in the title has a double meaning: first, *these two muscle groups are the most significant* for all women, and second, you must do these *specific* exercises, in addition to any sport or aerobics program, to prevent problems. People who exercise aerobically, without stretching, tend to become inflexible. Bouncing and jogging can cause or worsen bladder control.

Prevention of dysfunction and disease is an urgent priority considering the astronomical costs of the sickness industry in the United States. The Department of Health and Human Services, for example, issued a statement followed by several booklets, recommending that health care practitioners be proactive in questioning women about urinary incontinence. It was also advocated that non-surgical treatments such as exercise, biofeedback and electrical stimulation should be tried before surgery for this condition. As a result, numerous devices are available to help women regain continence. However, most of this equipment also rewards the user for incorrect muscle action because internal pressure is measured, and this pressure can be increased rightly (on exhalation) or wrongly (with breath-holding). To perform any exercise with care requires attention and understanding, as this entire book on just a few exercises shows. A trained health care provider is often necessary to help guide the integration of breathing and muscle action, at least initially. Physical therapists have the ideal background for this work.

Always understand the reason why.

I continue to caution readers to choose only books that provide a clear rationale for the specific exercise. It's easy to publish a book these days, and yoga instructors, childbirth educators, schoolteachers and other laypersons occasionally do. Some of these well-intentioned authors simply do not have the necessary training, experience, and skills to bring together and impart correctly the various aspects of exercise, anatomy and physiology during the childbearing year. Many of these manuscripts cross my desk. Only a couple of years ago, I was asked to provide some words of praise for a book wherein the author (amidst many other serious errors) recommended being upright for an active birth because this "decreased the drive angle of the uterus."[4] Actually, being upright **increases** the drive angle of the uterus; she had it exactly backward!

In a 1994 edition of a magazine[5] for childbirth educators, the "bow" position in yoga was recommended for postpartum exercise, because it "helps your abdominals." In fact, it stretches them, and breastfeeding mothers will not enjoy "see-sawing" on pubic bones and lactating breasts! I was about to delete the bow from this edition because I thought that people had the message by now. Apparently not, and so it can be found on page 43. In a 1995 booklet[6] for postpartum mothers I found double-leg lowering from a vertical position to the floor with straight legs all the way! This amount of leverage overpowers the ability of the abdominals to protect the lower back. I still see the "cat-back" recommended as a pelvic tilting exercise. This creates an ugly hunchback (see page 98), a tendency which women in general, and mothers in particular, already have. This movement just makes the hump worse! The adjustment is simple—lengthen your spine by increasing the distance between your hands and knees so that you can localize the movement to your pelvis instead of your upper back.

Other information may be simply erroneous rather than harmful. In a 1995 book on swimming in pregnancy,[7] the author describes how legs astride exercises stretch the pelvic floor muscles. (These muscles lie deep within the pelvis and are not attached to the legs, and when they are stretched, internal organs drop down!)

The persistent repetition of incorrect information continues to shock me. I receive a strong signal that important components of a position or movement must be made clear and obvious. I've found it an enjoyable challenge using the latest computer technology to present the facts to the best of my ability.

When I started with these exercises in my twenties, I did not realize their universal application. I still do them regularly at fifty; my children are aged 14 and 7 as I write this. The partner exercises in Chapter 8 were the foundation for a *Back Class* I developed. This program also included many of the same relaxation concepts that are helpful for pregnant women. Partner exercises will remain on my agenda for the rest of my life, and, I hope, on yours too.

Say Good-bye to "Don't" and "Try"

As a writer for more than two decades, I have learned the power of specific words. The unconscious mind hears no negatives; therefore, when someone says, "Don't . . . ," part of you immediately **wants to do just that.** Children provide many examples of this ambivalent negation. They often end up doing exactly what you have said—so many times—**not** to do! I have trained myself over the years to phrase my advice and instructions in positive terms—whether for patients, students or my own children. "Keep every drop in the glass" is much more helpful than "Don't spill your juice." "Knees at ease" gives you an immediate picture, whereas "Don't lock your knees" is confusing because your mind hears "Lock your knees." Why would anyone say "Don't forget your lunch" rather than simply "Remember your lunch!"

"Try to . . . " is another counterproductive phrase you won't find in this book because it embodies the unconscious suggestion that you might not succeed. "Try" adds nothing to the instruction; it encourages undue effort and raises anxiety that your performance will be inadequate. Most people want to do their best. I prefer to say "Raise your leg as high as you can." Not only does it work better, but a positive sentence requires fewer words than **"Try to** raise your leg as high as you can."

New Additions

Two new chapters explain principles of exercise, and address the needs of women on restricted activity or bed rest. The enormous growth of interest in health and fitness during the past two decades motivated me to write about exercise precautions and progressions. The regrettable increase in the rates of preterm birth in this country led me to discuss common pregnancy complications and how to prevent diseases of recumbency.

- ✦ There is an **Appendix** on painful syndromes in pregnancy and simple remedies you can try yourself.
- ✦ The **Table of Contents** now includes chapter sub-headings for easy reference. I have added a **List of Illustrations**, and extensive **footnotes** because *Essential Exercises* is used in physical therapy, midwifery and childbirth education training.
- ✦ Photographs have included added to link the body mechanics with real-life action and images. The postpartum bellies will motivate you to get started right away!
- ✦ The **Summary Sheets of Prenatal, Postpartum and Post-Cesarean Exercises** at the end of the book, as well as individual chapters, may be bought in bulk for distribution in classes or clinics.
- ✦ The **Resources** list has been expanded to reflect the ever-growing demand for products and services during the childbearing year. **Order Forms** can be found at the back of the book, with information about my other books, audiotapes, and videotapes, as well as basic equipment that I recommend, such as gymnastic balls and Flo® tubes.
- ✦ A **Reader Response** card is enclosed. Please let me know your opinions, suggestions and experiences.

1

Pregnancy Creates a Special Need for Exercise

The Childbearing Year

Over the past twenty years, I have watched the number of prenatal exercise classes grow around the country, although there are still many areas where no programs exist. There are also many women who are simply too busy to take the time to make sure that they are in their best physical condition before and after birth. Other women focus on childbirth classes alone and overlook the needs of the whole body, which undergoes vast adaptation during the entire childbearing year from conception through postpartum adjustments. Physical preparation is important during pregnancy, but postpartum restoration is even more important. Whether you plan a hospital or home birth, with epidural or no regional anesthesia, your muscles, joints and tissues will be challenged by the changes that occur in the childbearing year. If you want to prevent future problems, it is essential that you strive to improve your physical condition and emotional state to meet these challenges. This advice applies to all childbearing women, whether they are having their first or fifth baby. Even if you are reading this book in the last months of pregnancy, you can and should begin the essential exercises.

Your body undergoes tremendous hormonal and physical changes during the nine months prior to birth but afterwards these changes must be reversed within days and weeks. Your abdominal muscles in pregnancy, for example, feel toned because they are stretched taut over your growing uterus. Then, in one day, Baby is born, and these same muscles are now in a lengthened state without the resistance of the uterus to keep them tight and responsive. Isometric exercises must be started immediately to shorten these muscles to their original length and to avoid laxity for years to come.

Labor and delivery signify both an end and a beginning. The months of waiting and preparation are over, and so is the physical effort and excitement of the birth. But the greatest change and stress of the childbearing year occur after the arrival of your baby. Your physical, emotional and psychological needs will be more pronounced than in pregnancy, yet many women tend to neglect rehabilitation because of the demands of their newborn. The rapid return of your physical efficiency and stamina must be a priority, especially if you are planning to resume work soon or have other children at home.

Muscles Must Meet the Challenge

Childbearing is a natural physiological event, but this creative process is a challenge that may place your body at risk. Just as you would equip your car with snow tires if you expected heavy winter conditions, so should you ensure that your body has extra help in its physical development at this time. You must provide support for your growing baby and avoid undue strain or gynecological problems. Inevitable changes that occur during pregnancy include stretching of muscles, softening of ligaments, and loosening of joints in order to make more room inside for your baby and to help in the birth process.

Figure 2. Stretching and strengthening prevent most of these typical problems of pregnancy.

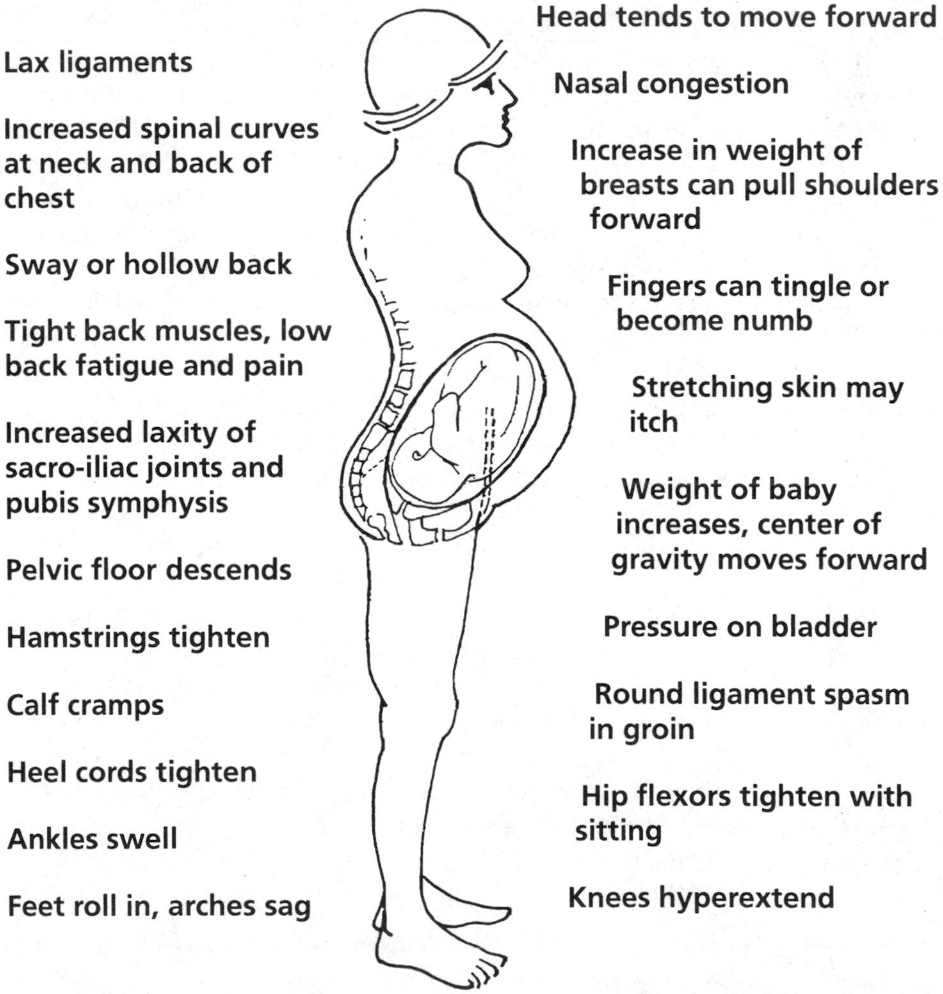

HORMONES < *soften tissue* / *joints loosen* — *BACKACHE*

EXERCISE < *stretching* / *strengthening* — *NO BACKACHE*

The muscles supporting your backbone, and those in front of and beneath your pelvis, all carry an increasing load during pregnancy, which alters their function if care is not taken. It is far from inevitable, in our sedentary society, that the structural supports of your body are adequate to meet and recover from these changes without exercise. Such exercise will provide significant benefits not only throughout the maternity cycle but for the rest of your life as well.

During birth, your uterus works by itself to ensure that your baby is born with or without additional expenditure of your voluntary muscles. It is more important to be in a position where your pelvis is free and to trust the process enough to let go. Preparation for the actual birth, then, is more for coordination and release than for maternal physical exertion. Stated another way, you will have confidence in your uterus to do its pre-ordained work. After delivery, your uterus will continue to have involuntary contractions, and by six weeks it will return to its original state. Neither the contractions nor the reduction in uterine size are under your control. Quite in contrast, only your physical efforts will return the other muscles to their former size and function.

Popularity of Exercise

In the last decade, the value of exercise has been increasingly promoted. Fitness clubs, the neighborhood "Y," adult education centers, community hospitals and even many hotels provide equipment, pools and classes. Unfortunately, competition (or just keeping up the pace) is often emphasized at the expense of enjoyment, body-building at the expense of flexibility, or pounding the pavement at the expense of damage to knees and ankles. Although women are becoming more visible in sports and physical exercise, most pregnant women are as sedentary as the rest of the population. Three-quarters of adults exercise less than three times a week, and half of them exercise on weekends only.[7]

The role of movement in preventing diseases associated with inactivity (obesity, stroke, diabetes, heart ailments, emotional problems) is now widely acknowledged. Research performed by Professor Hans Kraus[8] of New York University showed that 80 percent of cases of back pain are due to lack of adequate physical activity. Despite this awareness, many people still merely undertake seasonal fits of activity, such as tackling the winter flab before venturing out in beach attire or limbering up as the ski season approaches. Although we know that all of us would benefit from daily physical exercise, we are more likely to take the body for granted and to worry about making special efforts only when it seems threatened in some way or when we have in mind a goal that requires physical preparation.

Preventive Exercise for the Childbearing Year

The childbearing year is both a season and a goal for which physical preparation and restoration are both essential and rewarding. Often the special needs of pregnancy are recognized only when they have **not** been attended to. The new mother may look aghast at her "ruined figure" after childbirth. Her self-esteem feels as collapsed as her sagging posture, extra folds of flesh, and fallen arches. Some women, on the other hand, accept their "lot" with resignation and the typical excuse of "that's what having a baby does to you."

These external changes are well-recognized, but the frequent internal disturbances are far less understood. Even if you are not concerned with appearances, any impaired function of your mind or body is upsetting. A floppy belly is one thing, but problems with pelvic organ support, urine control or comfort during intercourse are as unnecessary as they are common. These symptoms, arising from childbearing, may be slow to develop and may subtly manifest themselves as pelvic pressure, fatigue and frustration. If some of these signs are ignored initially, with the passage of years and subsequent pregnancies, surgical repair may be necessary. Unfortunately many women put off mentioning incontinence to their health care provider, often for years.

This book emphasizes three important points: the first is the need for women to understand their bodies; the second is to enjoy being female while living and working in a man's world; and the last, and perhaps most important, is to find empowerment that can come from the mothering experience.

A woman's place is in her body. —*Jeannine Parvati Baker*

Healthy living is not something that arrives in a neatly-wrapped plastic package. The key concept for any healthy woman's continuing good health is prevention. Gaining knowledge about preventing unnecessary problems is the best approach. Since the childbearing year is not a time of illness, developing a better understanding of the essentials of health maintenance must be seen as an educational process. It is your responsibility to yourself during a natural, although challenging, process of many inevitable bodily changes. You can establish a lasting pattern in which exercise:

- ✦ Maintains optimal muscle length and strength;
- ✦ Relieves nervous tension;
- ✦ Enhances the benefits of good nutrition;

✦ Becomes an essential component of healthy living.

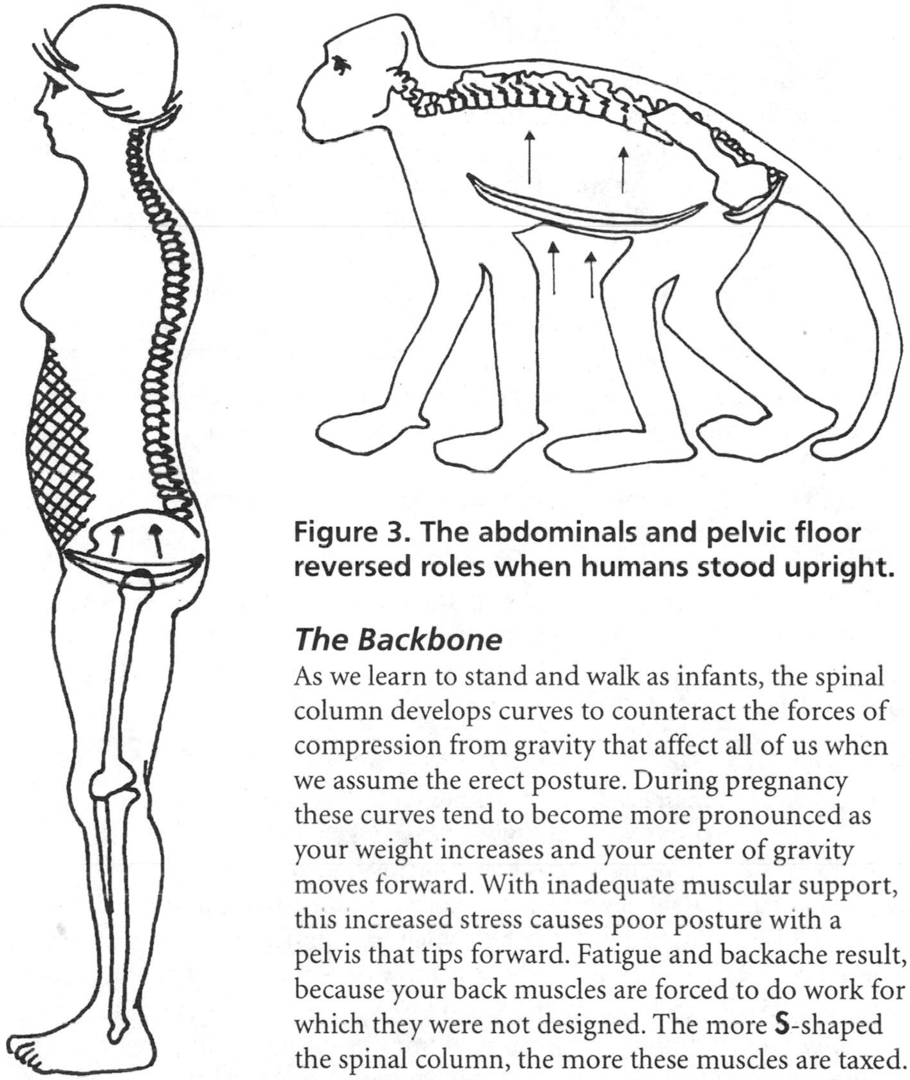

Figure 3. The abdominals and pelvic floor reversed roles when humans stood upright.

The Backbone

As we learn to stand and walk as infants, the spinal column develops curves to counteract the forces of compression from gravity that affect all of us when we assume the erect posture. During pregnancy these curves tend to become more pronounced as your weight increases and your center of gravity moves forward. With inadequate muscular support, this increased stress causes poor posture with a pelvis that tips forward. Fatigue and backache result, because your back muscles are forced to do work for which they were not designed. The more **S**-shaped the spinal column, the more these muscles are taxed.

The abdominal muscles, on the other hand, which support the spine against gravity in four-legged animals, do very little in the vertical position that humans customarily assume. They do even less work in our industrialized society because we mostly sit or stand. These essential muscles, during pregnancy, have the task of supporting the growing weight of your baby; consequently they must be stronger and more elastic than usual. Just as a tomato plant, laden with fruit, tends to droop forward and needs to be splinted to a support, so the abdominal muscles become stretched over the pregnant uterus and may be further weakened through neglect or incorrect use. Strong abdominals will support the backbone just as a stake will keep the tomato plant upright and allow it to branch without sagging.

Your Pelvic Floor

The pelvic floor is one of the least understood areas of the human body. It has many names and includes several muscle groups.[9] The main function of the pelvic floor is to keep the abdominal and pelvic organs from sagging down. In contrast with the abdominal muscles, and in response to gravity, more physical stress has been placed on the pelvic floor since we became upright. The pelvic floor must withstand increased pressure within the body during straining, lifting, elimination. In four-legged animals these muscles are much more extensive, arising from the whole of the pelvic brim. Even though we don't have a tail to wag, we do have the power to move our pelvic floor muscles to counteract the forces to which they are subjected. However, this necessary muscle action is poorly developed in most modern women. Pregnancy further jeopardizes the vulnerable pelvic floor because of the increased weight of the enlarging uterus. During vaginal birth the baby passes through the pelvic floor, greatly stretching and occasionally injuring it. Women who suffer a miscarriage, or who are delivered by Cesarean section, may also develop pelvic floor problems. The actual birth, then, is one factor that causes pelvic floor problems, but the long-standing pressure of the uterus on the hormonally softened tissues has a major influence, too.

Modern Life and the Upright Position

The course of human evolution, together with the cultural and technological developments that relieve us of physical exertion, explain why women today, more than ever before, need to exercise during and after pregnancy. Pregnancy accentuates the potential problems inherent in human evolutionary development. Unlike the brain and the hand, which have undergone remarkable refinement, the larger, more basic parts of the body have progressed little in evolutionary terms. When humans first stood on two legs, the structural supporting system became modified and the role of muscles in supporting the bony framework and the body cavity contents in the upright position became paramount. Unfortunately, our modern way of life, which allows the under-use of most muscles and the persistent overuse of others, causes certain parts of the body to merge as points of structural weakness and potential trouble. The vulnerable areas in women are, most significantly, the backbone, the abdominal muscles, and the layers of muscles forming the floor to the pelvic cavity.

Pregnancy taxes the weakest parts of a woman's body and exposes the liabilities of a sedentary lifestyle.

Of course, our forebears had to contend with these potential problems in human architecture and babies have always come out the same way. What, if anything, has changed? Only our physical condition! The key muscles involved in childbearing are just not adequately exercised during housework, neighborhood strolls or even during most aerobics and sports. Significantly, pregnancy worsens the potential structural weaknesses of the muscles in upright creatures. The comforts of modern life have more and more removed us from the routine physical work that compensates for these structural weaknesses by muscular development. We sit too much. We use clothes dryers instead of bending and stretching at the line. If you ever drive a car without power steering, or use a manual typewriter after an electronic keyboard, you have felt how labor-saving devices make us weak.

If that were not enough, leisure activities today are often not physical at all. For example, it seems to me that the major family recreation these days is to stroll at the local mall, eat fast food that bodies don't welcome, and buy more possessions that people don't need. Movies and video games are further examples of sedentary recreation. Obviously our muscles are underutilized when compared with those of women who work in fields or perform domestic functions, such as washing, preparing and cooking food while squatting, or sitting without the support of a chair. If you've ever dined on the floor of a traditional Japanese restaurant, you know how accustomed your body has become to furniture!

Understanding the Benefits of Exercise

Clearly, our cultural and personal habits have as much or more effect as evolution or inherited factors on the physical state of our bodies. The best way to meet the physical challenges of the childbearing experience is to understand them and to act in a manner to prevent damage. Waiting until you are forced to react may mean putting yourself in the hands of orthopedic or gynecological specialists. Recuperation then can be a real problem, since so many of women's household chores are often unavoidable and will aggravate conditions such as backache.

Preparation for childbirth and restoration afterward is not complicated or strenuous. Nor are athletic skills required as some books on prenatal and postpartum exercises seem to imply! Actually, you need to do many more of the easier exercises and far fewer of the harder ones. Moreover, you need to know the **rationale** for the exercises that you are doing or not doing. It's like selecting the most nutritious items in the supermarket when many other items of dubious dietary value may look or taste good. A decision is involved; however, in order to make an informed choice you need to know certain facts. As there is plenty of material that provides information on a general keep-fit regime, this manual will focus on the essential aspects of female physique that many fitness books overlook, especially during the childbearing year.

The responsibility of women today is to become informed consumers, especially when they become mothers.

I have designed an effective program for the woman with little time or little inclination to exercise, or one who has doubts about what is wise and safe in her condition. This program also works for every woman, whether she would normally exercise at any other time or not, who realizes that special needs must be met in pregnancy and postpartum. It is even useful for athletic women who may have a high level of fitness, but may have difficulty relaxing or suffer from pelvic floor dysfunction. *Essential Exercises for the Childbearing Year* is for every pregnant or postpartum woman, especially those whose activity level is restricted.

Throughout the book, there are detailed explanations to help you evaluate your body at the various stages of the childbearing year. If you learn to recognize early signs of weakness and dysfunction, you can usually reverse these problems with corrective exercise. You will notice that the muscles that you prepare before birth are the same ones that you restore afterward.

No exercise program is complete unless it includes ways to achieve good breathing habits and relaxation skills throughout the sequence of pregnancy, labor, delivery and postpartum. Your mate, other family members and friends can benefit from learning these skills of lasting value with you (see Chapter 8, Partner Exercises).

Physical Changes During Pregnancy

An obvious goal of prenatal exercises is to help your body better carry the load of pregnancy. In the most general sense this means developing good posture. Exercises for the abdominal and pelvic floor muscles maintain adequate support of the pelvis and its contents, including your growing baby.

The Vulnerable Midline

Your baby's growth puts a strain on a "central seam" that extends from the lower border of your breastbone to your coccyx, uniting the two sides of your abdominal muscles, pubic bones and pelvic floor. The union of the abdominals may stretch and bulge, pain may be felt between your pubic bones, and pelvic floor laxity is common.

While some relaxation of the pelvic joints is normal in pregnancy, the extent of joint instability and discomfort varies. There are techniques to help resolve these problems which can be found in the Appendix.

Posture

Postural problems are frequent in pregnancy for two reasons. First, the body adapts to structural changes, which alter its center of gravity; and, second, it responds to hormonal changes which affect the stability of joints. As a consequence, the alignment and balance of all body segments must adjust along with these changes. These adjustments occur mostly at an unconscious level because of automatic righting reflexes. Together these reflexes form a complex mechanism that enables your body to know its position in space, so you can get around without looking at your feet, holding onto things or falling over. Poor postural habits, often developed over years, tend to restrict the adjustment process and poor posture will need evaluation and conscious ongoing correction. Stretching tight muscles and strengthening weak ones is the foundation of improved body alignment.

The childbearing state certainly does not mean that you must suffer poor posture. On the contrary, exercise and re-education are of great value in preventing this. Obviously, unlearning bad habits, which may have existed for a long time, requires more effort than simply learning and maintaining good posture.

You'll learn how to align the parts of your body in whatever position you assume (particularly your habitual posture in standing and in working). Good posture protects your joints from strain, and energy from using unnecessary muscles is saved. Proper exercises also help prevent much of the discomfort, backache and fatigue that plague many women—pregnant or not—who spend much time leaning over counters and sinks, peering into the oven and fridge, and reaching down to children and objects on the floor.

Changes in your center of gravity

During pregnancy, women tend to stand farther back on their heels because the center of gravity moves forward with the weight increase in front. Some women compensate for this backward stance by tilting the pelvis farther forward and increasing the hollowing in the lower back, or else by swaying back from the waist. Whatever the form of compensation, it is uncomfortable and unattractive. Most of us don't realize our posture is faulty until we experience some symptoms of pain or deformity. These may not arise for many years, by which time muscles and other tissues will have shortened or stretched, often to a significant degree. In pregnancy, however, symptoms resulting from poor posture appear much more quickly, whether from a latent weakness, a disturbance of posture or from the normal hormonal softening of ligaments.

Pregnancy is a time to become attuned to your body and your baby.

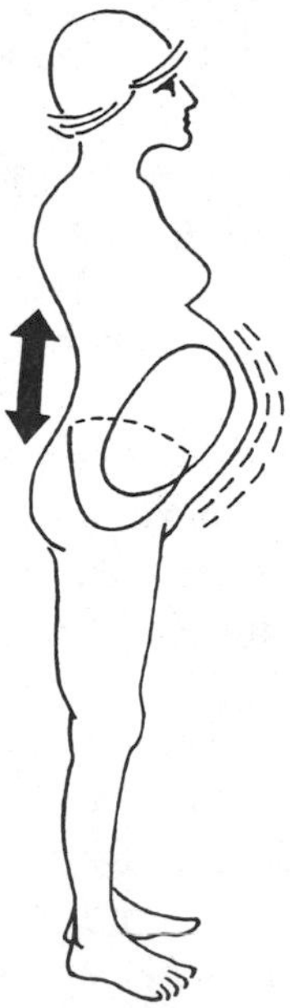

Figure 4. Like a bowstring, the back muscles tend to shorten as the abdominals lengthen.

As your center of gravity shifts forward, your back muscles work harder. Your muscles may become so stretched and weakened in front, and tensed and shortened in back, that they do not respond to the stretch stimulus that normally helps maintain good posture at a reflex level. When the muscles don't do their share, joints and ligaments become overloaded.

The general aim of exercises and postural training is to enable you not only to **see** the difference but to **feel** it. When postural awareness is achieved at a conscious level, it must be adequately reinforced to cause a transfer to unconscious levels of control. This way you can protect your body against sudden backache occurring from even a minor trauma.

Cultivate a variety of positions

A discussion of positions and body mechanics will help you avoid poor working habits, strain and injury. We have seen that joints become loosened during pregnancy because of softened fibrous tissue. Keep the muscles of your lower abdomen and buttocks strong to compensate because they are attached to your pelvis. Squatting to floor level rather than leaning from your waist maintains mobility of the joints, but at the same time protects them by a stable position of minimal strain.

Your Abdominal Muscles

Your abdominal muscles need to be as elastic as possible, because they must stretch to accommodate your baby. Indeed, their fibrous union in the midline of the body is often stretched wide toward the end of pregnancy or during labor. Weakness of your abdominals reduces your ability to push out your baby. Backache can occur in a first pregnancy or subsequently, because your back muscles are forced to compensate for your abdominals in holding your spine erect. Gas and constipation are more frequent when sluggish intestinal activity results from a slack abdominal wall and insufficient exercise. In the worst possible case, the muscles do not come back together after birth and a hernia can result.

Relaxation

Relaxation skills that you develop now will prove valuable for the rest of your life. Relaxation is more than just rest. It is also body awareness and tension reduction—muscles are frequently tense and tight as well as weak. Since we express emotions as well as carry out movements with our muscles, even the most subtle mental irritation can influence our muscular state. Most of our anger and annoyance from the hassles of daily life is suppressed; however, this process often accumulates stress in our body systems. Regular relaxation helps things to go more smoothly during the childbearing year and later when you have to cope with more distractions and anxious moments. Exercise and relaxation obviously are most essential on those frustrating days when you feel the most pressed and are likely to skip them. Indeed, studies show that regular exercise and relaxation helps depression (and chronic pelvic pain[10]) as much as any medication.

Breathing

Good breathing habits are necessary, especially while exercising, since both you and your baby benefit from an optimal supply of oxygen. Slow, deep breathing aids your blood circulation and its soothing rhythm helps you to relax. Of equal importance, knowing when to inhale and when to exhale is essential for the proper performance of exercises in general, and of the pelvic floor and abdominals in particular.

Breathing patterns requiring mental concentration have been commonly taught in childbirth classes as distraction techniques during labor contractions. (For some women this is a way of coping—but I have a simpler preparation that is much more effective. See Chapter 6.) Any control of an involuntary process, such as breathing, interferes with awareness and leads to effort and tension. Most of us quicken our respiration under stress, but over-breathing (hyperventilation) during contractions must be prevented. Excessive breathing results in an oxygen surplus for the mother (if carried to extremes this will cause her to faint) and has the **reverse** effect on the baby—whose oxygen is **decreased.** Easy, relaxed breathing maintains the best physiological balance, keeps you in a psychological state of calm and confidence, and conserves your energy.

Labor and Birth

Being in good physical condition enhances your relaxation and cooperation during the first stage of labor (when your role is passive and your uterus works by itself) and helps prepare for effective bearing-down during the second stage (when you may need to work actively to assist your uterus in pushing out your baby). If you are physically fit, you'll cope better with both mental and physical stress. You will have greater stamina if your labor is long or arduous. Your confidence will be increased when you know that your body is strong and healthy, and you can welcome the power of the birth process.

Childbirth Preparation

Childbearing is a fundamental biological process, but it is also a social and cultural experience. As such, it has been distorted by fear, ignorance, superstition and myth over thousands of years. These essentially negative influences should have no place in modern society, where opportunities for information and education exist and childbirth is substantially safer than crossing the road.

Birth is as safe as life gets. —*Harriette Hartigan*

Unfortunately, the increasing medicalization of the birth process causes many couples to doubt that the process is natural. Indeed, for some people, the very meaning of natural childbirth today has been reduced to a vaginal delivery, usually with an epidural, versus a Cesarean!

Preparation classes for childbirth are commonplace now. Guidance and group interaction are positive factors in any education. Emotional and psychological preparation are just as important as physical preparation. You feel less isolated when you discuss experiences with other expectant parents, and there is always something to be learned from others. A partner who accompanies you is of great value in sharing your emotional growth through this passage, boosting your morale, and providing reassurance as well as comfort measures and physical assistance in labor. The educated expectant mother, with or without a support person, is better able to attend to her body's messages, whatever kind of labor and birth she may experience.

Women must feel secure and self-reliant, and trust their bodies and their own resources.

Labor is a **process** that must be appreciated and trusted; it is often obscured by techniques and interventions. Preparation and active participation in the birth process reduce the need for medication and/or obstetrical interference. The actual birth generally takes less than a day and the nature of specific events is outside your control. Preparation for this occasion may seem more important than prenatal exercise. However, pregnancy and the postpartum state, with their immense changes that endure for months, have far-reaching effects. It seems logical, then, to view training for these adaptive phases as equally important as the birth itself. Significantly, those muscles that require preparation and restoration, unlike the uterus, are under voluntary control.

When to Start Exercises

The essential exercises can be begun at any time and **continued throughout life** as they also will maintain your health and comfort through the coming decades. Ideally, begin exercising as soon as possible, even before conception. You can always modify the exercises in later pregnancy, if necessary.[11]

If you have established a regular program before your baby arrives, it will be much easier to continue after birth, with the added distractions. It will also be easier on you mentally, because you have already made the commitment and established a pattern of regular exercise. Finally, it will be easier physically, because a healthy, active muscle regains its shape, elasticity and function much sooner than a neglected one.

Exercises after delivery should be begun as soon as possible—certainly within 24 hours. The greatest changes occur in the first week. The muscle work that you need to do in the immediate postpartum is not strenuous or in any way potentially harmful. Patients who have had major surgery do such exercises the first day. You must exercise for short periods and very often, to coax the stretched muscles back to their former length and tone. **This initial step must be achieved before starting any strengthening programs involving resistive exercises.** If you pull in your abdominal muscles isometrically and consistently, you will be ready to advance to movements after the first few days.

After birth you will concentrate on rehabilitation. Physiological changes normally occur in hours and days; in contrast, exercises need days and weeks to show results. The whole process takes 12 months—the childbearing year. However, it is not uncommon for women to take up to another nine months if they ignore the **early** postpartum phase.

Good postural habits need to be re-established. You must consciously contract your abdominal and pelvic floor muscles to balance your pelvis again after the sudden loss of its load. Your joints remain at risk for some weeks, even months, because of the hormonal effects of pregnancy. Good body mechanics are absolutely essential to protect your joints and ligaments while your muscles regain their former length and strength.

Figure 5. The belly is still very large right after birth.

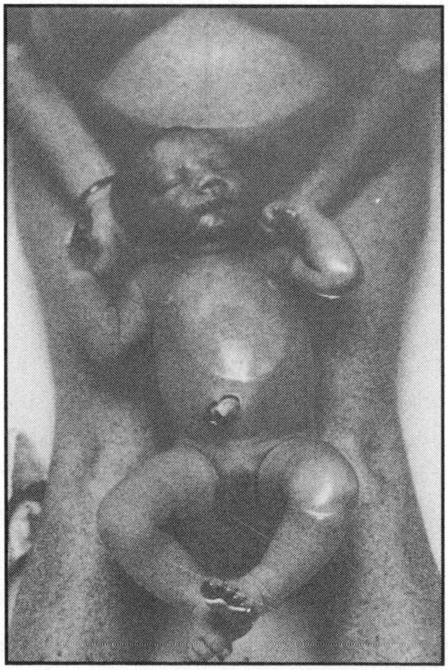

HARRIETTE HARTIGAN

After birth, the abdominal muscles display the most obvious need for immediate attention. Exercises are designed **first to shorten** and eventually to strengthen them. Your pelvis must be realigned in its correct relationship to your spine. With regard to the contour of your belly, please note the absence of straight lines in nature! However, in the United States, where two Barbie dolls are sold every second and Miss America gets thinner every year, a body with curves is not viewed as desirable. The art and sculpture of other cultures, nevertheless, attest to a more natural and realistic female body than the skin, bones and skeletal apparatus featured in American fashion magazines!

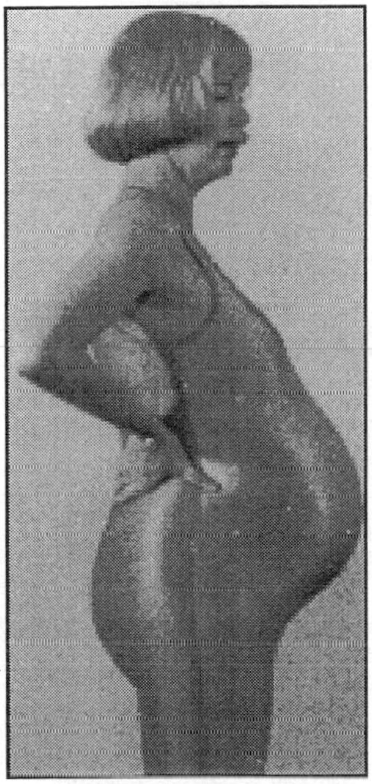

Figure 6. Curves are sensuous; who wants to look like a hat rack?

The first task postpartum is to shorten your stretched abdominal wall. Sucking in your belly on outward breath accomplishes this during the first few days—if you do it **constantly.** Before you attempt stronger exercises, a self-check, described in Chapter 4, must be made to check that your abdominal muscles are parallel again at your midline.

Pelvic Floor Exercises

After birth your vagina will feel slack and stretched. Pelvic floor exercises tighten muscles to re-establish control of your bladder and bowel. The longer you delay rehabilitation, the more muscle wasting or atrophy will take place. Because the pelvic floor muscles are internal and invisible, your most reliable guide is how well they function. Pelvic floor weakness has far greater ramifications for a woman than does weakness of the abdominal muscles, although laxity of the abdominal wall is more visible to the entire world. It is vital that you fully comprehend the function of the pelvic floor and any indicators of trouble.

You need to assess the state of these muscles before progressing with abdominal exercises. This is critical, because strong abdominal work can cause increased pressure on the pelvic floor, which can strain and further weaken muscles with inadequate withstanding power. Your breathing must be coordinated so that you are **always breathing out during effort.**

Exhale as you exert — every time.

Rest and Relaxation

After delivery you will need much sleep, rest and "true" relaxation. Lying on your front (on your stomach) with a pillow under your hips is a particularly comfortable position for relieving the pain of vaginal stitches. However, if you had a Cesarean, wait until you feel comfortable lying on your belly, even though it is a good position to relieve backache. In the early postpartum, you may need to place two pillows under your hips and one under your chest to avoid pressure on tender breasts.

If you have practiced the specific exercises in pregnancy, your muscles are prepared—and so are you. Nature takes care of internal changes like returning your uterus to its pre-pregnant size, but only you can bring about a change in the slackness of your voluntary muscles. The return in muscle strength varies from woman to woman, and from muscle to muscle in the same person. A program that states, "On Day 3, repeat Exercise B 10 times," is just not personalized. Arbitrary instructions, furthermore, make no allowances for any midline defects. Invariably such programs overlook the interaction between the breath, the abdominal muscles and the pelvic floor, which means that one group of muscles gets stronger at the expense of the other.

I have supplied detailed information to help you understand your key muscles and the essential role they play not just in this childbearing year but your childbearing years and later. You can avoid exercises that are pointless or harmful, such as double leg-raising. You will recognize that muscle length and tone must be restored before the muscles can be expected to perform strongly. Signs and symptoms of strain and weakness are described so you can evaluate your own abdominal and pelvic floor muscles and progress or modify exercises accordingly.

The Art of Prevention

Women, by the very nature of their reproductive system, will always be more involved than men in the use of health care. The more women understand and evaluate their own needs with a view to prevention, the less they'll rely on others to provide a cure. In the case of exercise during the childbearing year, judgments involve personal body awareness and feedback. Besides—how often is any muscle-testing included in a medical check-up? Women themselves must become qualified to make these subjective assessments, on the basis of objective physiological facts.

In sum, the formula for the best possible total birth experience must be conscious participation throughout the complete sequence—pregnancy, labor, delivery and postpartum. You are not the director in the drama of your birth—the uterus calls the cues. However, assisting nature to provide the best physical props and the tidiest dismantling afterward is your responsibility, and yours alone. Keeping your body in top form during pregnancy, and ensuring its successful restoration postpartum, is completely within your power.

2

Principles of Exercise

Now that you have understood the value of exercise during the child-bearing year, let us look at some general points about exercising. Exercise means different things to different people. It includes yoga, ballet, weight-lifting, running and contact sports, to name just a few. The essential exercises here are simple and do not require the precautions that some aerobic exercise does.

The exercises are described first by starting position, then by the movement, and finally by progressions which increase the challenge. It is important to move smoothly and safely from one exercise to the next (transitions) and to emphasize the quality of your performance rather than the quantity.

Basic Safety Measures

Warm-up Program

I recommend doing range of motion at each joint, that is, move in all possible directions. Circular and spiral movements of your shoulders and hips, wrists and ankles, promote energy flow. This sequence is a grounding experience, as you work toward your feet, becoming more aware of the components of your body and how they are connected. It is a great way to start the day, takes less than ten minutes, and is particularly helpful in cold climates where you tend to awaken feeling stiff.

Begin with your head and progress toward your feet, moving from the center of your body to the periphery. Shoulder movements are performed only in a backward direction to counteract the daily forces that bring them forward.

Suggested Scheme

Head

- ✦ Circle your head slowly.
- ✦ Move your head forward and back, slowly. Keep your mouth closed as you move your head backward for a nice stretch of your throat.
- ✦ Look straight ahead and bend your neck from one side to the other. Keep your nose facing forward as you increase the distance between your ear and shoulder on that side. This will relieve tension in your neck and shoulders.

Shoulders

- ✦ Move them back and down in circles, together or singly.

Elbows

✦ Fingers on shoulders, circle your elbows backward.

Arms

✦ Stretch open your arms and make backward circles. Imagine you have colored paint on your fingers and each circle is larger than the one before.

Wrists

✦ Keep your arms extended and circle your wrists. This helps any swelling in your hands.

Trunk

✦ Hold your outstretched arms at shoulder level and twist your trunk from side to side. Keep your feet still.

Pelvis

✦ Raise your arms for balance or rest your hands on your hips and do pelvic movements, like a belly dancer does:

✦ Circle your hips as if you were standing in an empty peanut butter jar and cleaning off the sides!

✦ Hike one hip up, and then the other, toward your shoulder.

✦ Suck in your abdomen, tilt your pelvis back, tuck your buttocks under.

Pelvic Floor

✦ Tighten your vaginal muscles, holding to a count of three before releasing.

Hips

✦ Balance exercises on one leg. Alternate legs between each exercise.

✦ Swing the other leg from front to back.

✦ Bend one knee and, as if a pencil were on it, draw a figure eight on the ground.

✦ With the leg straight swing it in front and behind the standing leg.

Feet

✦ One leg outstretched and off the floor, circle your foot to help return fluid to your heart.

You may be tempted to skip warm-ups or to make some short-cuts. If you do recreational aerobics, inadequate preparation will more than likely set you back a few days with a pulled muscle. Slowly build up to the more demanding exercises and taper off gradually. One way to taper off is to work back through progressions in reverse order.

Starting Positions

Before beginning any movements, always check that you are in the correct starting position, such as knees straight, feet flat, lengthened spine or pelvic tilt. The pelvic tilt is the key focus during the childbearing year; and when you read and hear pelvic tilt it means to orient your bony basin in a backward direction. The images "flatten your lower back/lumbar spine" or "press your waist to the floor" are helpful to recruit your abdominal muscles. However, a correct pelvic tilt is actually a neutral position, see pages 109 to 111, as the spinal column has three normal curves.

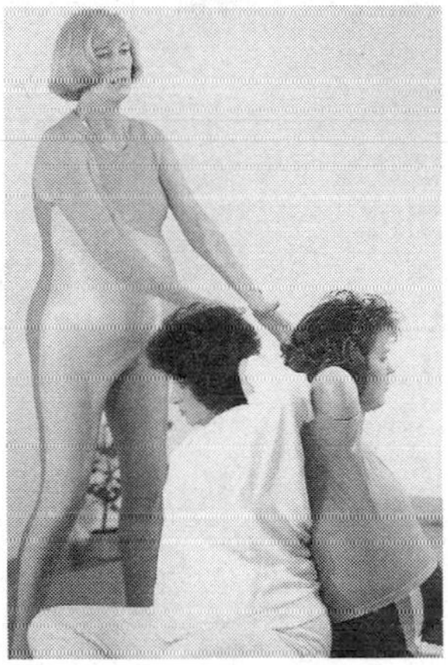
DOUG LONG, LONGSHOTS

Figure 7. Check the starting position before you begin a movement. Twist only if your elbows stay pressed together.

Frequently, people lose alignment also when they perform exercises, or the point of fixation moves during stretching. Precision is the whole point of the exercises that I teach; to establish and maintain the starting position despite progressions. This requires awareness.

Often, the starting position itself may be enough of a challenge; for example, holding the body in a modified push-up, without risking the movement if the arms and abdominal muscles are too weak.

In the illustration below, the pelvic tilt may have never been aligned to neutral before beginning, or it may have been lost during the action of raising the leg. The elbows are used here for support, but they are hyperextended which is undesirable, see below.

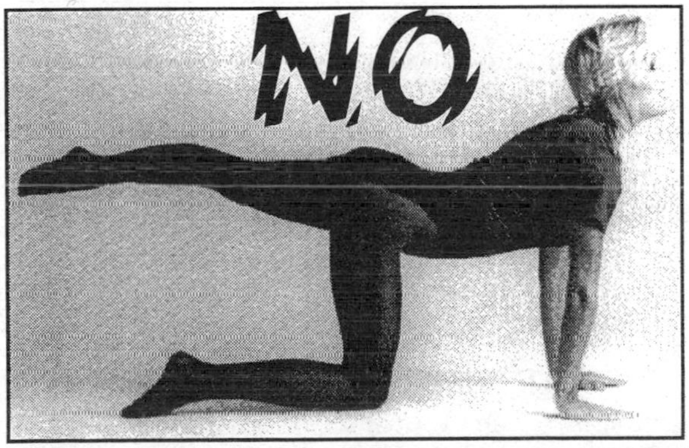

Figure 8. Loss of alignment: the elbows are hyperextended and the lower back has sagged. And she is not even pregnant![12]

Moderation Is the Idea

Obsessive behavior is not healthy. Some compulsive athletes actually look and get sick! Deepak Chopra, MD. warns that doing exercise that you don't enjoy can have more harm than benefit.[13] It is a Zen proverb that the enlightened person eats when she is hungry and drinks when she is thirsty. Most of us need to look at the clock! The same should be said for exercising. But no one has written a book called the *Joy of Exercising* in a society that considers it something that is good for us because it doesn't naturally occur in our daily activities!

Athletes like to perform against competition, but during the childbearing year, competitiveness is not appropriate. I advise pregnant and postpartum women to avoid classes where they have to keep up a fast pace. Not wanting to seem a wimp, you tend to keep pushing yourself even if you are out of breath or have wet your pants.

It is easy to do too much physical activity because your muscles may not protest until the day after. Muscles need rest in order to recuperate. (In fact, for athletes in training, it is during **rest,** not during exercise itself, when muscle growth occurs.) Exercise takes many forms; explore the different possibilities and alternate activities—a concept known as cross-training.

Pregnancy is a time to become more firmly in tune with your body; the exercises are an opportunity for increasing your awareness of your breathing, muscles, joints, and posture. Work within **your** own limit of comfort and tolerance; rest briefly between exercises. Stop before you are tired or if your muscles start to shake. You should not experience stiffness the next day. (If you do, the remedy is more of the same exercise but a small and gentle amount.)

The benefits of exercise accrue with consistency and careful progression.

Breathing

If you feel breathless, dizzy or tired—stop and rest.

Take your time. Toxic chemical waste products build up during physical activity; these can cause muscles to quiver or bring on general fatigue until your body adapts. This is called the training effect. Gradually you extend your limits.

Before arising from the horizontal position, especially after relaxation, stretch your whole body a couple of times and take one or two deep breaths. If resting on your back, roll onto your side first and wait before sitting up. Remember that in late pregnancy, you may get low blood pressure if you remain flat on your back for more than five to ten minutes (supine hypotension) and you can become dizzy arising too quickly from any recumbent position (orthostatic hypotension).

Keep breathing while exercising.

A position or movement that causes you to hold your breath is too strenuous. This increase in pressure can strain your abdominal wall and pelvic floor. If you are a chronic breath-holder, you will need to reverse the way you breathe while exercising.

Breathing is easier when coordinated with movement, such as pulling in or contracting the abdominal muscles on **outward** breath. For some movements it is arbitrary whether you breathe in or out, but for your pelvic floor and abdominal muscles, exhalation is imperative. To keep it simple, remember to exhale on exertion as a routine.

Perform the exercise smoothly and safely

Jerking, or the use of momentum, often cheats you out of the full range of movement. Usually it is a sign that the starting position or the action is too difficult, and that you should be doing a modified version. In many of the exercises, the biggest movement is not always the best one. Accuracy is more desirable—focus on the process rather than the end-point or goal.

Environmental Benefits

Common sense guides us not to work out in a hot, humid environment. I often wonder why people jog on sidewalks, inhaling car exhaust. I don't even like to pound the pavement, but prefer to run on grass or sand. The most enjoyable part of exercising for me is to be outdoors, in a place of natural beauty, to smell the fresh air, to listen to the birds, and to let my mind drift.

Adequate Fluids

Make sure that you have adequate fluid intake. Your urine should always be almost colorless. A couple of liters of fluid (10-16 glasses a day) is needed, more depending on your activity level. I have observed two safety valves for exercising pregnant women: they will need to have a drink or empty their bladders before their heart rates are raised to any significant degree!

Postpartum, thirst prevails as a safety measure. For as long as I breastfed, I needed a drink after only ten to fifteen minutes of vigorous exercise.

The Dangers of Hyperextension[14]

Joints at risk are those not protected by overlying muscles, and these are very few. One is the union of your pubic bones, which is part of what I call the *vulnerable midline.* Another "middle" area, the middle joint (knees or elbows) of each lever (arms and legs) is also at risk. Knees and elbows hyperextend in many people, especially pregnant women. This means the joint "locks" in an open position; the lax ligaments permit the straight lever to sway in the opposite direction of bending (flexion). The more you permit hyperextension, the more you weaken your ligaments. While it is common to see people standing with their knees hyperextended, the same problem with the elbows is seen only when the body weight is taken through the arms during exercises on hands and knees. The triceps muscle at the back of the elbow isn't used much in daily life, and hence it is much weaker than the biceps muscle which frequently bends the elbow.

Remember: knees at ease . . . elbows soft.

Exercises on the hands and knees are my favorite, because in this position women must be mindful of their elbows, which otherwise lock and hyperextend. The triceps has poor control when it is at its shortest (elbow straight). Women can thus strengthen their weak shoulders and arms and stimulate bone density, especially in their wrists—a common site of fracture in older women. The many other advantages of this position are described on page 98.

Harmful Exercises

The few movements that I consider inherently dangerous include double leg-raising, full sit-ups and the inverted knee-chest position **after birth.** I'll warn against other exercises because they are pointless or counterproductive.

Double leg-raising is always a dangerous exercise. This leverage is even more dangerous in pregnancy and postpartum.

Raising both outstretched legs from the horizontal to strengthen the abdominal muscles is not justified by the anatomical facts. **The abdominal muscles do not raise the legs.** They stabilize the lower back—but at a great mechanical disadvantage considering the length and weight of the legs. It is very difficult for the abdominal muscles to protect the vertebral joints against the stronger pull of the hip flexors, which lift the legs and are attached to those joints in the spine. Invariably, the backbone arches under this strain, and, if this happens repeatedly, back pain is inevitable. Strangely, some people just keep on repeating this exercise, believing the fallacy of "no gain without pain." Pain is actually an important warning signal.

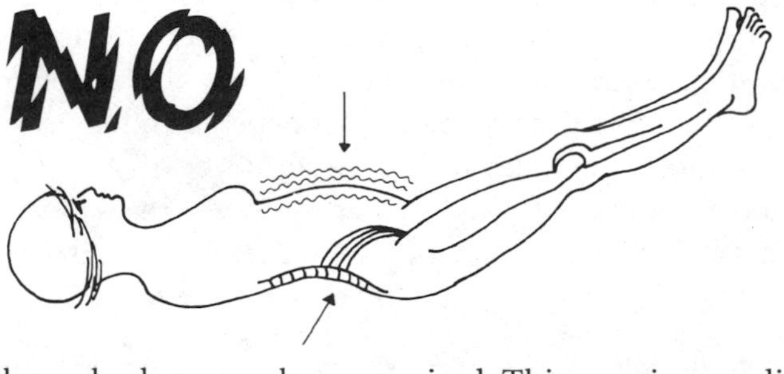

Figure 9. Raising outstretched legs can strain the lower back.

During and after pregnancy, your stretched abdominal muscles are unable to stabilize the lower back as your legs are raised. This exercise can distend the "central seam" of your abdominal muscles and cause pain in your spinal joints. **Therefore raising both legs from the horizontal, or lowering them with the knees straight all the way, must be avoided during the childbearing year, and at any other time.** Even if you are not pregnant, your abdominals cannot maintain a normal pelvic tilt during such exertion. This is a simple law of physics, that of the see-saw. This exercise can be reversed, however, and end, rather than begin, at the point of maximum difficulty. Safe double leg-lowering is described on page 105.

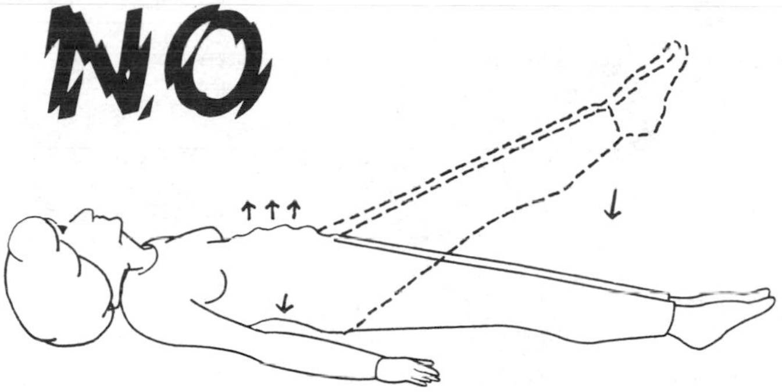

Figure 10. Lowering outstretched legs is also dangerous.[15]

Full sit-ups, likewise, work your hip flexors predominantly. They take over from a curl-up at about a 45 degree angle, to raise your trunk to vertical. People who orient themselves to the goal of sitting upright usually jerk right through the first half of the movement, which skips the abdominal work that needs attention. Double-leg raising and conventional sit-ups—both with straight legs—are commonly taught, although they are ineffective and undesirable. Many a person is proud of his or her ability to do a series of sit-ups or double leg-raises; however such actions depend primarily on the hip flexors.

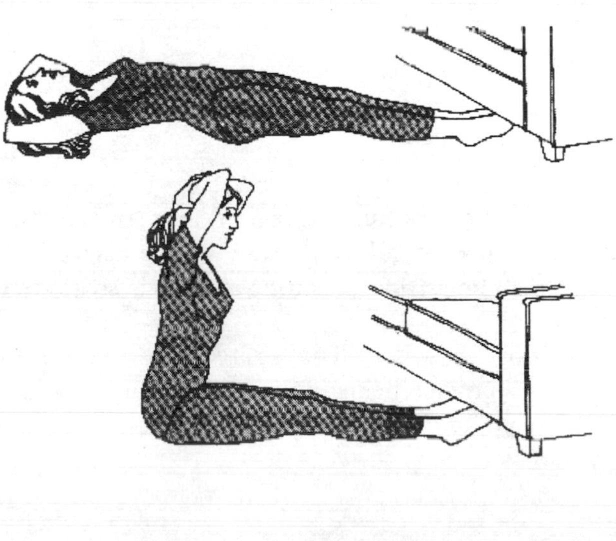

Figure 11. Full sit-ups, especially with the feet fixed, must be avoided, too.[16]

Figure 12. The "bicycling exercise" in this position favors round shoulders and a head that pokes forward!

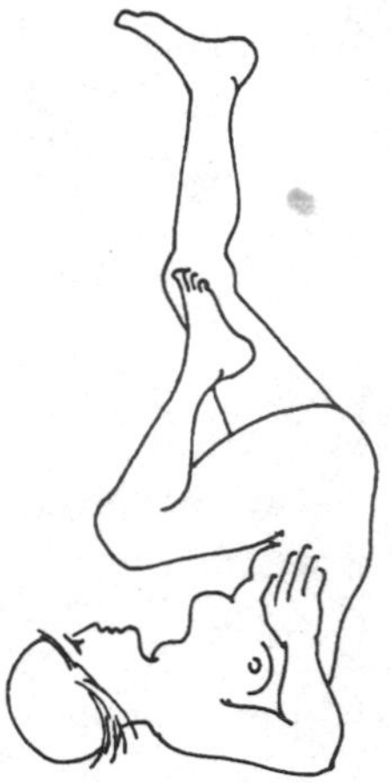

The "bicycle" (left) and the "candlestick" also known as the "plow" (below) are difficult to get in and out of during the childbearing year. They are potentially harmful as you could lose control at any point.

Figure 13. The Candlestick.

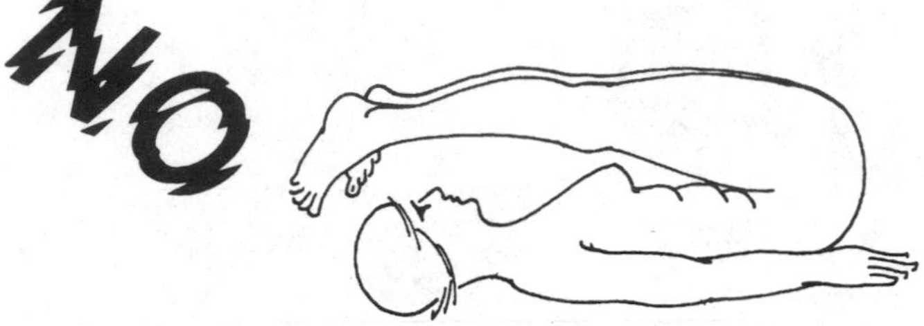

During the first few postpartum weeks, passive inverted postures such as resting with hips elevated and knees to chest put you at risk for fatal air embolism.[17] Wait until all bleeding has ceased before resuming such postures. However, the exact same knee-chest position is often recommended during pregnancy if your baby is a breech presentation! This position offers an advantage in labor in the rare event of cord prolapse as it reduces the likelihood of compression.

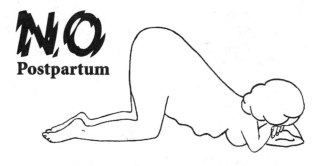

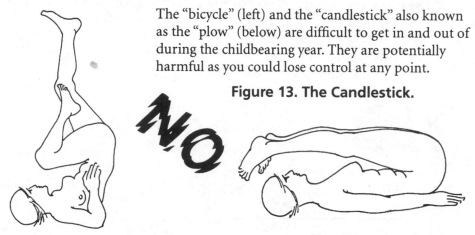

Figure 14. The knee-chest position may turn a breech during pregnancy.[18]

Avoid positions and exercises that increase the hollow in your back. Excessive hollowing of the small of the back (lumbar region) puts stress on the already-stretched abdominal muscles and compresses your spinal joints. Your back muscles tighten like a bowstring; squatting is a good way to stretch them in the opposite direction.

The "bow" exercise still hangs around as a postpartum exercise. It's clear that the abdominals, being in the front of your body are stretched, (which you want to avoid) and rocking on your tender pubic bones and full breasts is uncomfortable.

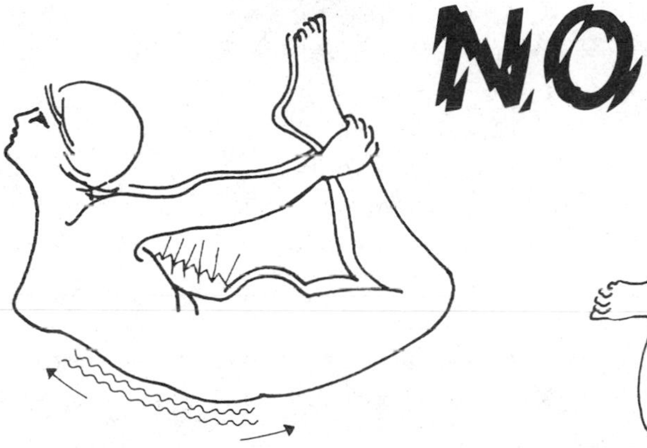

Figure 15. The "bow" strains the weakest points in the childbearing body.

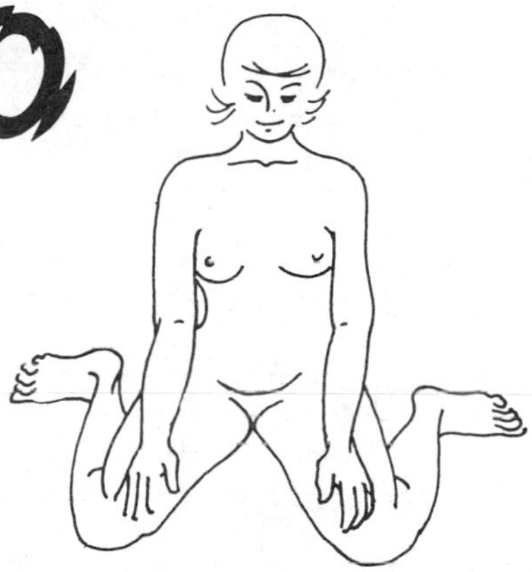

Figure 16. The W position can injure your pubic symphysis.

The **W** position causes your hip joints to turn inward, which can cause pain at the union of your pubic bones. This is a pointless exercise because women generally sit with their legs together and often crossed; therefore, these muscles are already tight. Quite obviously for birth we need to open our legs and roll our hips outward!

During pregnancy avoid forward bending in standing—it's fine postpartum. When you touch your toes a few times you tend to get dizzy from the extra blood volume traveling to your head, or heartburn occurs. You can get the same stretch in a seated position. See the partner exercises on page 187. Lifting with a forward bend is quite dangerous, see page 133.

If your ligaments are persistently stretched during the postpartum recovery phase, the shortening that normally occurs at this time may be compromised. Some of the positions shown above are used in yoga and may be resumed after the childbearing year when your joints feel normal again.

Supine Hypotension

Supine hypotension is low blood pressure that develops when lying on your back. Most pregnant women have no problem lying on their backs; they may even prefer this position for sleeping and relaxation, until the day they deliver. Occasionally, however, lying on the back can cause low blood pressure if the increased weight of the uterus interferes with circulation. In these cases, the women feel dizzy or light-headed, and they automatically roll to one side. In my experience, such symptoms come on only toward the end of pregnancy, when a woman is literally "heavy with child." The American College of

Gynecologists and Obstetricians (ACOG) Guidelines for Exercise in Pregnancy caution pregnant women about **vigorous** exercise in this position after the fourth month. This possibility of supine hypotension during exercise in pregnancy has stirred almost as much publicity as Jane Fonda's pregnancy workout! I have received phone calls from from women all over the country who had been exercising and sleeping on their backs, who were worried that they had harmed their babies. The media and ACOG would better serve the public by publicizing harmful practices, such as neonatal circumcision and the over-use of epidurals and Cesareans. No one who can freely change position, and does so when she feels light-headed and dizzy, was ever harmed by supine hypotension! I speak from thirty years of clinical instruction and treatment of pregnant women.

It is much more likely that when a pregnant woman wants to roll off her back, she is experiencing sacro-iliac joint pain, not supine hypotension. This pain is felt in the upper quadrant of typically one buttock and unlike supine hypotension, comes on **immediately.**

If you are in late pregnancy and are one of the **few** who experience supine hypotension, limit exercises on your back to less than five minutes. I alternate upper and lower trunk exercises and I intersperse supine exercises with side-lying ones. For example, you can do half a dozen curl-ups followed by half a dozen bridges. You can then roll onto one side and do some pelvic tilting and pelvic floor exercises. Next, on to your back again for some mini-curl-ups and heel sliding, and finally roll on to your other side and repeat the pelvic tilts and pelvic floor exercises. That's all you need to do to avoid supine hypotension.

In a group, I add more variations in side-lying, but I have confined the supine exercises to the movements that I feel are essential, and cannot be achieved in any other position. However, because back-lying exercises have received such bad press, a great many prenatal exercise programs omit abdominal muscle exercises completely and this is both absurd and unfortunate.

Ironically, the most vigorous exercise that many women will ever experience—labor—has been "managed" on the back for years! When I left Australia, even the low percentage of women who were having Cesareans were placed on a wedge to avoid supine hypotension. Regional anesthesia, such as an epidural, lowers blood pressure as well. Women today may be propped up for birth, but if they lift their legs up, or stirrups and instruments are used, they are obliged to lie flat.

Prior Level of Fitness

Most women, like most men, are not fit. Even if the cardiovascular system is in good shape, the pelvic floor usually is not. This is why I emphasize the essentials—what you must do, and what you must do **before** moving on to aerobics that may involve vigorous activity, heel strikes and momentum.

So much depends on how active you were before pregnancy. In Holland, for example, bike riding is a major form of travel, often against headwinds. In Australia, sports are very popular and accessible. Pregnant women enjoyed such physical activities for decades before medical guidelines approved them! When I was young, it was not unusual for someone whose labor began on the tennis court to finish the set! I went into labor while making a videotape of a prenatal exercise class which I intended to finish, cutting out my noisy contractions when it was edited. However, my baby came in less than one hour!

The weakest areas in women are the pelvic floor, abdominal muscles, shoulders, arms and wrists.

Progressions: Increasing the Challenge of Exercise

For prenatal exercises, progression occurs naturally with the advancing pregnancy, which provides increasing weight and resistance for the muscles to overcome, thus maintaining their strength and condition. Even for pregnant athletes, it is a matter of maintaining condition rather than improving it during pregnancy.

You may need to modify some of the abdominal exercises as you near term, going back to more basic movements from the progressions. If you have done the exercises from the beginning of pregnancy, you'll pick them right up again afterward. After birth, your muscles may be back to their normal length and strength easily within in a month—or six months. Then you are ready to progress, making exercises more difficult by certain established principles such as frequency, intensity (weight, leverage, gravity), repetitions and duration.

Frequency: How often should I exercise?

Regular exercise is important to gain the best results and to avoid sudden strain. Every day is better than three times a week. Think of it as your creative time; I have some of my best ideas while engaged in physical activity. Incorporate exercises into your daily routine activities. For example:

- Tighten your abdominal wall when standing or sitting.
- Contract your pelvic floor during intercourse.
- Get on all fours to pick up, wash floors, and so forth.
- Squat to lift any object—light or heavy.
- Sit on the floor like a tailor (knees out and ankles crossed) to watch TV.
- Rotate your ankles while your feet are elevated.
- Rotate your shoulders **backward only** after feeding the baby.
- Check your posture each time you pass a mirror.
- Circle your head and rotate your shoulders **backward** while sitting at the computer.

Intensity: How far should I push myself?

The longer the lever, the greater amount of power required to move it. For example, much force (and strain) is generated when you raise or lower both outstretched legs (which you should never do; as explained on page 40-41). Leverage is a principle by which exercises are progressed—not begun. One leg is easier than two, and a bent leg is a shorter lever than a straight leg.

Gravity is a substantial force. It makes walking uphill and lifting a bag of groceries hard work, and it is a potential help to you in labor. You still feel gravity when going downhill; in fact, you often have to brake your muscles against a fast descent, which can be tiring to your upper thighs. When you climb out of a swimming pool you feel the sudden impact of gravity as you lose the buoyant support of the water. Gravity can be used to assist weak muscles, too, especially when you do pelvic floor exercises in an inverted posture (such as the bridge, see page 143). Once your pelvis is elevated, the muscles can move to a higher position, but in a downward direction, with gravity helping.

Muscles work according to the weight they move. This can be as simple as a long lever—an outstretched arm against gravity. You could add a weight in your hand to increase the work for your shoulder and arm muscles. Often you can use the weight of your own body as the challenge, such as when doing modified push-ups.

Combining all these factors makes exercise more rigorous. For example, you could lift a heavier weight with your arm bent rather than outstretched. You could hold a lighter weight for longer and do more repetitions. Changes in position recruit different muscles. It is important to keep breathing because chronic breath-holding strains your midline.

During pregnancy, body awareness is the priority. Ideally, you will also enjoy recreational aerobics. If you do the essential exercises faithfully, then by the end of the childbearing year you will be in excellent shape to resume more demanding activities.

Repetitions: How many times should an exercise be performed?
Everyone is different, therefore it makes no sense to advise a set number of repetitions. Multiple repetitions often lead to mindless exercising that causes fatigue, stiffness and even injury. It is better to alternate muscle groups and progress to a more challenging position, leverage, or weight.

Ten repetitions of one specific muscle are enough. Then I prefer to change one of the other factors. You can total as many as Jane Fonda,[19] but do them in smaller bundles, changing muscle groups to avoid tiring both a specific muscle and also your whole body. For example, curl-ups (page 102) may tire your head and neck. When you feel fatigue coming on, switch to lower abdominal work (page 96) and rest your upper body. After those muscles begin to tire, change to bridging (page 143) which exercises the back of your body. Back-lying exercises in pregnancy are always kept brief and alternated with side-lying exercises.

Some modalities, such as the Flo® tube, allow extensive repetitions which are not fatiguing because you are alternating muscle groups. Spiral movements can be repeated more often than straight ones. When swimming, change from the crawl to backstroke to breast-stroke when certain muscles tire.

Duration: How long should each exercise set and the total session be?
Obviously it is important to develop holding power. But prolonged duration is the most difficult and unpleasant way to progress. If you lean your back against the wall and keep your knees bent for a few minutes, your body will quickly tell you when you have had enough! This is more tiring to your thighs than the complete movement of squatting up and down.

Muscles are composed of two kinds of fibers, fast-twitch and slow-twitch. Some muscles have a preponderance of one type, and so do some people. In the pelvic floor, for example, the fast-twitch fibers act rapidly when you sneeze. The slow-twitch fibers provide continual tone for this anti-gravity supporting muscle layer. From using biofeedback, I have seen that some women achieve a high score (of microvolts) with a quick flick, but cannot hold the contraction at all. Others can hold and hold, but never attain high numbers. Muscles, then, need to have all components—strength, endurance and the ability to relax.

Calisthenics and stretches lend themselves to interval activity—very handy to do when taking breaks from sedentary occupations. A stretch needs to be held for at least one to two minutes to achieve lengthening of the muscle.

On the other hand, the value of a run or a walk is in its duration as well as its intensity. For example, in order to get your muscles burning fat (after the childbearing year) you need to keep going for at least forty-five minutes. Twenty minutes to a half-hour burns more glycogen (sugar), which is why many people fail to lose their fat until they continue on for that extra fifteen minutes.

Pace: What speed is desirable?

Quality movements are slow and complete. You should be comfortable and in control of both the position and the movement. Avoid pushing, pulling or leaning in such a way that you could lose your balance or strain muscles. Rhythm is a wonderful encouragement but momentum can be risky if it takes you beyond your comfortable range of motion.

Stretching and limbering activities must be done gently and never forced. However, the definition of a stretch is to go to your limit. But rather than bouncing (which activates receptors in your muscles to make them contract), you surrender. This release on the outward breath allows the specific muscle to lengthen in its own time.

In general, most people are tense and tight more than they are weak, and men are stronger than women but women are more flexible. Even in pregnancy, the tight muscles which need stretching do not put the associated joints at risk. Typically, tight muscles are the hamstrings, heel cords, and the pectoral muscles in front of your shoulders. (Can you squat with your feet flat or shake hands with one hand over your shoulder and the other one behind your back?) Sensible stretching does not jeopardize any joints.

Aerobic Exercise

Aerobics refers to those exercises which make your heart pump faster and increase your breathing rate. The popular image suggests fast movements to loud music with a strong beat. At its beginning, the aerobics craze was primarily high-impact—jumping and bouncing. As a result of injuries, programs became less forceful and offered low-impact aerobics which did not put joints and bladders at risk.

All the exercises in this book are no-impact and sub-aerobic: they are not designed to raise your heart rate. This is because I emphasize understanding the whole picture—your entire body throughout the childbearing year. Body awareness programs are much less prevalent than fitness classes. I hope to increase your precision in body positions and movements, and to prevent not only injuries but dysfunctions that may have later, if not immediate, repercussions. The essential exercises focus on neglected muscles and are the priority during the childbearing year. If you have spare time for cardiovascular fitness, that's fine. If not, choose the essentials during and after pregnancy. Also, being pregnant is aerobic in itself: your heart and lungs work harder than before, even at rest.

Classes which feature aerobic exercises for the non-pregnant population[20] are usually too strenuous for late pregnancy and early postpartum, unless you have been following such a program for some time. However, modified classes specifically designed for childbearing women are becoming more common, but such classes may overlook some of the essentials that I emphasize in this book.

I advocate that you do recreational aerobics; this is possible without having to buy special clothes and club memberships. Walking, swimming, and bicycling are enjoyable activities that not only provide excellent general exercise but bring you into the outdoors and fresh air. They are the most popular forms of exercise because they are accessible and inexpensive. Regular exercise of this type combines many of the desirable features of prenatal exercise: to strengthen muscles; build up endurance; improve circulation and respiration. You'll adapt more easily to your increasing weight and changing balance. This promotes better overall function of your body and extends its limits of exertion. Such aerobics help burn calories if you are overweight[21] and relieve constipation. **Warning: Avoid impact aerobics if you have any pelvic floor weakness—at any time in your life.**

Aerobics During Pregnancy

So far, no human research exists on how much blood is diverted to working muscles and the effects, if any, of such temporary changes on your unborn baby. In fact, it is impossible to measure these differences. Regardless, we do know that reserve blood is stored in sinuses of the placenta called cotyledons. Initially, ACOG advised that vigorous exercise be limited to fifteen minutes with a heart rate of more than 140 beats per minute (which in pregnancy is about the equivalent of 160 in a non-pregnant woman.) However, clinical studies supported the anecdotal evidence that even strenuous exercise is not invariably harmful, as pregnant women competed athletically without adverse effects. James Clapp, M.D., at Case Western Reserve, has reported on the excellent perinatal outcomes of superior athletes.[22]

Despite what I have just said, strenuous exercise should stop short of increasing the body core temperature, which is different from peripheral temperature. Pregnant women have efficient cooling mechanisms from their expanded capillaries (which give them the wonderful rosy glow). Animal studies indicate that increased core temperatures may cause neural tube defects. Pregnant women should not exercise if they have a fever or in hot humid weather, when the natural cooling mechanisms of the body are reduced. Similarly, they should not sit in a sauna, which is an enclosed hot-box. In contrast, hot tubs permit cooling of your head and shoulders, and you can sit on the edge if you feel too warm.

Exercise should never be done to lose weight during pregnancy. You need to gain weight to grow a healthy baby! You are also growing a placenta and increasing the capacity of all your systems. Very active women require extra fluids and calories.

Women have run marathons while pregnant. Some women maintain a jogging program right through the ninth month and resume it a few weeks postpartum. Others, in contrast, experience difficulty and pain even just walking in late pregnancy. Most pregnant women give up jogging or similar impact exercise around the sixth month. High impact aerobics can strain the pelvic organ supports, as each heel strike transmits a jolt to the bladder. If you have no problems at all with your undercarriage, then it is fine to be as active as you wish. Just listen to your body and tune into your baby.

Unborn babies kick if they are disturbed by loud music, certain positions or sudden movements. Babies also kick if the uterus is tense—understandably they prefer soft stretchy surroundings. Content babies move slowly and gently.

Aerobic exercise differs from calisthenics, which focus on developing strength, flexibility and coordination of muscles, and improving joint mobility. Both dimensions are important for complete conditioning, but my priority for childbearing women concerns the essential exercises in this book—for the abdominals and pelvic floor muscles. I have spent thirty years treating women whose backache and urinary problems came on during pregnancy; rarely have I treated childbearing women with heart disease. The childbearing year is a special time with unique priorities; you have the rest of your life to achieve cardiovascular fitness.[3]

Aerobics Postpartum

After birth, you no longer have to worry about what may happen to your baby when you are physically active. Nevertheless, my focus is on preventing problems and I advise you to wait until your pelvic floor is in optimal condition before jogging or doing any impact aerobics. It takes six weeks for your uterus to return to its normal size and until then it is an additional weight on your pelvic floor. (My pelvic floor didn't feel ready for jogging until three months postpartum.) Also, your breasts are much heavier with milk in the early postpartum weeks and can feel very uncomfortable when you jog.

In the meantime, you can be quite aerobic on a mini-trampoline, or seated on a large gymnastic ball which also challenges your balance. Postpartum mothers have more problems with balance than during pregnancy, because of sudden postural changes after birth.

Aerobic exercise helps you feel good and is also important if you wish to lose weight later. Many women are concerned about the store of fat on their thighs, Nature's caloric reserve for breastfeeding. Covert Bailey,[23] the *Fit or Fat* expert, advises that if you want slim thighs, breastfeed! He writes that the hormones produced during lactation seem to the only mechanism that activates the release of fat from female thighs! The postpartum body is designed to breastfeed and you actually need additional calories, about 500 more each day, than during pregnancy.

The Benefits of Water

Swimming laps, or specific exercises in water, known as aquatics or aquayoga, are ideal in pregnancy because the buoyancy of the water takes 90 percent of your weight. You can lie on your back without any risk of supine hypotension and you can also lie comfortably on your front. Other than going to the beach and digging three holes in the sand, I never found another way to be in my favorite position during pregnancy! Water is a versatile medium that can be used for assistance, resistance, work-out (if it is cool) and relaxation (if it is warm). Exercises in water can be aerobic too, and thus increase your oxygen uptake (the measure of cardiovascular fitness) metabolism and overall endurance. Water is particularly useful when there are problems in pregnancy, such as high blood pressure, or preterm labor contractions. Relaxing in water diminishes contractions, and exercises in water reduce swelling.

Videotape Instruction

Videotaped exercise programs are available for home use during the childbearing year. I was the exercise consultant for a MGM/UA production starring Marie Osmond during her first pregnancy. This is a comprehensive one-hour program.[24] I also made a video *BabyJoy,* when I was twelve weeks postpartum with my son. This covers all the essential exercises, many involving your baby, plus activities on balls, in water and infant massage. (See Resources.)

"Post–Postpartum"

When does the childbearing year really end? Twelve months after conception is the theory, but in practice many women do not feel that their body has returned to its former shape, size and function at that time. Women often enjoy coming to postpartum exercise class for six months or so. Around this time, their babies begin to crawl, and they are not safe on the floor with a group of moving moms. This is another indication that it's time to move on. I've noticed over the years that women often form strong bonds with their peers in exercise class and will continue to meet for years outside class time.

Look for a class or an exercise tool that genuinely appeals to you, something which you will pursue because you **enjoy** it. A Flo® class is an ideal progression but not readily available because this is a fairly new modality on the market. However, you can learn from a video, and you can create your own movements too. The Flo® tube is a plastic sleeve with hand grips and wrist straps on each end. It comes in different lengths; you will need to state your height on the order form at the back of this book. When the straps are over your wrists, the tube should just clear the ground in front of you. Water is poured into the tube to provide weight, about a quart (2 pounds) is enough. The tube can be emptied, folded up and carried in a handbag, so you can travel with it anywhere. You do need adequate space to move the tube over, under, and around your body; it is ideal for exercising outdoors. The rhythmical, helical movements provide a workout that limbers and strengthens your body, and it also relaxing. Muscle groups alternate to avoid fatigue and the sound of the swooshing water is soothing. You need to integrate your movements mindfully **with** the flowing water, in quite a different way from, for example, lifting weights while attending to the television as I observe in gyms. In addition, there are many women who have neither the time, inclination, nor the money to join gyms or health clubs and would prefer a simple piece of equipment to use at home.

Desk workers especially can benefit from the many movements using the arms **behind** the back—backstroke, figure-8, the "overflo"—to name just a few. Wide arm movements challenge your balance, leg movements in unison increase your heart rate. You can also exercise with a partner using two tubes. The Flo® tube is a logical complement to a jogging program, which concentrates on your legs and cardiovascular system. However, if you wish to use the Flo® aerobically instead of jogging, that is possible, too. I developed a class called *Movement for the Middle Years* to offer a regimen of stretching, strengthening, and aerobic exercise for women aged 40 to 70 years. This combination of Flo®ing and gymnastic ball exercises, and the concluding relaxation session, is described in my forthcoming book, *Essential Exercises For the Rest of Your Life.*

3

The Pelvic Floor

Your pelvis is the bony basin that carries your baby. As the location of your center of gravity, it is the keystone of good posture. The flexible muscular base of the abdominal cavity is referred to as the pelvic floor. This region is also the seat of many emotions and experiences.[25]

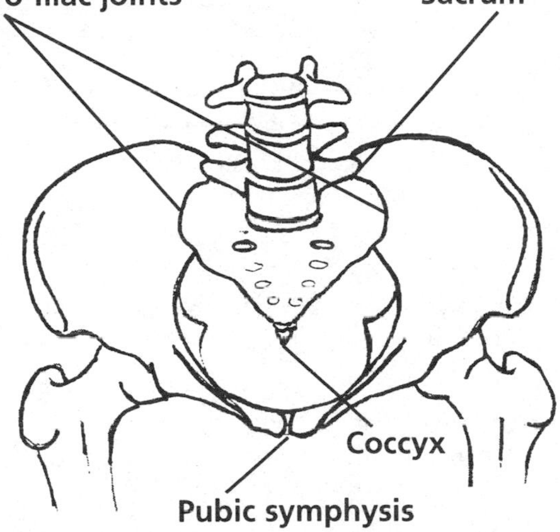

Figure 17. The bony pelvis.

Important landmarks:
✦ Your two *pubic bones* united in front by connective tissue, **not muscle**. This joint is known as the *pubic symphysis (PS).*
✦ Your *sacrum*, the triangular wedge of bone between your buttocks.
✦ Your *coccyx*, the tailbone, is buried deeply at the base of your sacrum, above your anus.
✦ Your *sacro-iliac joints.*

Each SI joint unites the sacrum with an ilium on each side. During pregnancy these become more mobile from the softening effects of hormones on your connective tissue. You can find the upper part of these joints easily by feeling for the indentation, like a dimple, above each buttock.

The Vulnerable Midline

Your pubic bones are part of the *vulnerable midline* where the muscles of your abdomen and pelvic floor on each side are connected by a fibrous union. We can think of your pubic symphysis as the only bony junction on this line running from your coccyx to your breastbone. Activities during which one leg moves differently from the other, such as walking or even turning over in bed, can cause pain if you have increased laxity of this joint. As no muscle spans this joint, we cannot rely on exercises to compensate for its vulnerability.

Pubic symphysis pain—a raw feeling—occurs at the exact center of this midline. It is different from adductor tendonitis which causes a tender area to one side. PS pain is also different from the benign intermittent spasm of the round ligament in the groin which all women experience from time to time in pregnancy. See Appendix for a simple treatment to resolve PS pain.

Sacro-iliac Pain

Sacro-iliac pain is felt in the upper quadrant of usually one buttock. Often the joint on one side is stiff (hypomobile), and this puts added stress on the looser one which may become increasingly lax (hypermobile). If you have a painful locking sensation in this joint, especially on arising from a horizontal surface, such as a hard floor, see Appendix for a technique to alleviate these symptoms.

Coccyx Pain

Coccyx pain occurs sometimes after birth, because the passage of the baby's head may push it outward or deviate it to one side. A fall on your coccyx pushes it inward; gentle mobilization via your rectum restores it to its correct position. (See Resources to find an OB-GYN physical therapist). Coccyx pain is most noticeable in sitting, but it can also be provoked by pelvic floor exercises, in the rare cases when the muscles are strong enough to pull on the coccyx. If sitting on a rubber ring relieves pain in your tailbone area, then you probably have a problem with your coccyx. Deep massage and polarity therapy[26] may help, but I would recommend visiting a physical therapist who can re-align your joint, and in the postpartum period administer some ultrasound as well. Sitting on a rubber ring also takes the weight off your sit-bones. Occasionally, there is tenderness over one of these deep bones in your buttocks, where your hamstring tendon inserts. Deep friction massage will help. Ultrasound may be used if you are postpartum.[27]

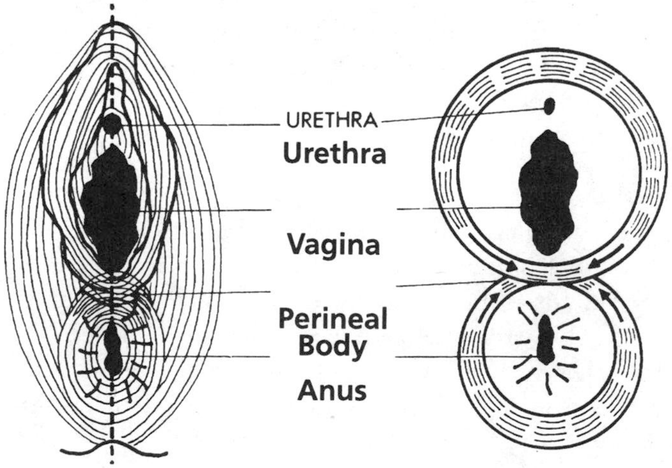

Figure 18. Three orifices penetrate the midline of the pelvic floor. The muscles form a figure eight around the perineal body.

Structure of the Pelvic Floor

The position of the pelvic floor is at a disadvantage in humans because of the effects of gravity in the upright position. Nature provided an excellent design to maintain the angles of the organs and their passages—as long as the muscles are in good shape. The most significant support is provided by your pubococcygci—a left and a right pubococygeus[28] musclc—which arc also known as thc levator or levatores ani. For simplicity we will refer to the PF from now on. This key muscle of the pelvis is suspended primarily at two points, the front and back. Also there are three orifices in the central seam of the PF. In most women the middle one, the vagina, is stretched during birth. These conditions, plus frequent daily increases of pressure within the body, when we lift or eliminate while holding the breath, explain why the pelvic floor is likely to sag, just as a hammock does.

Ideally, the muscle floor is firm and supportive, forming an upward curve between two bony points (pubis and coccyx). The healthy, active pelvic floor, has strength, endurance and elasticity. Once weakness or injury causes the flexible shelf to sag, it will continue its downward trend. Pregnancy and childbirth are the most common causes of pelvic floor laxity, but sexual abuse also causes damage. Excessive sagging over a long period of time can result in structural changes which disrupt bladder and bowel function as well as sexual response.

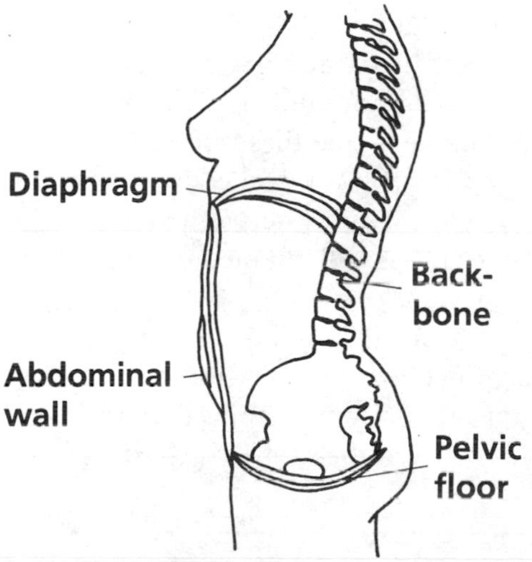

Figure 19. The pelvic floor is the base to the abdominal/pelvic cavity.

Functions of the Pelvic Floor

*The Five **S**s*

1. To provide Sphincter control of your bladder and bowel.

A sphincter is formed by a ring of muscle fibers that constrict and control pressure. Many sphincters are composed of involuntary muscles; for example, we don't have control over those placed in our gut. But like tightly closing an eye, we can squeeze our vaginal sphincter. Usually we don't think about keeping the anus closed, or the internal urinary sphincter at the bladder neck because they have muscle components that contract without our awareness. If we closed the open ends of the letter **S** we would have an **8**, representing the two sphincters in the female pelvis that control three orifices.

Good sphincter control is a crucial factor of pelvic floor integrity. Voluntary control can be superimposed, as when we interrupt the stream of urine, relax the muscles during vaginal or rectal examination, or grip the penis during intercourse.

2. To Support the pelvic organs and their contents, specifically bladder, uterus and bowel.

Except under anesthesia, there is always some tone in the sphincters and surrounding muscles. These sphincters can be closed more tightly than their normal state of partial contraction, and the pelvic floor can be drawn up into a more supportive position by the action of voluntary muscles. Slow-twitch muscle fibers provide this support.

3. To withstand all the increases in preSSure that occur in the abdomen and pelvis.

The forces may be intermittent, such as during laughing, coughing, sneezing, nose-blowing, lifting, straining, bowel movements and pushing during the second stage of labor. Faster-acting muscle fibers are needed for sudden exertion. During pregnancy the uterus enlarges from a capacity of 2" x 4" to 10" x 14", and causes long-standing and increasing pressure on the PF. Constipation and consequent straining also stress your pelvic supports. During urination or bowel movements, your PF relaxes, and afterward, the muscles return to their supportive state. Since most women are not informed of either the functions or the importance of their PF, it is unlikely that these are supple muscles over which you have awareness, let alone control. Your general fitness may be excellent, but this has no relation to the state of your internal structures. **The pelvic floor is not exercised during sports or calisthenics and, in fact, high impact aerobics will make a weak muscle worse.**

Pay special attention to draw up and squeeze your PF, simultaneously tightening your sphincters. The majority of women don't bother to develop the power in these muscles, especially if they do not suffer any symptoms that indicate weakness of the PF. Why, then, should they concern themselves with exercises? This bring us to the fourth reason.

4. To enhance Sexual response.

Another worthwhile bonus of PF exercises is heightened sexuality. Your vagina becomes more snug as your muscles improve in strength and thickness. Sensation in your vagina becomes keener because feeling inside depends on deep pressure, unlike outside skin which has different types of nerve endings near the surface for temperature and light touch. Your ability to contract the PF also enhances your sexual arousal, your orgasmic platform. One can read in such books as the *Kamasutra* or *The Arabian Nights* of cultures where the ability to contract the vaginal sphincter, was encouraged and highly rewarded. Sex shows, particularly in the Far East, sometimes feature vaginal muscle skills such as cigarette "smoking" and ping pong balls being drawn in and ejected. I mention this simply to show you that your muscles can be a lot stronger than you ever imagined! Nevertheless, I have felt less than a few dozen strong PF muscles in all the women whom I have evaluated in the past twenty-five years.

Female ejaculation is a normal and powerful sexual response that occurs in about ten percent of women—those with the strongest muscles. *The G-Spot* by Alice Ladas, John Perry and Beverly Whipple was the first book to describe female ejaculation extensively. (See Further Reading.)

Sometimes these "gushers," their partners, and also their doctors, confuse female ejaculation with urinary incontinence. However, the ejaculate does not smell or look like urine and it is chemically similar to the prostate secretions in the male. During sexual arousal, fluid builds up in the Skene's glands on each side of the urethra and is ejaculated during orgasm, **through the urethra,** not the vagina. Medical authorities are not only, for the most part, ignorant of the existence of female ejaculation, but many even deny it. They should just ask women! Unfortunately, operations have been performed needlessly because the woman's physician thought she was suffering from stress incontinence (and some women do indeed lose urine during intercourse) instead of recognizing her to be a sexual athlete.

5. To help your baby's head Slide out during birth.

The deep nerve endings in the PF provide the means of vaginal sensation during intercourse, and they also play a significant role in the second stage of labor. During the actual birth, your PF links the descent of your baby's head with the power of your contractions. Stimulation of these nerve endings (proprioceptors) causes uterine contractions during orgasm, and in labor the descent and pressure of your baby's head increases the power of uterine contractions. Registration of this pelvic pressure is relayed to your pituitary gland, which pours out oxytocin, the hormone that makes your uterus contract. The lower your baby's head descends in your pelvis, the more it presses on your PF, and the more oxytocin is produced. The most powerful contractions are those that actually bring your baby into the world. The urge to push is a reflex that unites nerve sensation with hormone production—**only if you have no anesthesia.** Local anesthesia, such as a pudendal block, and regional anesthesia (epidural and spinal) knock out both the proprioceptors and the high oxytocin levels. This combined loss causes the contractions to wane. As a result, epidurals, which are usually given in the first stage of labor, are allowed to wear off by the time the head is on view to allow this natural reflex.

As Dr. Arnold Kegel,[29] (whose name has been attached to the muscle and exercise), pointed out decades ago, a strong supple PF will slide out of the way as it distends over your baby's head. In contrast, a thin one will be forced to stretch past its limits and perhaps be compressed against the pelvic bones, causing some damage.

Eight Additional Benefits of Pelvic Floor Exercises

You want to avoid pessaries,[30] pads, and surgery; positive motivation is even better. Here are some more reasons to get your PF so strong that your partner will say "wow." (I have never heard of a case of "ouch"!)

1. Relief from pelvic congestion via improved pelvic blood circulation. Together with general aerobics, PF exercises relieve menstrual cramps. You may think of the childbearing year as a year without bleeding, but menstruation can return within the three months postpartum.[31]
2. Exercises promote quicker healing of stitches if you had a tear or episiotomy.
3. Pelvic floor exercises and relaxation reduce painful muscle tension or spasm that may be related to an incision, generalized tension or simply too much sitting.
4. Pelvic floor exercises can help diagnose coccyx pain, and also relieve some cases of it.
5. Exercises promote more abundant vaginal lubrication through improved blood circulation. After birth, your vagina may be dry for a few months, and, as we age, our estrogen levels fall—especially after natural or surgical menopause.
6. Exercises relieve constipation if your rectal proprioceptors respond poorly to a full bowel.
7. Exercises reduce *varts*—air being sucked in and expelled from the vagina. Varts may occur in various sexual positions and inverted postures for yoga.[32]
8. PF exercises promote optimal outcome if you have future pelvic surgery, such as hysterectomy, anterior repair (cystocele) or posterior repair (rectocele).

Causes of Pelvic Floor Problems

Not all inefficiency of the PF is associated with the "trauma" of childbirth and not all childbirth is associated with later inefficiency of the PF. The months of pregnancy may play as much of a role as prolonged pushing during labor. Leaking urine, discomfort from sagging or prolapse of internal organs can result from other factors as well. The cause may be congenital or simply poor development of the nerve and muscle circuits. Injury or disease involving the nervous system or specific nerves may be the reason. Pelvic floor dysfunction follows the muscle and tissue degeneration that occurs with aging. After menopause, estrogen, which facilitates the function of involuntary muscle, may be deficient. While PF problems are more common in women over forty who have borne children, they can also be found among adolescents and young mothers. In fact, a study of Norwegian students at a college for physical education found that about one quarter of them had stress incontinence.[33]

Dr. Kegel observed that the predisposition to urinary control problems begins frequently in childhood, when the muscles are developed before the nerves that supply them. There is no control of the PF until connections are established between the muscles and the central nervous system. Until this occurs (around eighteen months) the child's PF is in a relaxed or emptying position. Thus earlier "success" at toilet-learning is parent-training! When the circuits between the PF and the brain are complete, the child is then able learn voluntary control according the customs of family and culture.[34] Habitual posture and patterns of behavior in childhood account for variations in development, which by adulthood may be less than complete. Problems may persist, or go away only to recur in pregnancy or later life. Dr. Kegel stated that one third of women reach adulthood with immature bladder control. Dr. Moyses Paciornik[35] in Brazil has correlated continence and good PF support with the constant use of the squatting position. Australian gynecologist Robert Zaccharin[36] concluded from his studies in China that frequent squatting and the absence of obesity enhanced PF function. I made the same observation when I was touring medical facilities in China and other countries where people squat to rest, eliminate and perform many tasks.

Common Problems with Pelvic Floor Function

The onset may be subtle; you may not experience clear-cut symptoms but the condition often worsens over time if it goes unchecked. Many women wait years before admitting to anyone that they suffer from problems "down there." For example, you or your partner may feel nothing during intercourse, due to the laxity of your PF muscles. You may have difficulty retaining a tampon for the same reason. Sometimes vaginal walls are so slack that other pelvic organs or the intestines protrude and cause discomfort.

Figure 20. The pelvic floor supports internal organs.

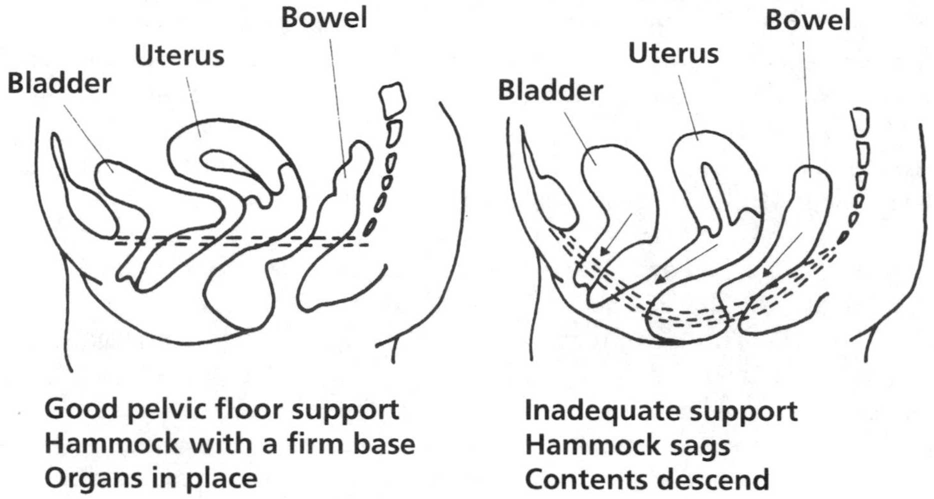

Pelvic Organs Out of Place

One such condition is *prolapse of the uterus,* which progresses through several stages before it actually bulges through the vaginal outlet, similar to the way upholstery padding protrudes through a chair when its supporting base is defective. If your bladder bulges into your vagina, it is known as a *cystocele,* and if it is your bowel, the term is *rectocele.* There is an area between your vagina and rectum where a portion of intestine can slip down. This herniation is known as an *enterocele.* Many women have one or more of the above conditions existing together. If you suspect such a condition, squat over a mirror and take a look. Put one of two fingers in your vagina. If the shiny, pink, ridged bulge is above your fingers, it is your bladder. If it is behind then the rectum is prolapsing.

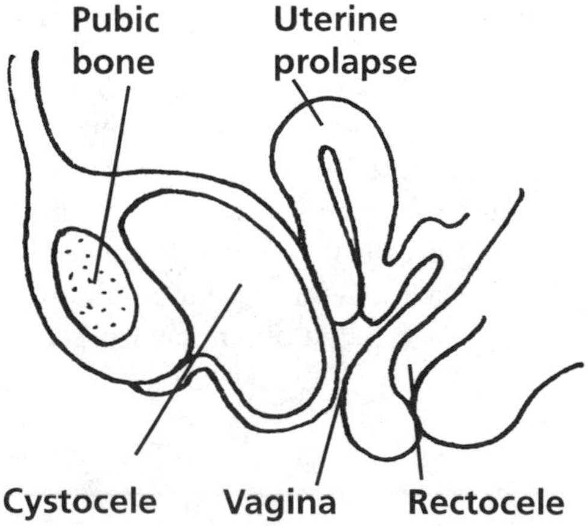

Figure 21. Pelvic organs protrude when support is inadequate.

The uterus and bladder are in the optimal position when the main body of the organ has a well-defined angle to its exterior passage. The uterus is sometimes "tipped" or retroverted—that is, angled backward instead of forward—but it is nevertheless positioned safely away from possibility of descending into the vaginal canal. The normal axis of the vagina, as you may well know from inserting tampons, slopes **backward** toward the hollow of your sacrum. Uterine prolapse occurs when the uterus lines up with the vagina and can slide down into it, and even all the way through so that your uterus hangs outside your body. Any increases in intra-abdominal pressure (such straining during elimination, breath-holding during exertion, persistent coughing) will, in time, cause its progressive descent. Your uterus should be high enough that feeling for your cervix is difficult. If you insert your longest finger into your vagina and feel your cervix readily (it feels like the tip of your nose), then it is too low.

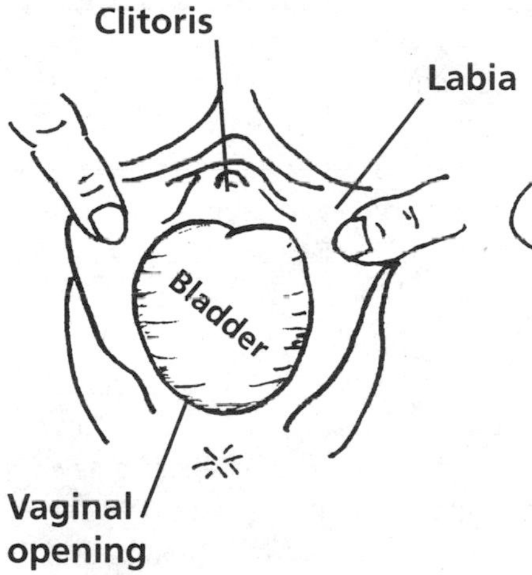

Figure 22. Cystocele is the bladder bulging into the vagina.

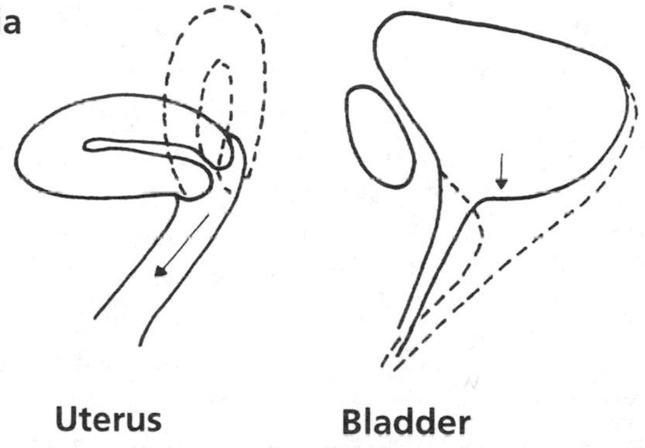

Figure 23. A well-defined angle is the key to organ stability. The dotted line represents abnormal alignment.

The bladder normally joins the urethra at an angle of about 90 degrees. When this angle is lost, the bladder neck area becomes funnel-shaped. The back of the bladder is now aligned with the urethral passage, similar to the way the prolapsed uterus lines up with the vagina. This bladder neck angle may take years to increase; like most pelvic problems it is usually slow in onset. **Early restorative exercise should be commenced at the first sign of malfunction.** Whether incontinence is because of general PF descent or specific damage to the bladder neck, re-education of the voluntary muscles is always necessary. Improving the function of this supportive muscle sheet will enhance the success of any surgery, if required.

Incontinence

Incontinence is commonly defined as the involuntary loss of urine and/or feces at inappropriate times in socially inconvenient places. Stress urinary incontinence, the most common and the most distressing PF problem, is the involuntary escape of urine when you laugh, cough, sneeze, lift, run or otherwise suddenly increase the pressure within your abdomen. Chronic leaking of urine is even more embarrassing and depressing than vaginal herniation. The afflicted woman must cope with odor, skin irritation and tissue inflammation, all of which are aggravated by the need to wear absorbent pads or diapers. Sometimes when there is a cystocele or rectocele as well, urine or feces collects in the bulging hernia that forms, causing incomplete voiding and elimination. She then must press against the pouch with her fingers inside her vagina to complete emptying.

In the absence of increased pressure, urinary control is usually present. This is because pressure in the narrow urethra is naturally higher than in the bladder, until there is an additional sudden push from above which overpowers the weakened structures below. However, in some cases of severe weakness, just the combination of gravity in the upright position and the pressure of a full bladder is enough, for example, to cause a woman to dribble all the way to the bathroom on arising in the morning.

Sometimes urine leakage occurs during pregnancy and seems to clear up after the baby is born; however, the basic weakness has manifested itself. Unless exercises are done postpartum to strengthen the muscles, the problem gets a little worse with each subsequent pregnancy, and recovery of good urine control after each birth takes longer. Decreasing hormones after menopause and increasing age hasten PF deterioration. Also around menopause, an additional symptom may develop—urgency.[37]

Anal incontinence may also exist, especially after fourth degree tears during birth. Even without extensive tears or episiotomy, damage to the anal sphincter and its nerve supply is not uncommon.

Professor Ralph Benson of the University of Oregon once estimated[38] that at least 50 percent of Caucasian women suffer from incontinence at some stage of their lives, and 20 percent of all gynecological surgery is done to correct this unfortunate problem. The increasing population of the elderly will raise the incidence even higher. We have only to think how often we laugh, sneeze, cough, lift, strain, and run, thus putting pressure on the PF. Our PF is obliged to work consistently, with additional intermittent stress, and at a mechanical disadvantage against the force of gravity. Yet, how often do we consciously draw up this hammock to counteract these effects? It's no wonder that over the years the floor and the organs that it is supposed to support become displaced. When a bed gets progressively softer and less supportive, we tighten the springs as far as we can and may eventually place a board under the mattress. Likewise, we must tighten our PF muscles.

Lack of awareness and conscious control may be compounded by weakness and injury through childbearing. If we don't keep the PF supple and strong, it will sag, and extraneous aids such as a pessary may be required. Early symptoms and mild descent of internal organs can be alleviated by exercise, but in severe cases, surgery is the only alternative to a lifetime of diapers. I have noticed with alarm the strong growth in the sale of these products in drugstores and supermarkets.

The Prevalence of Pelvic Floor Dysfunction

Problems with the PF are so common that it seems that our society takes them for granted. At least half of the female population has some laxity of the PF with or without symptoms. Doctors tend to think of the firm efficient PF as the exception, if they check your muscle strength. Reports and confessions of these afflictions are still surrounded by shame and secrecy. Many sufferers accept this is as just part of the hassle of childbearing, or growing older, or else it "runs in the family." Although increasingly more medical journals publish articles on the non-surgical treatment of PF problems, the lay press rarely deals with these subjects. Television ads feature movie stars promoting adult diapers rather than informative messages about how to resolve the problem.

Dr. Kegel was an unusual surgeon who laid down his scalpel and invented the first vaginal biofeedback device, the perineometer. He found that 80 percent of the women sent to him for surgery resolved their symptoms simply with exercise. Although many health care providers today are following Kegel's pioneering work, postpartum restorative exercise remains rare rather than routine, and the need for prevention during pregnancy, and **beginning in early childhood,** is not emphasized at all. Part of the explanation is that most gynecologists are surgical specialists and, until recently, males. (Presently equal numbers of women are entering OB–GYN residencies.) Some male physicians routinely performed a stitch called the "husband's knot" when suturing the episiotomy—a surgical incision in the vagina during birth. This "knot," which is actually an extra stitch or two, does not restore any PF function for the woman; it merely makes the vaginal entrance a little tighter. The name is significant since it reveals not only a sexist bias but implies that the female vagina is quite passive and therefore improvements need to be structural instead of functional. The woman's needs, as the name indicates, are totally secondary! Sometimes an actual tuck is taken as the birth canal outlet is sewn up "as tight as a virgin" after an episiotomy or perhaps during later gynecological surgery. This can cause pain to the woman during sexual penetration. As long as doctors cling to an architect's view of the vagina, the value of exercise will be overlooked. Instead, surgical enlargement and closure of the opening for childbirth will continue, along with future reconstruction.[39]

Many doctors, and their patients, believe that PF exercises do not work. I have learned this over the years, because the women tell me that they were **not instructed in exactly how to do the exercise correctly.** Some are simply told to "go home and do 300 Kegel exercises a day"!

The Pelvic Floor During Pregnancy

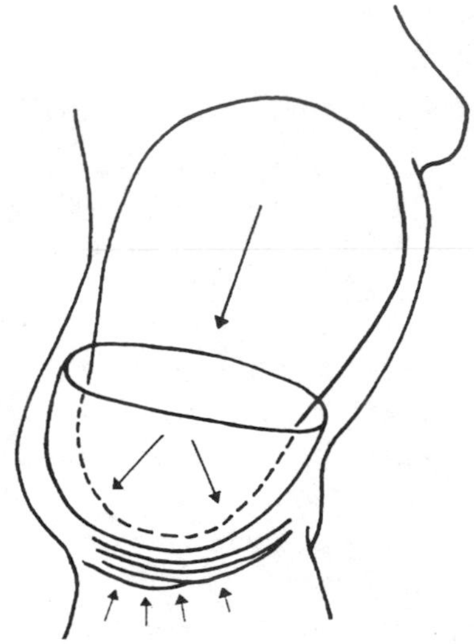

Figure 24. A large load leaves little room within the pelvic basin.

The PF is the supporting hammock of the pelvic basin and its contents throughout the entire lifecycle. Obviously it is vulnerable to internal stress. This includes prolonged pressure leading to weakness and inadequate support for the pelvic organs, or the temporary distention of the birth canal during birth. The passage of the baby does stretch the PF—just as you stretch a tight sweater neckline when you push your head through. The ability of the PF to stretch for the actual birth is increased not by structural slackness but by suppleness and elasticity. The vagina is designed to distend; it accommodates the penis during intercourse, and with the preparative hormonal softening of your tissues during pregnancy, the passage of your baby. The PF should be firm and supportive at all other times.

The uterus, which is suspended between the bladder and bowel, relies particularly on the PF. It is not a fixed organ and the significance of its attachments by ligaments is minimal compared with muscular support. During pregnancy, the increasing weight of the uterus creates additional, continuous and increasing stress on the PF. It's like a shelf that bows if you put too many heavy things on it. Furthermore, hormonal effects cause the tissues to soften in preparation for delivery. It is normal for the PF to have descended about an inch by term.

Pelvic Pressure and Constipation

The result of the increased pressure of the pregnant uterus, together with typically infrequent muscle action in the supporting floor, slows down blood circulation and causes congestion. Unless the PF gets occasional relief through changes in position and unless the PF muscles undergo active contractions which pump venous blood on its way, varicose veins may result in the rectum (hemorrhoids) or even in your vulva.

Toward the end of pregnancy, when your baby drops lower and its head engages in the pelvis, compression of the pelvic organs and symptoms increase. Straining during elimination is always undesirable because of the stress placed on both the PF and the abdominal muscles. This is particularly worrisome during the maternity cycle. Constipation[40] should be relieved with increased fluids, fiber and exercise. Elimination may be easier if you support your feet on a stool or better still squat, and allow the gentle interaction between abdominal compression on outward breath and PF release. Contraction and relaxation of the PF stimulates the proprioceptors that were described above and wakes up sluggish bowel muscles. Normally, additional increases in pressure are not necessary during elimination because involuntary muscles work by themselves. If you ever need to make an effort to empty your bowels, make sure that you are exhaling. (See Chapter 4 for pushing in labor.) Chronic constipation and straining with the breath held can cause, as well as aggravate, PF problems.

The Pelvic Floor During Labor and Birth

The strong supportive role of the PF in pregnancy is temporarily relinquished during birth. Your muscles need to relax and stretch. Tension, which is inevitable if you hold your breath, will slow your baby's progress through the birth canal, and must be released. In the second stage of labor, your PF undergoes extreme distention to permit first the delivery of the presenting part of the baby, which is the head in 96 percent of cases. With subsequent contractions, the shoulders are delivered and the rest of your baby slides out. The delivery of the placenta and membranes then follows, after which there is no further expansion of your vagina.

Unlike the cervix, which is gradually thinned-out (effaced) and opened (dilated) over a period of many hours in the first stage of labor, your vaginal canal receives considerably less preparation for the passage of the baby. In particular, the outlet is stretched very quickly in comparison. Of course, hormonal changes in pregnancy make tissues softer and more elastic (your cervix feels as soft as your lips when it is *ripe* at term). Your baby's head thins out your perineum, causing it to become numb, although until that point you may feel prickling, burning, and/or a build-up of tension like the feeling prior to orgasm. The greatest stress from the stretching is at the margins of your vagina, near your anus in the back-lying position (which is why you want to avoid that position) and also in the area of your bladder neck.

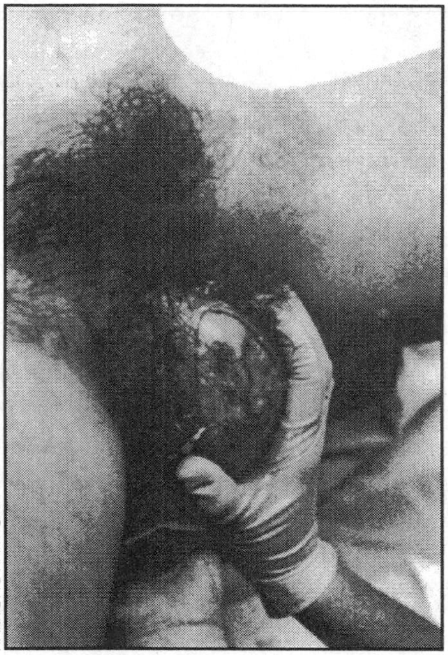
HARRIETTE HARTIGAN

Figure 25. Squat to open for your baby, allow the outlet to slowly s-t-r-e-t-c-h.

Episiotomy

When the baby's head is crowning and scalp and/or hair can be seen, an incision is commonly cut to enlarge the outlet and decrease the stretch on the tissues. The advantages claimed for episiotomy include minimizing stretching and nerve damage, preventing perineal tears, and reducing compression of the baby's head. It may also shorten the second stage of labor when there is tough resistance from the PF. (The mother is tensing the muscles to counteract the pressure and stretching, resisting rather than releasing and giving birth.) Episiotomies are also performed in instrumental deliveries, and even when the mother has been given anesthesia, (which results in total relaxation of the PF anyway.)

In general, a midline incision is easier to repair and heals better, although some birth attendants are afraid of involving the anal sphincter and prefer to cut toward one side. In these cases there is more blood loss and greater postpartum discomfort. More importantly, muscle function is harder to regain when scar tissue forms on one side; the fibers have to reunite randomly on the bias rather than in the central perineal body. Many women have some difference in strength between their right and left PF muscles to begin with. This is then exacerbated by an episiotomy on one side.

Episiotomy is clearly justified in cases of fetal distress—an emergency situation when the doctor has reason to "get the baby out." The other usual reasons are just "maybes." Maybe you will tear, maybe you will be stretched and have a prolapse in later life . . . maybe not. Dr. Leo Sorger, my husband, is one obstetrician with an episiotomy rate of 2.7 percent, and yet he does mainly high-risk births. In contrast, 55 percent of women in the United States had episiotomies in 1993.[39] There is always a chance of a perineal tear. However, women who have experienced both episiotomy and a tear (in different births) usually prefer the tear even though suturing it may be more difficult. Doctors who perform episiotomies as a matter of course do so because they prefer not to risk a tear. However, once the perineum is cut, the incision may be extended further during the birth. This results in greater damage than if the tissues had torn only the amount required and following natural lines of stretch. Episiotomy causes blood loss: it is minor surgery and your informed consent should be given. A first-degree tear heals spontaneously and so may a second-degree tear, which is usually sutured. Third-degree tears into muscle definitely need suturing, and especially fourth-degree tears since they involve the anal sphincter. Many physicians also feel that even if a tear were avoided, the muscles would be irrevocably stretched. But it has never been demonstrated that routine episiotomies reduce damage to the PF structure. In fact, incision and repair may lead to poor results later.[40] Exercises to prepare and restore a temporarily stretched—but intact—perineum are preferable. Even if there is nerve damage after delivery, the intact nerve fibers will form new connections as the muscle is rehabilitated with exercise. It has never been proven that episiotomies benefit the baby in any way, in the absence of fetal distress. Furthermore, the squeezing of the baby's chest by the intact perineum helps to expel mucus from its lungs and reduces the need for suctioning after birth. The intense concern that women feel about this intervention is revealed by the number of questions they ask about this subject in prenatal exercise and childbirth education classes.

My advice is to shop around for a midwife or physician whose episiotomy rate is no more than 5 percent and who has a very low tear rate. Many midwives consider it a matter of personal skill and pride to avoid both tears and episiotomies in the mothers they assist.

Preserving an Intact Perineum

If the second stage of labor is advancing rapidly, the sidelying position will eliminate the force of gravity and provide for a smoother birth. Sometimes the position of the baby's head is posterior (the back of the baby's head instead of the baby's face is against the mother's sacrum); it often helps if the mother goes on all fours for a while, or lies sideways, with the back of the baby's head uppermost and the mother's upper knee drawn close to her chest. If progress is slow in the second stage and there is difficulty with rotation of the baby's head, she can help by squatting. In this ideal position the force of gravity together with the weight of her torso between her spread thighs further opens her pelvic outlet. Squatting also changes the forces on the perineum so that any tears tend to involve the insignificant labia rather than deeper tissues. Also you can best protect yourself from an unwanted episiotomy in this autonomous position!

AVOID

- Pulling on your legs or pushing with your feet against resistance. This causes jack-knifing and muscle tension which spreads to your perineum.
- Placing your body weight on your pelvis, especially in a semi-recumbent

or backlying (supine) position. This constricts your pelvic diameters.
- Holding your breath to push. This causes reflex tightening of your PF.

Optimal Positions for Birth

During the descent and birth of your baby, your pelvis must be free of your body weight, as in squatting, standing (also known as "the dangle") and kneeling. Such positions have the added benefit of gravity. On your hands and knees is a neutral position. Women who are free to choose will find a position that feels instinctively right. Touch your baby's head as it emerges for important feedback. Massage and hot compresses (chamomile tea is popular) may help, too. You must psychologically want to "open up" your sexual organs. As during orgasm, there is a time to **let go** and trust. With all your senses intact, you will easily by guided by your body and your baby.[41]

The Postpartum Pelvic Floor

During birth, your vagina is greatly stretched, with or without an episiotomy. The tissue connecting the two sides of your PF can stretch further apart from the midline (*diastasis*, which can also occur in the abdominal muscles, see pages 89-92). Stitches will cause discomfort for a few days until they dissolve. Your tissues may be bruised and swollen, and the whole area tender to any pressure from thighs or buttocks, or internal strain from coughing, sneezing, and lifting (which you must avoid). For bowel movements, support the sutured area with your fingers wrapped in tissues to minimize "fecal distress." Clots will be passed through your vagina for the first few days after birth.

Sexual response can be impaired because the vagina becomes too tight or there are lumps and ridges as a result of the suturing. Most women strongly dislike the thought of their vagina being deliberately cut, suffering stitches and perhaps future scar tissue. Ultrasound (the type used by physical therapists, not the scans used in obstetrical diagnosis) relieves pain and reduces scar formation in my experience. When you first try to squeeze your vagina after birth, you may feel absolutely nothing and have difficulty controlling urine. However, your vaginal sphincter is capable of amazing recuperation—if you take the trouble, and right away. If not, you may join the majority of modern women, who suffer from some form of gynecological problems such as laxity of the vaginal walls, incomplete elimination, stress incontinence, constipation, and painful intercourse. **Exercise must start at once before muscle wasting or atrophy sets in.** If labor and birth have gone smoothly, with only stretching of your PF, recovery will be easier. But if you tore, or nerve cells were disconnected from the muscles they supply, you will have to do more exercises. Suturing, while restoring the structure of the PF, will not by itself return adequate function. **You must exercise to make the muscles efficiently supportive**

again. The nerve connections to injured muscle fibers can be re-established. This re-education means that the stronger muscle fibers help the weaker ones along until the whole muscle is working together again.

Exercising Your Pelvic Floor Prenatally

You gain a great advantage if you exercised your PF before delivery. There will be better support for your uterus and other pelvic organs during pregnancy, and an easier release during birth because of your increased awareness and supple muscles. Muscle responds to the demands made upon it and progressive exercise increases the size and power of each muscle fiber. At the same time, the blood circulation improves so your PF will be elastic enough to stretch over your baby's head with minimal damage. Then more muscle fibers will survive under distention because their nerve connections and blood-circulation remain intact.

By training your muscles before your vaginal outlet is distended, you'll know better how to re-educate them afterward. Restoration of a healthy muscle is quicker and easier than a neglected one. You'll be able to compare your present and past performances, and the comparison will increase your motivation to exercise after birth.

Pelvic floor exercises, above all others, should be part of every program for expectant mothers.

Exercising Your Pelvic Floor Postpartum

The process of learning is more difficult postpartum, when the muscles are stretched and slack, and feedback is poor. The longer you wait, the less muscle memory you have, and the more muscle fibers waste (atrophy). However, there are all kinds of devices to help you learn PF contractions. Exercise is always necessary—especially when severe functional deficit is present.

Exercise alleviates discomfort from any stitches you have. As you squeeze your vaginal muscles, the edges of the incision are pulled together rather than apart. Be assured that this exercise will help the healing no matter how sore you are or how scared you feel about doing it. Circulation to the wound will be increased; the blood brings fresh supplies of nutrients and carries off the accumulated waste products. Pelvic floor contractions relieve the pain not only of the tear or episiotomy wound, but of hemorrhoids or varicose veins of the vulva made swollen and tender during birth.

Comfort can be increased by:

- Ice packs
- Soaking in water with sea salt or comphrey leaf
- A heat lamp (a desk lamp will do)
- Castor oil, vitamin E oil
- Air and sunlight

Sexual intercourse can be resumed as soon as you feel like it after the discharge (lochia) from the site of the placenta has ceased. An episiotomy repair is usually healed by the second or third week, but sensitive scar tissue may make intercourse painful. Friction massage across the healed scar at right angles will help as well as just pressing hard for a few minutes on the nodule and then letting go. Experimenting with different positions, using lubrication, and releasing your PF on outward breath helps the first few attempts at sexual penetration. Breastfeeding mothers often need lubrication for vaginal dryness.

The comfort measures for an episiotomy also minimize symptoms from hemorrhoids, although if you are using a heat lamp for the episiotomy, you may want to cover any hemorrhoid(s) with a gauze pad. These distended veins are commonly caused by the pressure of delivery and will disappear postpartum. You can also try gently pushing them back inside, using a finger with some lubrication while your hips are elevated on several pillows. Remain in this position for a little while and perform some PF exercises to keep your anal sphincter tightly closed. Ultrasound, given by a physical therapist, brings quick relief to episiotomies, tears, and hemorrhoids.

Exercise returns the PF to its supportive role, which provides relief from the "low-down achy feeling" or the sensation that "everything is going to fall out." Exercises also minimize the likelihood of future pelvic problems. During the first few days, until your muscles resume their elasticity, tighten your buttocks and sphincters and draw up your PF, while exhaling, each time you get up from the bed or a chair. This will avoid any unpleasant sensations of "spreading"

If exercises are not done, your muscles may remain stretched and become further weakened as you resume your activities. Since muscles atrophy when they are not used, their eventual recovery will require more time and effort. By starting PF contractions immediately after birth, you will be doing them routinely by your six-week appointment. Let your midwife or physician check and, you hope, confirm the success of your exercises at this time, rather than disappoint you with the news of your vaginal shortcomings. However, seek treatment **before** your six week check up if you have any problems such as pain or urine control. Urinary retention, or infections, must be treated right away. Voiding may be a problem particularly after spinal or epidural anesthesia. Straining makes it worse.

Postpartum Voiding

After birth, when compression from the heavy uterus is no longer present; the stretch reflex of the bladder must suddenly adapt to the increased room in the pelvis. This adjustment is complicated by the large amount of urine that accumulates after delivery because the increased blood volume reduces quickly now that it is no longer needed. Waste products are excreted from the uterus and from the general bodily activity involved in labor and delivery.

You may need a urinary catheter to empty the urine if your bladder becomes over-distended, but some simple suggestions may help. Stand up, or put your feet on a stool when sitting on the toilet, or on a chair if you're using a bedpan. Gravity, the backward tilt of your pelvis, plus compression of your abdominal cavity combine to help voiding. (Actual squatting is best.) Some deep breathing and PF contractions compensate for the loss of intra-abdominal pressure and stimulate the bladder reflex. Gently massage your lower abdominal wall and turn on a faucet so you hear water flowing. Some women find it easier to void in the shower.

You may feel no need for a bowel movement for several days after birth. Stitches break down only if there is an infection or if there were not enough stitches. It's better to find that out earlier than later. **Exhale** slowly to avoid straining.

Technique for Pelvic Floor Contraction

During exercises, the muscles on each side of your PF move up and in toward the midline, which provides a squeezing and lifting effect. The floor works as a unit, with tightening of the sphincters and elevation of the inside passages occurring together.[42] Correct use of the PF requires some understanding of how the muscles are arranged and work. Inside feedback, which I'll describe shortly, is also essential. Your opinion as to how you are doing may be mistaken and it's impossible for an outsider to tell merely by looking whether you're doing the exercise correctly.

Your PF contracts when you hold back gas or a bowel movement, or interrupt your urine flow; this is one way to gain both awareness and control of these muscles. Stopping and starting the urine flow is an objective test of muscle power and can be done as an exercise to improve the strength of the PF. This action involves the front half of the muscular figure eight, which is the sphincter shared by both the urinary and vaginal passages. Dr. Kegel called this the "master sphincter" of the pelvis. This "mistress sphincter," in my terminology, needs development more than the stronger anal sphincter. It is easiest to concentrate on constriction of the vagina when there is something inside, particularly when you are first learning the art. You can check the muscle action yourself inserting one or two fingers; the bath is a clean and convenient place to make this investigation, or squat over a mirror.

The Role of the Pelvic Floor in Sexual Response

Analogies to defecation are a common way to explain and encourage PF function. But it is more pleasant and just as effective to condition the birth canal and its supporting structures with sensual squeezes. Unlike our fingertips, for example, which easily discriminate a pinprick, the stroke of cotton, and fine degrees of temperature, the vagina responds to deep touch, pressure, and stretch. This proprioception is also the way we get messages from other muscles in the body and is linked with the urge to push in second stage.

Nature provides for increasing resistance during intercourse by the engorgement of the tissues during sexual arousal. This building of the orgasmic platform decreases the amount of space in the vagina. The amount of stimulation relates to the extent of the orgasmic platform, and the snugness offered by the vaginal walls (PF muscles) which as well as being passively engorged also respond with active contractile efforts. Sexual response thus becomes conditioned with pleasurable experience as the PF muscles grip the penis.

Erotic interest is most intense during the second trimester of pregnancy, because your pelvic tissues are in a constantly engorged state quite similar to sexual arousal. This is an ideal time to work on your sexercise skills. Toward the end of pregnancy, spotting of blood during and after intercourse is not uncommon and there may be medical reasons that cause your midwife or physician to advise against coitus. Any prohibitions should be fully explained to both partners. Unless sexual activity is contraindicated for medical reasons, there is no reason to give it up. Considering that there may be several weeks postpartum when you may not feel like sex in any form, continue beforehand for as long as you desire. Sexuality is rarely associated with pregnancy in our puritanical culture although sex is the activity that puts us in that condition! *Susie Bright's Sexuality Book,* has a realistic and entertaining chapter about her sexual desires while pregnant. In addition, the sexuality of birth has been well-described by Jeannine Parvati Baker in her book *Conscious Conception* (See Further Reading).

One advantage of sharing PF exercises in a sexual situation is the benefit of feedback and encouragement that your partner can supply. In this way, the quality of your PF can be evaluated and improved. At first the contractions may be weak and fleeting, but if you are diligent they will be come more pronounced and last longer. The PF muscles are thinner than bulky muscles like your biceps and the muscle in the front of your thigh (quadriceps). These larger muscles have enough endurance to be exercised repeatedly against resistance. The PF, on the other hand, is more sheetlike, similar to the muscle that makes the front of the neck taut when we grimace. The PF's ability sustain a series of strong or prolonged contractions is less than other muscles. It becomes numb as it is stretched during birth, just like your jaw when it is forced wide open at the dentist.

Your partner can inform you of your progress because your subjective interpretation may be unreliable. You may think that your seventh and eighth muscle contractions were just as strong as the first six, whereas your partner will feel if your squeezes started to fade away after, say, the fourth.

Work within the number of contractions of equivalent strength that you can do, plus one. If you try for ten in a row, you'll just fatigue the whole structure. As you improve, add an extra contraction before resting so that you slowly build up the series. (Ten is enough.) Prolonged holding is tedious and tiring, like continuous standing, and not the aim of the exercise. Ten seconds is enough; those with weak muscles find this seemingly impossible. Frequent contracting and relaxing of the PF is more beneficial, and fatigue is avoided, by working within the inherent physiological limits of this muscle.

Common Errors in Exercising the Pelvic Floor

Holding your breath and bearing down strains and bulges the PF downward instead of drawing it upward. The abdominal and buttock muscles are frequently tensed instead of the PF. It's acceptable to exercise the abdominal and buttock muscles at the same time, but you must take care not to substitute these muscles for the PF muscles. The beginner has difficulty discerning the sensation of PF tightening when there is also tension from the stronger and more familiar muscles of the thigh, abdomen, or buttocks. For this reason I recommend **isolating** your PF first **and later integrating** PF contractions with those of your abdominal muscles for pelvic stabilization. This combination of muscle bracing is very important for lifting and other activities of daily life when you must protect your lower back as well as your PF.

Tensing of the inner thigh muscles at the expense of a PF contraction usually happens when the exercise is taught in the ankles-crossed position. This can interfere with your understanding of the specific action of the PF and its exact sensation. Furthermore, you may be encouraged to squeeze your thighs together to hold back urine—an ineffectual remedy for real muscle weakness. This extra effort in no way aids the weak sphincter. Control must be developed at a higher, deeper level of the pelvis. Your PF muscles are at the middle third of your vagina. To perceive the feeling accurately you need to practice with legs apart and think "high."

Another common misconception is that positions in which your legs are forced astride will stretch the PF. The positions claimed to achieve this include tailor-sitting, sitting with the soles of your feet pressed together, squatting, or sitting with your knees pulled up and apart toward your ears. The PF is not stretched simply because the muscles are not attached to your legs. However, some of these positions may promote awareness of PF function because you are not confused with the contractions of other muscles. Therefore, it is good psychological preparation to learn PF release for delivery in legs-astride positions. Furthermore, some of these positions are excellent for stretching other muscles, such as those of the inner thighs and the calves.

Learning Difficulties

Squat a Lot

Attempts to stop and start the urine flow usually teach the correct action of the PF muscles. Interrupting urination reinforces the specific sensation so that the muscles can be contracted the same way at other times; it also provides an objective test to measure how effectively you interrupt the flow. But some women have insufficient muscle strength even to slow down the flow and they usually also have problems starting and finishing. It merely adds to their despair if their gynecologist cheerfully tells them to practice stopping and starting the urinary stream in order to strengthen the muscles. This is their fundamental problem! I once heard a urogynecologist lecture that such an exercise could cause "tremendous damage." Curious, I asked him explain what this "tremendous damage" might be. He was unable to give me any details at all. It was something that he had read or heard! Any woman who has given a clean-catch urine specimen knows that at her doctor's request she must start the urine flow and then stop it. I do agree that attempting to work weakened muscles in this way with a **full** bladder can increase anxiety and loss of control. During a urinary tract infection it could also irritate the urethra, and as an exercise it may become tedious. However, it is the cardinal check of bladder control and a means for women themselves to identify the correct muscle action.

Contractions must be done a **few at a time but often.** A PF that is undergoing re-education must be treated with care at all times. Make sure that you brace your PF before laughing, straining, coughing or sneezing. If you dribble when walking to the bathroom in the middle of the night, or upon arising in the morning, it will help to do a few PF contractions before you stand up.

You and your partner can practice and check vaginal contractions:

- Begin lying down; the force of gravity in upright positions is considerable when the muscle floor is weak. Lying on your front (in early pregnancy or after birth) is often easier because you are more aware of the front, weaker part of your PF. If muscle response is still lacking, use gravity to assist.
- Raise your hips and buttocks on several pillows (lying either on your front or back), so your PF sinks down into your body, becoming closer to the organs it supports. Inverted yoga postures achieve this, but beginners should not attempt head and shoulder stands during the childbearing year and **they should never be done in the first postpartum month for fear of air embolism** (see page 42).
- Treatment may be sought from a physical therapist specializing in obstetrics and gynecology. (See Resources.) This will involve manual assessment and facilitation of your vaginal muscles and probably a biofeedback device and/or electrical stimulation. With a vaginal perineometer you learn the correct isolated action of vaginal constriction. Once a woman learns to identify the PF muscles increased awareness and function are readily developed. A biofeedback device is most helpful because diminishing scores indicate that the PF is fatigued from too many contractions or insufficient rest intervals. You'll be encouraged to see the higher scores as you become able to contract the muscles more strongly. The success of exercise depends on motivation—commit yourself to repetition and regularity, perhaps with one of the various devices for PF training listed in Resources.

Pelvic Floor Exercises

All the following activities concern the action of raising the PF and tightening the sphincters. These exercises involve lifting up and drawing in the muscles (no bones move); they are not only safe but absolutely essential. Exercises 1 and 3 also teach you to recognize the lower position of a relaxed PF and the sensation of voluntary release in preparation for the second stage of labor. While the learning process, especially **exhaling while tightening,** may be a challenge at first, with regular practice PF tightening becomes easier and finally habitual.

Exercise 1: Contract, Hold, and Release

Your muscles need power, endurance, and the ability to relax. Ideally, you are equally skilled in all three components which are covered in this basic exercise.
Position: Lying down on back, side or front. (On the front is the most comfortable position postpartum if you have stitches.) Legs apart and chest relaxed for normal breathing.

Action: Draw up your PF, feel the additional squeeze from the sides as your sphincters tighten and the inside walls become closer together. Concentrate particularly on the front portion of your PF—the mistress sphincter surrounding the vagina and urethra. Place one hand over your pubic bones and think about lifting your PF to the level of your hand. From time to time, insert a finger inside your vagina as well to localize the muscle contraction. Press with your finger successively against the contracting muscle in four quadrants: upper, lower, right side and left side. Most women have a stronger PF contraction on their dominant side. In this case, spend extra time working the weaker side against the pressure of your finger. A partner can help with this.

Hold for two to three seconds and then allow the muscles to relax completely. Note the sensation as your PF lets down loosely. Allow it to slacken a little more, releasing any residual tension. Drop your jaw, too. The jaw and pelvis, vagina and mouth are interrelated—especially during birth. In the beginning, do just two or three in succession before resting for a couple of minutes and always end with a contraction to return the muscular floor to its supportive level.

Progressions:

- ✦ **Positions:** Sitting, Standing, Squatting.
- ✦ **Muscle Interaction.** When you have learned the correct action, combine and alternate PF contractions with those of neighboring muscle groups (buttocks, inner thighs, abdominals) to test your awareness and control.
- ✦ **Increased time interval.** In the beginning you may be able to keep your PF tight for just a second or two. Gradually increase your holding time while you keep breathing. Longer than ten seconds is not necessary.
- ✦ **Increase the number of repetitions**, up to ten.

You can provide effective exercise of the muscle by doing this frequently, 50 times or more a day, but for example, in a series of 5, holding each contraction for 5 seconds. If you have a feedback device you might aim for holding 10 seconds, repeating 10 times and reaching a score of 10. Remember the physiological limitations of the PF and the importance of rest intervals.

Exercise 2: Quick Flicks and Sensual Squeezes

Commonly, women either reach a high score momentarily or else they hold for a substantial number of seconds at a low score.

Position: Any.

Action:

- ✦ Practice a couple of **quick** flicks—anticipate a sneeze!
- ✦ R E S T
- ✦ Increase the number. (Remember, ten is plenty.)
- ✦ Increase the duration. (Ten seconds is enough.)

- ✦ Focus on **slowly** squeezing, feeling the ring of muscle becoming concentrically smaller, holding it.
- ✦ Alternate these two activities, allow as much time to rest between them.

Exercise 3: Sexercises
Position: Your choice of coital connection[43] with your legs relaxed.
Action: Grip the penis as firmly as you can with your vagina and hold for a couple of seconds before relaxing. At the same time allow your buttocks and abdominals to be slack. Focus on the constricting sensation of the ring of muscle in the middle-third of your vagina. Repeat a few times until your partner feels that the strength of the contractions is diminishing. Rest and repeat in a few minutes. Practice holding longer at the same power. During this pleasant exercise your partner may remain still, although small adjustments of penetration may coordinate with your muscle contractions. This, in turn, will encourage your muscle action, providing for greater mutual pleasure. With practice, vaginal sexual response can be conditioned so that orgasm occurs without direct clitoral stimulation. For deeper internal sensations, experiment by lying or sitting on top of your partner so that you can increase the penile pressure on your G-spot. Side-to-side sliding movements also stimulate the exquisitely sensitive side walls of the vagina which are neglected with straight in-and-out intercourse. This exercise provides for progressive increase in muscle strength as you learn to make the contractions stronger, more consistent, and more numerous. Focus on the sensations of post-orgasmic release in your PF as well.

Exercise 4: The Elevator
Position: Any position, although it is easier at first to eliminate the force of gravity by lying down.
Action: Imagine that your PF is an elevator. As you ascend to the next level, draw up the muscles a little more. keeping the tension progressively accumulating. (It's like making a fist; keep squeezing until you feel that you have recruited every single muscle fiber.) After you reach your limit, gradually relax the muscles in stages as you descend "floor by floor." When you arrive at the basement—the resting level of tension in the PF—allow your PF to slacken a little more so that you feel the finer degrees of muscle tension release.[44]

Blow out through pursed lips or a partly closed glottis to the increase the pressure in your abdomen. Feel that there is no strain on your PF below, because air is being released from above. During birth you want to breathe your baby out with no interfering resistance from your PF. Holding your breath to push creates a closed pressure system, like a balloon, and your PF sphincters automatically tighten as a protective reflex. Remember—keep breathing, stay loose, jaw slack.

Exercise 5: The Faucet

Position: Seated on the toilet, legs spread apart for urination. Your feet may be supported on a stool if voiding is difficult to start or incompletely finished.
Action: Stop and start the flow a few times. Break it off smoothly with no dribbling.
Progression: Do this exercise squatting. You can position yourself with your feet on your toilet seat, but it is much easier for your balance to squat outdoors. Always concentrate on a strong uplifting contraction or two after bladder and bowel elimination. This will provide both frequent opportunities for muscle exercise and serve as a reminder.
Tip: Let some urine out first. Do this in the middle of the day rather than first thing in the morning or late at night. If you have a urinary tract infectio skip this exercise as it may irritate your urethra.

Exercise 6: Passive Weights

I have observed that women using an internal measuring device will invariably try too hard. They often hold their breath, bear down, tense their shoulders, clench their jaws and in general use just about every muscle in their body except their PF! In contrast, the placement of a smooth object inside the vagina (while standing) is an excellent stimulus for the right muscle action. For example, you insert a tapered plastic vaginal cone and take a few steps. If its starts to slide out, you will automatically squeeze your vaginal muscles and suck in your belly with an audible gasp. This is the right response. Passive weights can clarify the correct breath and muscle integration at an unconscious level because your reaction is spontaneous. These weights can also increase muscle strength, as you retain heavier weights for longer periods of time. You'll know if you are overworking neighboring muscles because your lower abdominals or lower back may get tired and achy. When your muscles tire, the passive weights drop out (wear underpants), so you are not tempted to overwork a tired muscle. Remove the weight and rest before those signs of overuse.

Vaginal cones can be purchased in a set of 5 for less than $100, see Dacomed in the Resources. An alternative, usually costing less than $20, are the *Chinese balls* sold in health food stores or New Age bookstores and catalogs. In contrast to the narrow tapered cones, they are larger and spherical. A disadvantage of the lighter cones is that they can be tucked away in a cul-de-sac of a roomy vagina without needing any PF support—just as well there is some fishing line on the end to pull it out! Thus cones are only helpful when they can slide out. The Chinese balls are at least twice the diameter and with their greater weight offer some women increased awareness. Furthermore, if you place both of them in your vagina, you will stimulate your G-spot, an area which needs specific cultivation in most women.

The cheapest device is a fishing-line sinker in a condom. You can tug gently on the condom to educate your vaginal muscles to hold the sinker inside. This exercise can be done in a semi-recumbent position whereas the challenge when using other passive weights is to retain the object while walking and doing general exercises.

Home Trainers

Various devices with internal sensors are available for rental or purchase. (See Resources.) Some units display EMG biofeedback, which measures the electrical activity in the muscles. Others feed back information about your PF power and endurance with air or water pressure, or a manometer gauge like the kind used for taking blood pressure. Only EMG biofeedback measures and facilitates relaxation which is a priority in chronic pelvic pain and tension syndromes. Yet other devices provide electrical stimulation. You should definitely seek out a physical therapist specializing in PF rehabilitation if you are not progressing with the instructions in this chapter. Many women simply need one lesson—to identify the correct muscle action and to integrate it with exhalation.

Figure 26. Exercise your pelvic floor in these three positions.

Bridging (page 143)

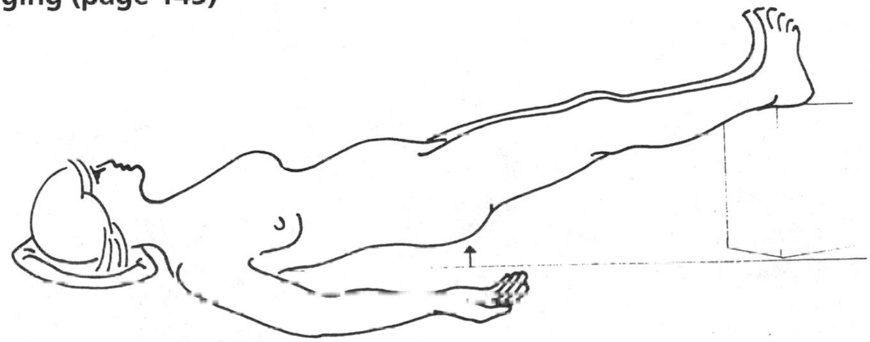

Pelvic tilting (page 96)

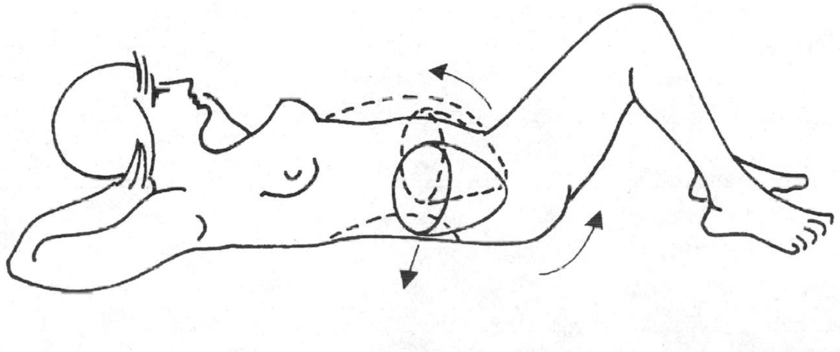

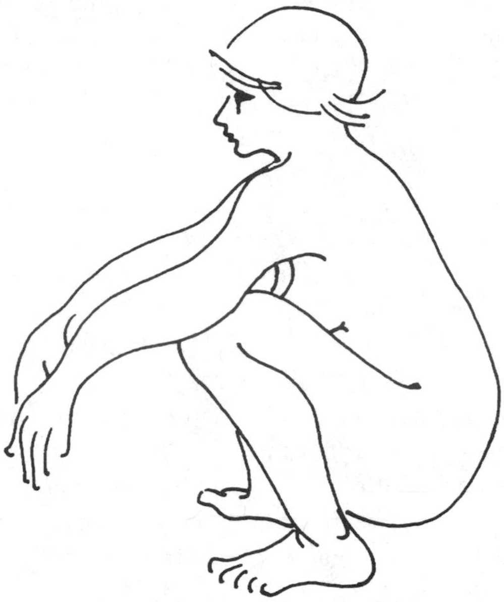

Squatting (page 129)

Unlimited Opportunities for Pelvic Floor Contractions

Pelvic floor contractions are entirely private and can be performed at any time and in any place or position.

- ✦ At red traffic lights.
- ✦ On the telephone.
- ✦ During boring conversations.
- ✦ While stirring food on the stove.
- ✦ During TV commercials.
- ✦ Anytime you have to wait (especially standing).
- ✦ While brushing your teeth.
- ✦ When coughing, sneezing, laughing, and, climbing stairs, straining.
- ✦ For sexual arousal.
- ✦ Any other time that you think of doing them.

Remember: Quality is more important than quantity. About 5 in a series, holding each contraction for about 5 seconds—then rest a while. Always end with an uplifting contraction. Fifty a day, at least, during pregnancy and postpartum. Fifty a day, at least, **for the rest of your life.**

4

The Abdominal Muscles

In contrast to the pelvic floor, the abdominal wall is quite a noticeable body part, sometimes outstandingly so! The state of these conspicuous muscles is readily observable through our clothes, whether there's a trim waist to be admired or a "spare tire" to be disguised. Unlike the pelvic floor, we're usually more concerned about appearance than performance, since the personal features of one's abdominal area significantly determine the size and type of clothing we choose, and how others see us.

Many people fail to realize that the abdominal muscles support the pelvis and lumbar spine, and it may seem strange that muscles placed in the **front** of the body may relate to discomfort or pain felt in the **lower back** region.

Most readers will be familiar with some kind of abdominal exercises, but certain modifications and precautions are required during the childbearing year. Some of the outward signs of a prior pregnancy may be obvious. Stretch marks, for example, if they occur, remain, despite numerous home remedies. Inadequate muscles are different because you can return them to healthier state. The central seam of the supporting muscle structure is vulnerable to herniation; this may have occurred during a former pregnancy. You should check for this continuously throughout pregnancy as the seam between the muscles can stretch wider and indeed is more likely to do so as pregnancy progresses.

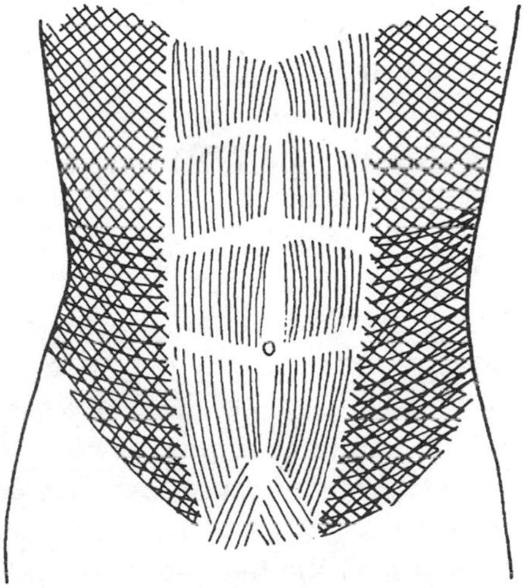

Figure 27. The abdominal muscles are like an elaborate corset.

Structure of the Abdominal Muscles

The abdominal muscles are arranged like an extensive four-way corset. They span the front of the trunk from the breastbone and ribs to the pubic bones, and then come around both sides of the pelvic ridge that you can feel at each hip. Their arrangement and attachments are quite complex, but we can compare them to an elaborate foundation garment. The extensive diagonal fabric around the sides of a factory-made girdle is similar to the two oblique abdominal muscles that overlap in such a way that each layer pulls in the opposite direction. The vertical panel down the corset's center represents the two straight *recti* abdominal muscles—an important point that will be discussed later. An extensive horizontal waistband is formed by the transverse abdominal muscles.

Functions of the Abdominal Muscles

Although each segment of the abdominal muscle corset makes its own contribution, the different parts are combined rather than isolated during exercises and activities. For example, the top half of the muscular corset is emphasized during movements with the upper trunk; the lower half works to stabilize the pelvis, or lower trunk, when the legs are moved. The functions of the abdominal muscles are varied:

- ✦ To maintain the proper positions of the abdominal and pelvic organs (including the enlarging uterus in pregnancy).
- ✦ To assist in deliberate breathing, singing, shouting, coughing, sneezing, nose-blowing, elimination, vomiting, straining, and the second stage of labor. The abdominals are the muscles that force exhalation—you can feel this when you blow up balloons or if you play a wind instrument.
- ✦ To control the angle of the pelvis. The downward pull of the buttock muscles, together with the upward pull of the abdominal muscles, maintain the correct alignment of the pelvis in relation to the backbone. The sideways pelvic tilt—hiphiking—is also abdominal muscle action.
- ✦ To flex the trunk to one side, which involves half of the muscles at a time.
- ✦ To raise the trunk upward from a back-lying position. Commencing the movement is the most difficult part since the force of gravity must be overcome. Even just raising the head will cause the upper layer of the abdominal muscles (recti) to tighten.
- ✦ To rotate the trunk; for example, bringing one shoulder toward the opposite hip, or moving the hips in relation to the chest.
- ✦ To brace the body when it is under stress—lifting, straining, or attack. This is a reflex protection during effort.
- ✦ To stabilize the lower back during leg-raising, knee-rolling and other limb movements.

Our habitual use of the standing and sitting positions provides little stimulus for the abdominal muscles, nor are these muscles exercised when we walk at a normal pace on level ground. Therefore, the abdominals are usually the weakest muscles among the general population and their weakness is one of the most common causes of backache. Maximal exertion of the abdominals occurs only when there is resistance, such as the leverage of the legs, arms and body weight. This is why appropriate exercises are trunk raising and pelvic stabilization during leg lowering. Running and lifting will call for some indirect abdominal activity, but not as effectively as specific exercises. Abdominal work can be done on all fours, but it also is not as effective as when lying on the back.

The Abdominal Muscles During Pregnancy

In order to accommodate the increasing size of the uterus, the abdominal muscles are capable of stretching to an enormous degree. Stretch marks are an outward sign of this lengthening and indicate that the skin has reached the limit of its elasticity. Smoothing out of the navel occurs around the seventh month.

During pregnancy you must keep your abdominal muscles in good shape to support the increasing load in front, which is placing increasing stress on your spine. A correct pelvic tilt that holds your spine in neutral is essential. Without it, poor posture, muscle strain, and backache are a foregone conclusion.

The abdominal muscles feel deceivingly fit during pregnancy because they are continuously stretched over the enlarging uterus—the resistance keeps them taut and responsive. However, without special effort after birth, you cannot be assured of a complete return to former tone and length. Your abdominal wall may resemble a girdle, but one that is made of worn out elastic, known as a jelly belly! Muscles, unlike girdles, **do** recover their inherent properties. Supple muscles, which have maintained optimal contractile ability and blood circulation with exercise, will lengthen easily during pregnancy and shorten more quickly afterward.

Back-lying During Pregnancy

The essential abdominal muscle exercises can and should be done at any time to maintain existing strength. The most effective exercises for your abdominals require you to lie on your back (supine). You do not want to be semi-recumbent (i.e., with your head and shoulders on pillows) because the abdominal muscles work during the first 45 degrees of trunk raising. In a sit-up the rest of the movement is completed by your hip flexors, working in reverse direction.

The Abdominal Muscles During Labor

Uterine contractions in the first stage of labor (that are not under your control) open your cervix as your baby remains inside your uterus. Relaxed abdominal muscles during this phase allow your uterus to tip forward with each contraction. This is part of the drive angle which helps your baby's head to enter your pelvis—two good reasons to be upright.

When normal breathing is accompanied by the gentle rising and falling of the abdominal wall, the muscles are soft. When you are fearful or anxious, you generate physical tension, which restricts breathing (the "tight chest" feeling). As labor becomes intense, simply let nature take over, continue your attitude of surrender, trusting your body. Your breathing will change. Just keep breathing: your way and your sound is the right way!

The first stage of labor is completed when your cervix is fully opened. Now your baby can leave your uterus and move down your birth canal but the actual urge to push **develops only when your baby's head is on your pelvic floor.** Your baby will be born from the combination of the expulsive contractions of your uterus and your bearing-down efforts. The second stage is the exciting part of labor! Your inside companion for nine months is, at last, on its way out, and you can actively assist. Knowing this gives you a new wave of enthusiasm after perhaps long hours of first-stage labor.

If you are unfortunate enough to be lying flat on your back, you will have the additional task in labor of raising your head and neck—**against gravity—** for each push. Rocking up and down on your spine like this can result in backache. Although you may be encouraged to pull up on your legs, as is illustrated in Figure 78, it is a waste of energy. **Get yourself upright and mobile, and use the considerable benefit of gravity.**

Birth is more a matter of letting go than mustering force, and only the woman herself knows what feels right. I gave birth to my last child underwater and during the pushing phase I squatted, with support from my bent arms on the edge of the hot tub. Being in water meant that I gave up any assistance from gravity. However, the comfort of the water, the freedom of movement and the knowledge that my son would just float into my arms (not needing to be caught) made the extra pushing effort worthwhile. I loved labor, and pushing especially.[45]

Direction of the Expulsive Force

The baby's path is down the birth canal, up to squeeze under your pubic bones, and then out into the world. (See diagram on page 110.) Women who deliver lying flat on their backs actually push uphill. If you are semi-recumbent, you have **even more** of your body weight compressing your sacrum and coccyx than if you are lying flat. These pelvic joints have loosened in order to expand during birth; it is counterproductive to compress them with your weight.

Side-lying may be preferred when the baby's progress is rapid. As gravity is eliminated, pushing is a little easier to withhold, if necessary.

Maternal Effort

Many people believe that natural childbirth is a major athletic event—total exertion and total exhaustion. Babies are born, with or without help of the mother or an attendant. Appropriate assistance, of course, is sometimes necessary and often very useful to mother and baby. Time, timing, autonomy and release are the most important considerations for second stage. Often there is a lull following complete dilation, which is physiological and allows the mother a respite. British author Sheila Kitzinger calls this the "rest and be thankful stage." Then the contractions build up again to drive the baby's descent. Let me state again, however, that **the actual urge to push is felt only when the baby's head is low enough in the birth canal to stimulate the stretch receptors in your pelvic floor.** You may be fully dilated for quite some time before this stage develops.

The Hurried Birth

Frequently, women are told to bear down **before** the uterus is ready, and an arbitrary time limit is set for delivery. The "active management" of labor is the current trend; this intervention excuses itself as a way to lower the Cesarean rate! There are kinder and gentler ways to facilitate labor than by routinely rupturing the membranes and giving pitocin to stimulate contractions. These interventions force the process instead of allowing mother and child to flow with their own integrated rhythm. Women must hold close to their hearts a vision of free birth.

When the urge to push is irresistible, you will **spontaneously** bear down. Only the mother experiences the inner cues. One cannot be taught how to push a baby out any more than one can be taught how to have an orgasm. At a certain point, the mind lets go and trusts in the physical response of the body. If you don't feel the urge to push, then just wait. When the urge comes, you will have no choice.

Women often ask, "How much voluntary effort is appropriate?" It's logical that the informed, prepared mother is the best judge of the answer. After all, it is she who can harmonize her response to second stage contractions just as she did in the first stage of labor. Often, however, a woman in labor is subject to a ceaseless chorus of those around her exhorting her to bear down. This well-intentioned enthusiasm is invasive and it does not allow for the differences perceived from woman to woman and from contraction to contraction.

Although such bossy behavior is slowly going out of fashion, many women have not forgotten the ***push–push–push–push–push–push*** they heard with each contraction in a prior delivery. At worst, such commandeering is defeating; at its best it is distracting for a mother who is trying to tune in to her uterus which she sensibly trusts more than she does any outsider. Pushing, of course, is necessary in slow and difficult labors, but many other factors play a role as well—such as the mother's position and energy level. (These can be changed, whereas such factors as the size of the baby's head, whether it is a first or fifth baby, etc., cannot.) Rather than push so hard, squat to make more room within your pelvis and let gravity exert its well-known effect. Especially if Dr. Leo Sorger needs to use forceps or a vacuum extraction, he asks the mother to squat and never uses stirrups. If he finds her flat on her back, he tells the nurse, "Only pancakes are flat!"

Relaxation may be all that is needed—the uterus can push your baby out without additional effort from you.[46] If your help is needed, you will experience an irresistible urge to bear down. Occasionally, women report no urge to push, even when they have not had an epidural. Usually the baby's head is still too high in your birth canal. Wait and walk. Squatting helps, and pressure on your pelvic floor from the attendant's finger(s) inside your vagina (as if the head were pressing on the proprioceptors) if there is no progress. Most often, feeling no urge to push is the result of medication and anesthesia; epidurals especially interfere with the bearing-down reflex if they are not allowed to wear off before the baby's head reaches the pelvic floor.

Your pelvic floor automatically relaxes during bearing down **as long as you're exhaling.** Holding your breath has the opposite effect. During elimination, you can observe the relationship between increasing the pressure within your abdomen on exhalation while at the same time releasing your pelvic floor muscles. Often the unprepared and apprehensive mother, upon feeling the enormous pressure on the pelvic tissues and the stretch of her distending vaginal outlet, becomes alarmed and tenses her pelvic floor instead. Other women are concerned about escape of bowel contents. Extreme rectal pressure (especially if you are on your back), more uncomfortable than painful, may be felt at this time. In any case your baby's birth is your priority—not the state of the sheets![47] Dr. Sorger explains "the four-opening push" (three orifices of the pelvic floor and the mouth) to women: "Let them all go!"

Prepare for birth by:

- ✦ Appreciating the principles involved;
- ✦ Learning what can happen;
- ✦ Anticipating what you might feel;
- ✦ Knowing how you can help;
- ✦ Taking every opportunity around the house to practice positions such as squatting, kneeling, tailor-sitting and legs-astride.

Premature Urge to Push

You would not drive your car out of your garage without the door being fully open, so pushing before complete dilation of the cervix is senseless. However, some women do bear down inappropriately, usually because they are supine or recumbent. In such positions, their rectal proprioceptors are stimulated because of the pressure from the baby's head. The solution is to stand, kneel, squat, or walk around and see if this urge diminishes. On the other hand, your baby could have made a lot of progress and be at a lower station in your pelvis than the attendants had realized. If your baby's head has indeed reached your pelvic floor, then it is not a premature urge to push, but a true "call of nature" because the time is ripe!

Crowning

At the moment of crowning you may be asked to "stop pushing," although it is always better to receive instructions in positive language, such as, "keep breathing" or "pant." Now, you simply let your baby's head (or buttocks) slide out just as you would ease your own head slowly through a tight neckline. First, your baby emerges from your bony pelvis. The back of his or her head extends up beyond your pubic bone; it cannot slide back anymore. Next, the baby must negotiate your perineum. You will feel intense stretching and burning sensations, followed by a natural numbness. (This happens at the dentist when your lips are stretched to their limits.) A calm, smooth delivery results in minimal trauma to your pelvic floor by allowing its gradual distention—without tearing or episiotomy.

Feel your baby's head emerging from your body with your hand because this keeps you focused on him or her. This may sound strange, but often in labor we feel so absorbed working with this tremendous internal energy that the presence of our unborn child fades in comparison. The rests between contractions are opportunities to reassure your baby, with your voice and hands, that this is a team endeavor.

It is often difficult to refrain from a hearty push at the moment of birth. You will have been pushing for perhaps quite a while, frequently with encouragement from those around you; and your uterus is still contracting expulsively. The next push will bring your baby into the world—yet ideally just let your uterus nudge your baby out by itself. Panting will help because you can't bear down at the same time; it will not take away the urge. Your diaphragm fluctuates, your ribs move and, since the abdominals no longer have a firm base to work from, your power to push is greatly reduced.

A general guideline for your effort in the second stage is to push only when you cannot resist the urge to do so. An alert woman, with abdominal muscles that she can effectively coordinate with the expulsive urge and a pelvic floor which she is able to release, often speeds along the second stage. However, the amount of maternal effort required will depend on the particular circumstances of your labor. You must be guided from within. Your partner can be most helpful at this time by affirming any sound, effort or movement that you make spontaneously, thus reassuring your faith in your body's natural response.

Remember

- ✦ **Flow** with each contraction, breathing **out** as you bear down.
- ✦ **Trust** your spontaneous breathing, grunts and groans.
- ✦ **Surrender** to the stretching of your pelvic floor throughout second stage. Allow all sphincters to relax—especially your mouth—with your lips and jaws parted as your baby is born. Spontaneous sound ensures this.

- Direct your effort low down and in front—increase the pressure in your abdomen, not in your face! Keep your eyes open.
- Push only as long and hard as you feel the urge to do so.
- Avoid prolonged pushes, which affect your breathing, circulation, and also your baby's heart rate.
- When asked to refrain from pushing at any time—immediately rest and pant. Make it light and brisk to disengage your abdominals.

The Abdominal Muscles Postpartum

During the first few days after birth, the abdominal muscles are the same size as before but they provide inadequate support for your pelvis and spine because they are no longer stretched taut over your uterus. As a result, these joints remain at risk. You must avoid spinal strain or further stretching of your abdominal muscles. Exercises, then, are performed in stable positions where support is maximal. Your ligaments gradually tighten back to their former state as your uterus returns to normal. All physiological adjustments during the postpartum weeks are beyond your control. Returning your abdominal muscles to their former shape, size and efficiency, on the contrary, **requires your active input.**

For best results**, commence exercises within twenty-four hours** after birth. Initially, you will only be tensing, retracting and pulling in the muscles to coax them back to their former length. These isometrics do not require any movement; indeed when the abdominals are lengthened, movements are done by other muscles. It is a simple matter of shortening your muscles by "sucking in." Think "bellybutton to backbone" frequently. This abdominal shortening is easy, completely safe and can be done in any position. **Strong exercises must not be attempted until there has been good recovery of the abdominal wall and the pelvic floor.** This will vary with each woman and relates to her physical condition before pregnancy, her labor and the immediate postpartum phase. Always remember to brace your pelvic floor for any anticipated increases in your abdominal pressure—otherwise your stitches (if you have them) will remind you!

Problems with the Vulnerable Midline (Diastasis recti)

In the diagram of the abdominal muscles (page 81), you will notice that there is a seam down the center of the front panel. Rather than one single band of muscle extending vertically along the midline of the abdomen, from top to bottom, there are two halves—the right and left recti muscles. The corset previously referred to is thinnest in this area since these broad flat bands form a single muscle layer at this point. This arrangement differs from the other abdominal muscles that overlap at the flanks. Simply stated, these recti muscles are covered only by sheaths of fibrous connective tissue from the neighboring muscles, which unite in a central seam called the *linea alba.* This seam is about half an inch wide and together with the horizontal fibrous bands, it can be readily observed in male athletes—the famous "washboard stomach." (Men have far less fat under their skin than women so their anatomy is more visible.) During pregnancy, the skin over this area turns dark in some women; this superficial line is known as the *linea nigra.*

The softening and stretching of the linea alba, which extends above and below the navel, makes the central connection vulnerable. This seam is part of the vulnerable midline and must be evaluated before starting abdominal exercises and continuously throughout pregnancy.

Most of the time the weight of your uterus falls on the front wall of your abdomen. The recti muscles in particular act to maintain pressure within your abdomen during any form of straining, such as undue bearing down efforts in the second stage. Habitual straining during elimination is also a contributing factor.[48] The umbilical or navel area is potentially weak because of our early development, and hernia can still occur at this point even in adults.

Your central seam can spread just like a closed zipper may open at the point of greatest strain. You may be quite unaware of this since you feel no pain directly from this condition (but you may have chronic backache). Although the muscles are still joined to their connective tissue, the effect is a wide soft space between them as if they had separated.

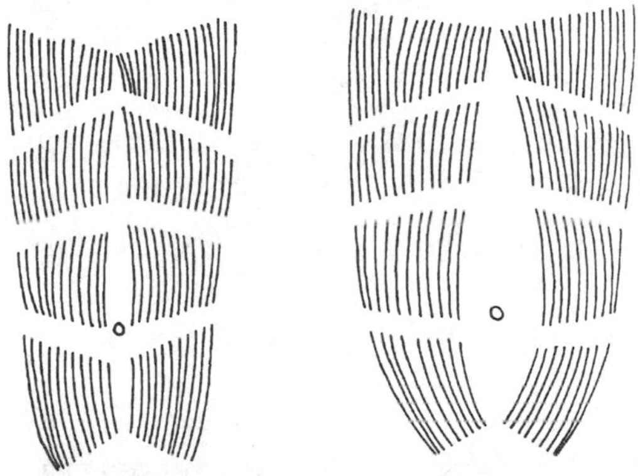

Figure 28. The recti muscles can stretch apart as a zipper opens under stress.

During pregnancy, this condition is seen typically in the last trimester, unless you developed a gap with a former pregnancy. The cause is a combination of the hormonal softening of tissue, the stretching of muscle and the sometimes excessive strain occurring in later pregnancy when the muscles are in a lengthened state. One of the many reasons for avoiding double leg-raising exercises (see page 40) is that they can cause or increase this gap between the recti muscles. "Jack-knifing" to sit up from a horizontal position is also a danger; always roll onto your side and use your arms for support and strength to get up from lying.

Any abdominal strain during pregnancy or labor will be registered at the central junction, just as a seam in your clothes will split before the fabric. Other predisposing factors include obesity, multiple pregnancy, a large baby or excess fluid in the uterus.

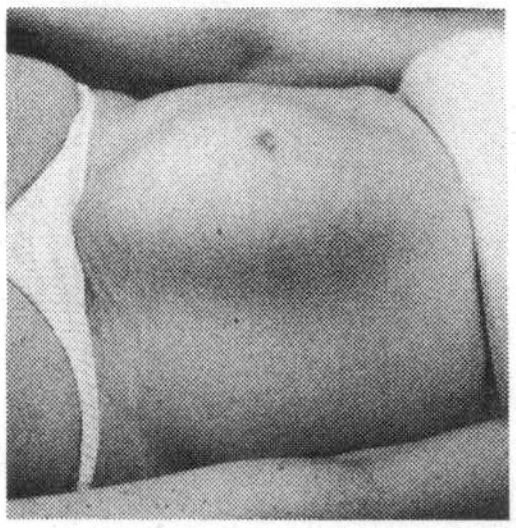

Figure 29. Sometimes the bulge is large like a watermelon, seen only when the head is raised.

Make sure that you investigate any bulging of your abdominal seam that you may notice when getting out of bed or the bath. The gaping of the muscles can be slight or so wide that the uterus or even abdominal contents postpartum can be felt through the space. If not corrected, a weakened abdominal will be less supportive for your spine or a subsequent pregnancy. As the recti muscles in the midline insert not into bone, but the central seam instead, this is the point of fixation from which the remaining abdominals contract. Since the recti muscles are important in controlling the tilt of your pelvis, which in turn supports your backbone, their weakness can give rise to poor posture and pain in your lower back.

Check for Recti Muscles in Pregnancy

During pregnancy, check your central seam frequently, and if it has stretched, take care to maintain or improve the position of your recti muscles. When you have a gap that bulges three finger-widths or more, curl-ups and leg-lowering exercises will make it larger, so you must avoid them. All the other exercises in this book can be done safely. If you are in doubt, observe your central seam for bulging while doing a particular movement.

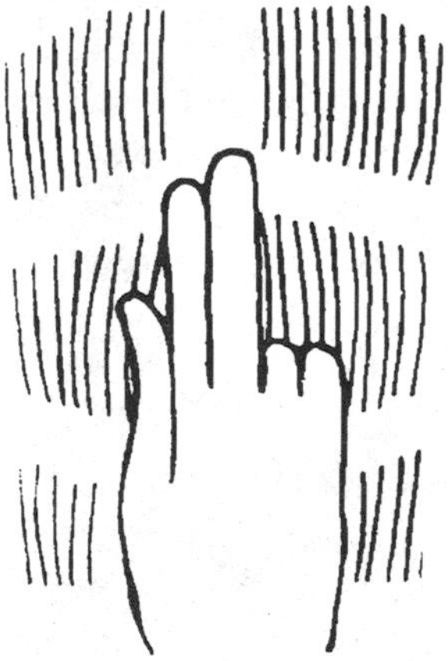

Figure 30. Place your fingers horizontally in the softened gap near your waist.

Position: Lying on your back, knees bent.
Action: Slowly raise your head and shoulders reaching toward your knees with outstretched arms.
Check: You may notice a **vertical** bulge in your central abdominal area. With one hand you can feel a softer region more than an inch or so in width between the taut recti muscles on each side. Check how many fingers you can insert **horizontally** in this gap. If you can fit in three or more fingers, do the following exercise.

Note: Everyone has a gap, the question is only how wide? One to two fingers is normal, since both gaps and fingers vary with individuals.

Corrective Exercise for Diastasis Recti during Pregnancy

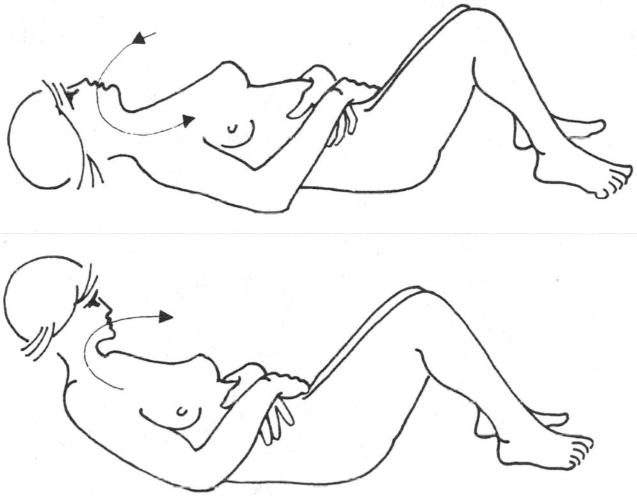

Figure 31. Support your recti muscles as you raise your head on outward breath.

Position: Lying on your back, knees bent, cross your hands, one wrist above the other, over your abdominal area so that you will be able to support the two muscles as you raise your head.

Action: As you **slowly** exhale, raise your head to your chest until just **before** the bulging begins. Pull in your abdominal muscles while breathing out. Keep your shoulders on the floor. Return slowly to the starting position. If your abdomen is large, it may be necessary to support the recti muscles with your wrists and to cup your hands, one above the other, to confine the central bulge.

This exercise should be done a few times, when lying on the bed in the morning and the evening, so that your recti muscles can be kept in maximum tone and to discourage further separation.

Postpartum Check for Recti Muscles

Evaluate your central seam around the third day. Before this time the whole abdominal area feels so slack that the test is not reliable. Besides, you will already have had two days of frequent isometric exercises to prepare you for closing the gap.

Position: Lying on your back, knees bent. Press the fingers of one hand (held horizontally) firmly into the area around your navel.

Action: Slowly raise your head and shoulders. Reach for your knees with your other arm. You will feel your rectus muscle on each side pull toward the midline, pushing your fingers out of the way.

Check: How many fingers remain in the gap? A slight gap, one or two fingers wide, is just tissue slackness and will tighten of its own accord. But if you can place three or more fingers between the taut bands of muscle, then you need to make a special effort to restore the integrity of this area. The bulge during pregnancy becomes a hollow postpartum.

Postpartum Corrective Exercise for Recti Muscles
Position: Lying on your back, knees bent. Cross your hands at your waist and guide your recti muscles toward the midline to stabilize them with your hands as you raise your head.
Action: Breathe in first. As you slowly exhale, raise just your head off the bed, at the same time pulling the underlying muscles together with your hands. Return slowly to the horizontal.

Head-raises activate only your recti muscles. Raising your shoulders as well includes your other abdominal muscles which insert into the central seam.

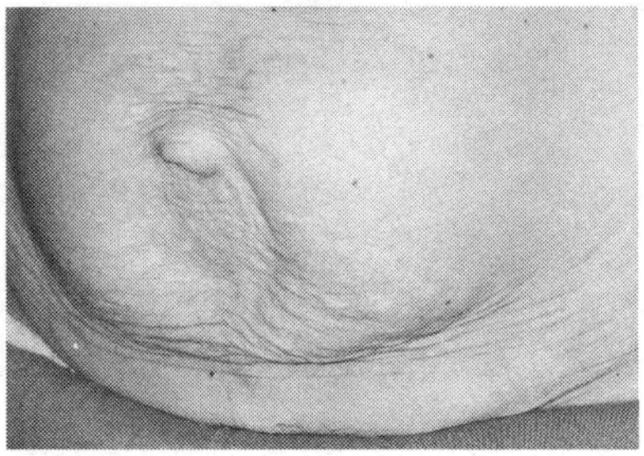

Figure 32. The recti muscles are four inches apart and there is an umbilical hernia, too.

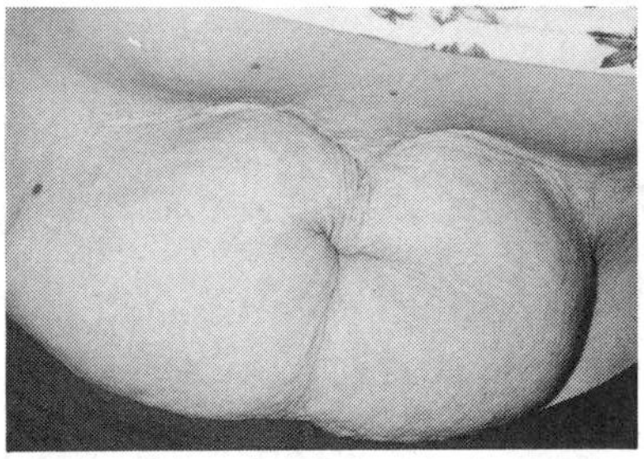

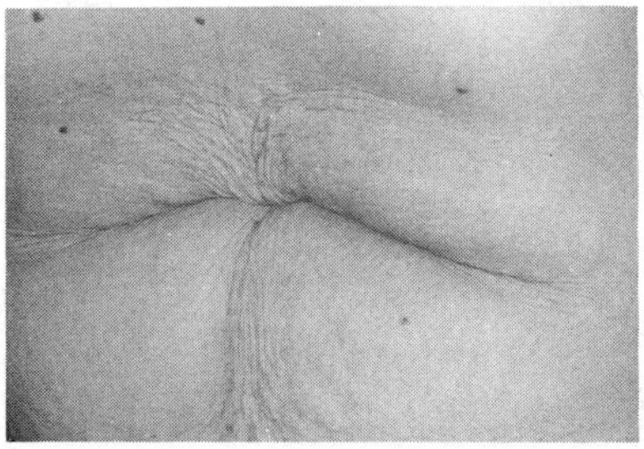

Figure 33. Bulging must be avoided at all times. Suck in your bellybutton.

To bring your recti muscles parallel, repeat this corrective exercise often, at least fifty times a day. Do ten each hour if you can, slowly and mindfully. Daily improvement will be noted if you are conscientious, and the gap should be back to the normal half-inch **within a week.** Even in the rare cases when a whole hand can be placed sideways in the gap, diligent exercise can close the gap in ten days!

If you exercise less consistently it will take longer. Until you have closed the gap, avoid exercises that twist your hips, or rotate or bend your trunk to one side. The other abdominal muscles are indirectly attached to the recti; therefore, the recti will be pulled further apart when other components of the corset shorten. Sometimes the gap widens again after progressing to curl-ups if your recti muscles are not yet strong enough. In this case, do a few more days of head-raises before attempting the curl-ups again.

Add your shoulders to the load only when your recti muscles can cope with a head raise without being supported. This is why progressive exercises will increase, not decrease, the gap. Remember, the movement must be done slowly in order for the recti muscles to stay aligned when these neighboring muscles exert their additional pull. Raising your head and shoulders on **out-**

ward breath requires your abdominal muscles to work without the fixation of your diaphragm, because it moves up in the chest, emptying the air. If you were to hold your breath, your diaphragm would move down and increase the pressure inside your abdomen. Weak muscles are unable to compress the abdominal wall if pressure within is increased, so they bulge outward.

If weeks, months or years have gone by and you find that you have a hollow in the center of your belly, you still need to go through the same routine.[49] Sometimes women become quite athletic and work out at a gym, doing very strong abdominal exercises that make the gap worse. You have to do step one first. Go back to head-raises and coax the muscles until they are parallel at the central seam. Then go through the abdominal progressions, watching carefully that the center seam can stabilize the pull of the other abdominal muscles.

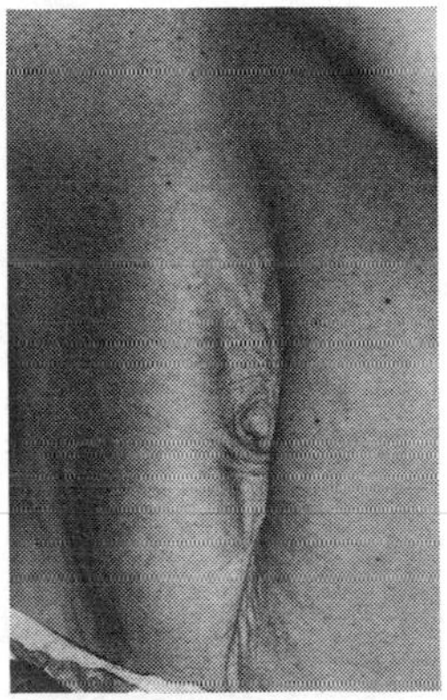

Figure 34. Postpartum, the bulge becomes a gap when the head is raised.

Hacking

There are two problems with the long-term jelly-belly even when the gap has closed. One is that muscles allowed to remain in a lengthened state after pregnancy now hang in a fold or pouch. The second concerns the proprioceptors, which are no longer stimulated because there is little tension, resistance or elasticity. The abdomen has a doughy feel because the nerve networks are almost lifeless. This condition is so easy to prevent—just a few days of isometrics after birth—but very difficult to reverse. Chronic jelly-bellies become "dead-zones."

A type of deep massage called *hacking* stimulates the proprioceptors, which are deeper than nerve endings in the skin. Use a relaxed chopping motion with the outer border of your hands. Go up and down as well as side to side. Hack with your head raised and muscles tense. Hack with your belly soft; hack with a pelvic tilt. In other words—hack both with and without muscle contraction.

Important Principles for Abdominal Muscle Exercises

The key to safe and sane abdominal exercises is, first, to protect the lower back from the adverse pull of the hip flexors, and second, to be in control of the leverage and resistance from gravity.

The essential exercises emphasize control of the pelvic tilt to improve posture and relieve back strain. They require minimal exertion and maintain the condition of the muscles as they expand over the enlarging uterus. Some degree of progression is naturally provided because muscles work more as the weight of your uterus increases.

However, stronger exercises that progress your abdominal muscles against the resistance of gravity as well are necessary to **improve** the condition and power of your muscular corset. Exercise in pregnancy, ideally, should begin before the muscles start to stretch—but it is **never** too late.

Abdominal muscles are exercised by the leverage and resistance involved in raising and lowering the trunk or the legs. Curl-ups emphasize action in the upper part of the abdominal corset as the muscles shorten to raise your upper body. Leg movements demand strong stabilization from your lower abdominal muscles to control your pelvic tilt. It is difficult to isolate the abdominal muscles because their action is complicated by the hip flexors.

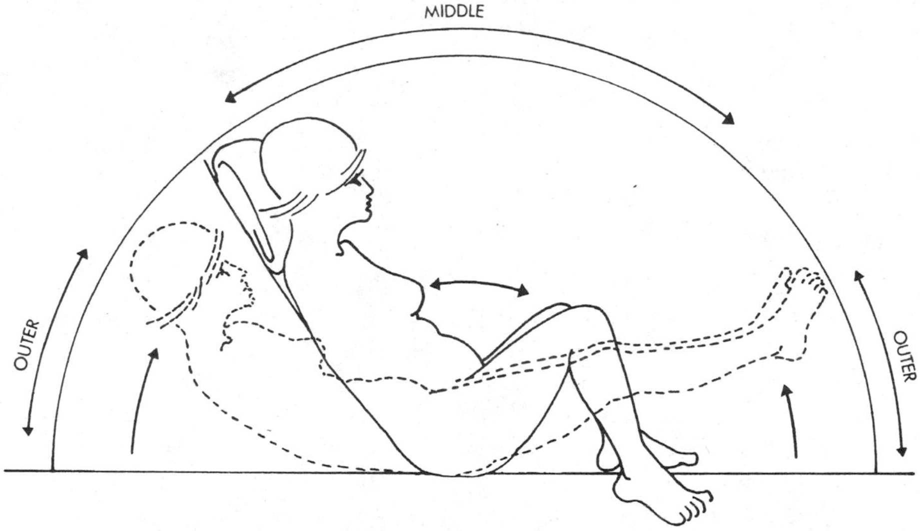

Figure 35. The outer range of muscle contraction is more difficult and the resistance of gravity increases toward the horizontal.

Normally, muscle activity occurs midway between the two points where the muscles are attached. Outer range movement, with muscles at their longest, is more difficult. Examples include raising your head from the horizontal, or standing tall and "holding in your dinner" as my dance teacher puts it.

Essential Abdominal Muscle Exercises

Exercise 1: Abdominal tightening on outward breath

This exercise works your transverse muscles, which compress your abdominal contents and prevent your abdominal wall from bulging. In pregnancy, think about hugging your baby.

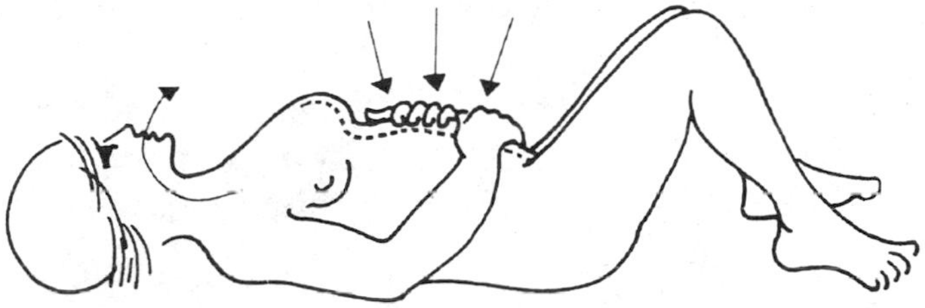

Figure 36. Tighten your abdominal muscles as you exhale.

Position: Lying on your back or side, knees bent. Place your hands on your abdomen until you have learned abdominal retraction. Then this exercise can and should be done in any position.
Action: Take a complete breath in through your nose, feeling your nostrils widen slightly. (Breathing through the nose warms and filters the air.) Allow your abdominal wall to expand upward. Then, lips slightly parted, blow the air out through your mouth, slowly but **forcibly,** pulling in your abdominal muscles until you feel out of air. It's like sustaining a note while blowing a trumpet or singing. The resistance of your lips is important to recruit your abdominals—the muscles of forced exhalation. Rest between efforts to avoid becoming dizzy.
Progression: Other positions,[50] such as sitting or standing. Sitting in a rocking chair is ideal—blow out and tighten your tummy as you rock back.

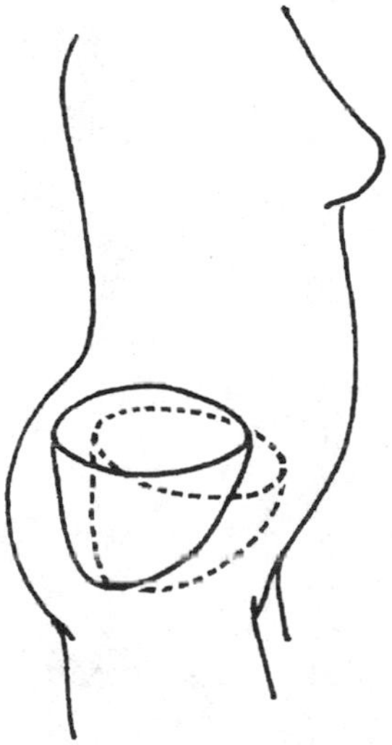

Figure 37. The pelvic basin and its contents must not tilt forward.

Pelvic Tilting

Pelvic tilting improves posture and relieves a stiff and aching lower back. The abdominal muscles in front pull up your pelvis; your buttock muscles pull it down. Belly dancing is pelvic-tilting in its most elaborate form: the movements are from side to side, front to back, and in circles. Many women move their knees or trunk instead of the pelvis—standing is a difficult position unless you remember the days of the hula hoop.

An analogy may make this clearer. Imagine that your pelvis is a basin, in fact, the Greek word for basin is *pelvis.* Place your hands on the bony crests at each hip—this is part of the upper rim. Just as you would tip back a basin that is leaning forward, to contain the contents, so you tilt back your pelvis and baby. Feel the movement with one hand in the hollow of your back and the other just above your pubic bones.

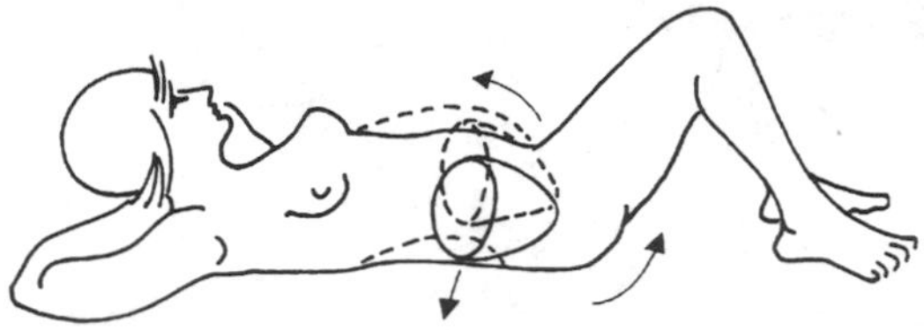

Figure 38. Active pelvic tilting strengthens your abdominals.

Lying on your back with bent knees puts you in a complete pelvic tilt; then you add the abdominal muscle action. Your shoulders and hips are stabilized and gravity assists your abdominal muscles as they press your pelvis backward.[51]

Exercise 2: Pelvic Tilting

Position: Lying on your back, knees bent.
Action: Rest your hands on your lower abdominal muscles to feel them shorten as you roll your pelvis back to press your waist on the floor. Hold the position for a few seconds as you exhale.

Make sure that your buttocks and shoulders stay on the floor and think "bellybutton toward backbone." Postpartum, think about "making yourself thin" from front to back.

Progression: Diagonal Pelvic Tilting

Place your right hand on your lower abdomen as if it were in a pocket. Tighten the underlying muscles in a diagonal direction from your left groin to your right wrist. Then place your left hand in the same manner and tighten in the opposite diagonal direction. Buttocks stay on the floor at all times. This is a subtle exercise to enhance your abdominal awareness.

Exercise 3: Heel Sliding

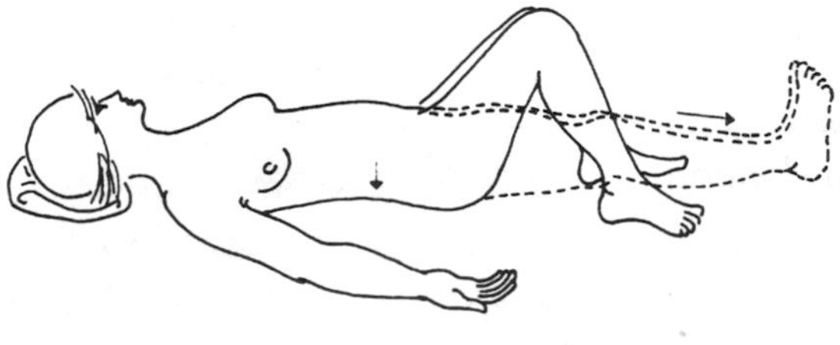

Figure 39. Control your pelvic tilt as you slowly extend your knees.

Position: Lying on your back, knees bent to tilt your pelvis backward.
Action: Hold your pelvic tilt ("bellybutton to backbone") while you slide your heels away from your buttocks. Just **before** you lose your pelvic tilt, draw your knees back **one at a time,**[52] to the point where your spine began to arch. Work in this range of motion until your abdominal muscles control your pelvic tilt with both legs outstretched.

Modification: If sliding both legs is too difficult, just slide one heel down.

Pelvic Tilting Can Be Done In Many Positions

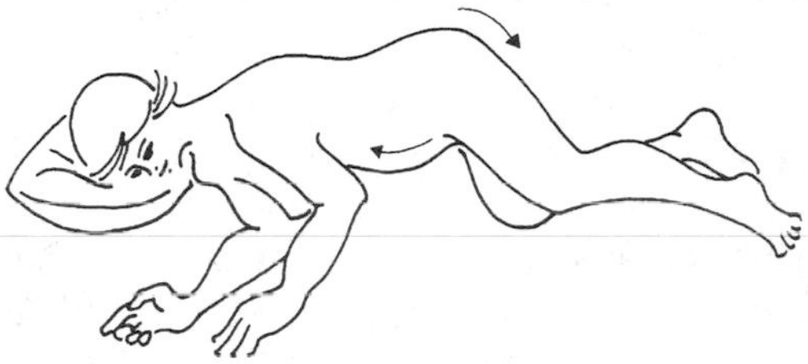

Figure 40. Pelvic tilting while side lying.

Here, as in other positions, pelvic tilting is easier with bent knees; more movement can be felt than with your legs outstretched. A pillow between your legs can be used for comfort.

Figure 41. Pelvic tilting while sitting.

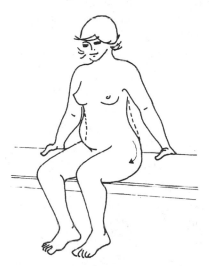

Figure 42. Balance on the ball, keep your pelvic tilt, add arm or leg movements.

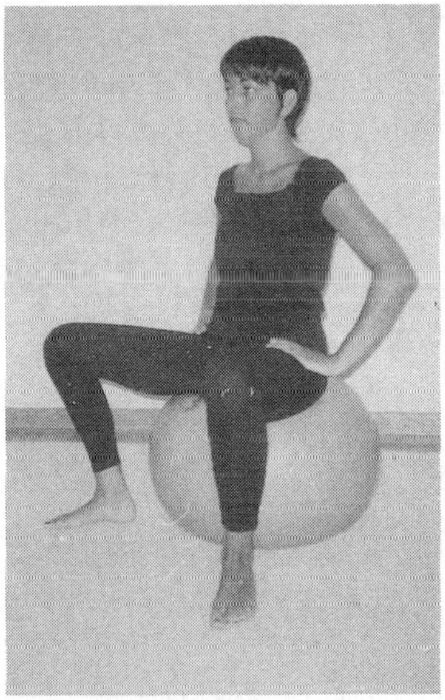

Do this exercise when seated on uncomfortable chairs or on a bench. Reaching behind with your hands to grasp the back of the seat may help to localize the action to your lumbar region.

If you have access to a large gymnastic ball,[53] you can do pelvic tiling in all directions: "round the clock," front and back, and side to side. Arm and leg movements can be added for extra challenge.

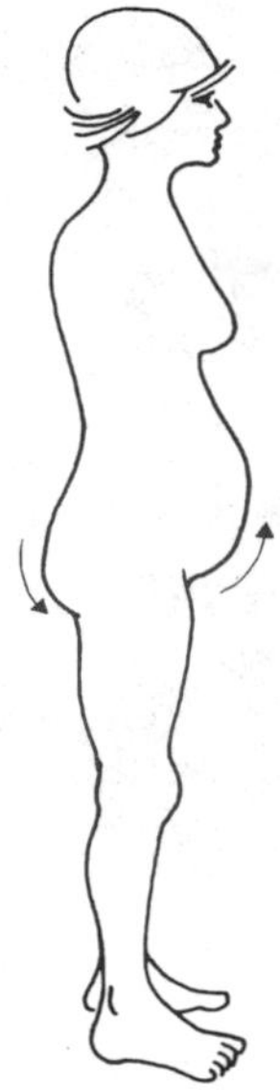

Figure 43. Pelvic tilting is tricky while standing.

Hold your pelvis in the correct position while standing, without moving elsewhere. Keep your upper body erect, with knees at ease,[54] shoulders in neutral position, raise your breastbone, your palms forward. Check your posture, side view, in a mirror. (See page 40.)

All Fours

The force of gravity when you are on all-fours tends to make your back sag, as does the weight of your uterus below. Pelvic-tilting on your hands and knees works your abdominal muscles against gravity. Supine hypotension is avoided. Your shoulders and knees are stabilized, which, unlike standing, localizes the action to your spine. Pelvic tilting in this position is frequently called the "cat back" or the "angry cat." Unfortunately, this name influences women to raise their upper back, rounding it just like they do most of the day. Hunchback posture (known as thoracic kyphosis) is a major problem in our sedentary society.[55] If you are exercising with a partner, he or she can help by placing a hand over the **small of your back,** providing guiding resistance so that you raise **only your lower back.** Hollowing the lumbar spine in this position is only necessary for a woman with a flat back, and they are rare.

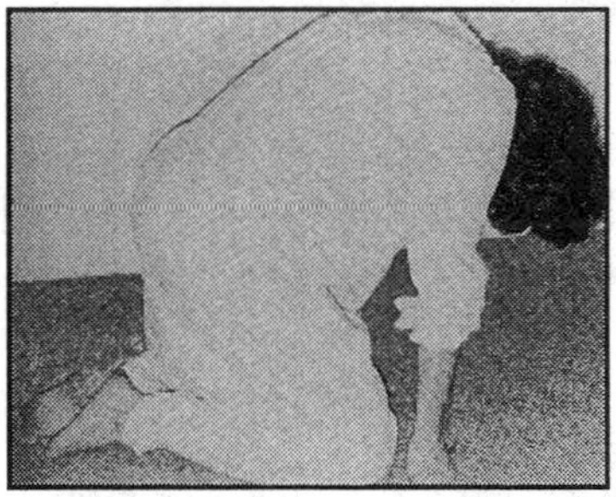

Figure 44. No one need practice "dowager's hump"!

NO

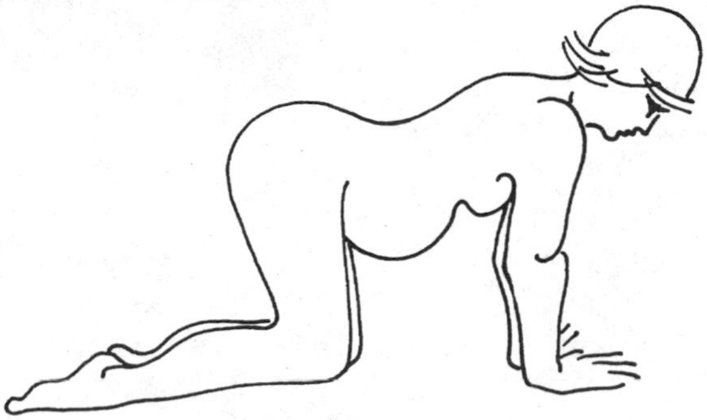

Figure 45. Align your spine instead.

NO

Figure 46. A flat back is better than a cat back![57]

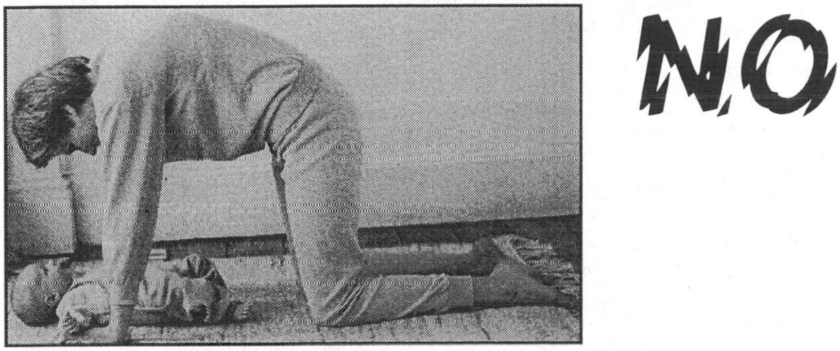

Figure 47. Take the weight off your spine during pregnancy and labor.

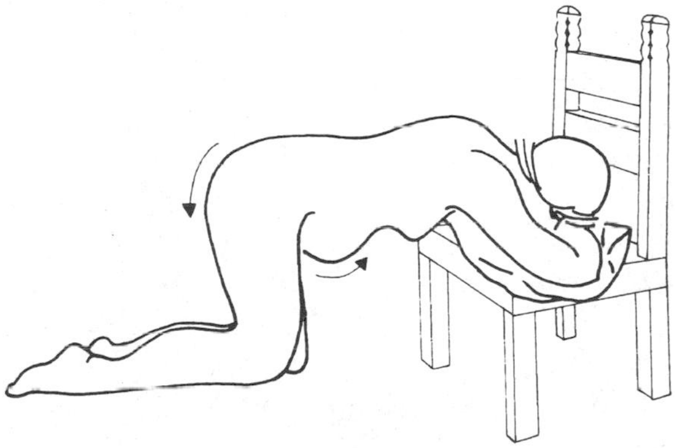

Unweighting your backbone allows your uterus to move partially out of your pelvis, where it compresses major blood vessels. This provides relief from blood congestion, nerve twinges, and pelvic pressure. The baby often decides to adjust position, too. During labor, going on hands and knees alleviates "back labor"—the bony back of the baby's head, instead of the soft face, lies against your pelvis (posterior position or occiput). The all-fours position can assist rotation of the baby's head to a more comfortable position for you, and will speed the process of birth.

In the postpartum phase, pelvic-tilting on hands and knees is highly motivating because slack abdominals really droop!

Exercise 4. Pelvic Tilting on Hands and Knees

Position: Hands directly under shoulders, and knees under hips is the basic four-point position. However, because you, like most people, may round your upper back, I recommend that you **lengthen your spine**. Increase the distance between your hands and knees, feeling the point at which you can localize the spinal movement to your **lower** back.

Action: Pull in your abdominal muscles and buttocks, raising your **lower back** toward the ceiling. Hold for a few seconds—then relax a little so that your back returns to **neutral** only. This means that you will still be holding the muscles needed to maintain this antigravity position. Keep breathing!

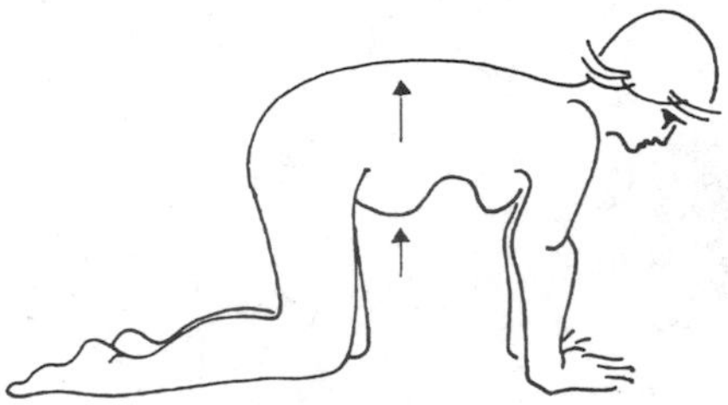

Figure 48. Raise your pelvis to be as flat as a table top.

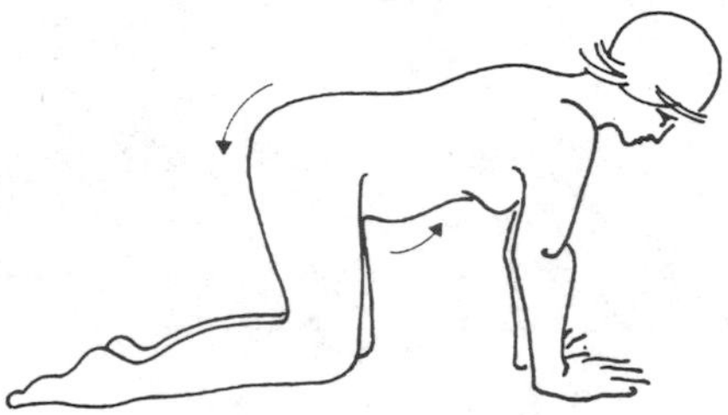

Figure 49. Relax only to neutral.

Progressions: Keep your back as flat as a table top (= neutral pelvic tilt, no sagging) and alternate from side to side as you:

- ✦ Reach out with **one arm.** Check that the supporting elbow joint is at ease. (Women frequently hyperextend their elbows when weight-bearing through their arms.) Hold the outstretched hand at the same height as your shoulder.
- ✦ With your weight on both hands and one knee, raise **one leg,** keeping your pelvis parallel to the floor. The heel should be on the same plane or lower than your buttock.
- ✦ Raise the **opposite arm and leg,** so that you balance on two opposite points.
- ✦ Extend one arm, and **add movement** by bending and straightening the opposite leg.

These progressions primarily challenge the starting position—your abdominal control of your pelvis. Stretching, strengthening, balance, and coordination movements are added when you raise your limbs.

Exercise 5. Side-Bending on Hands and Knees.

Also known as *tail-wagging,* in this movement you tilt your trunk and pelvis sideways. The same position and principles apply as with the prior exercises. The aim is to work your front abdominals against gravity while bending from side to side as well. This relieves ribcage compression and helps the muscles on the side of your abdomen to remember there was once a waist!

Action: With a neutral pelvic tilt, bring your head and hip toward each other on the **same** side. Alternate sides, exhaling as you bend, inhaling as you return to the midline.

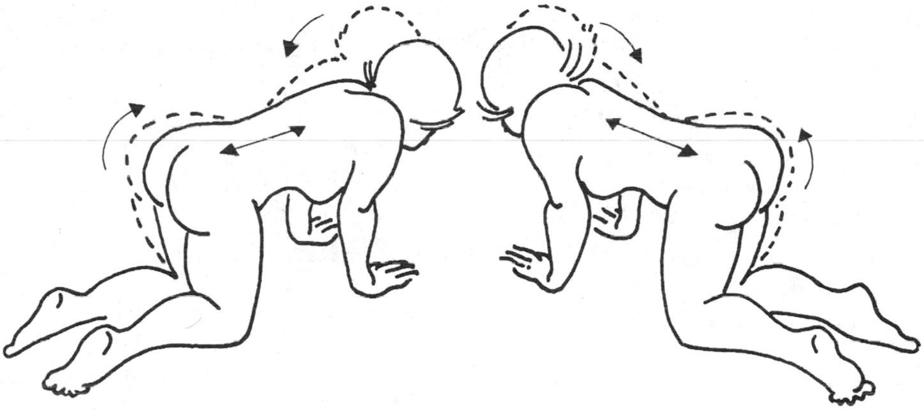

Figure 50. Bend from side to side, keeping your spine neutral as if a glass were resting on your back.

Important Points About Performing Curl-ups

- **Always check the midline of your abdominal wall** first. If the gap is three fingers' width or more, from this or a previous pregnancy, postpone this exercise. Concentrate on supporting your recti muscles and limit yourself to head raises as described on page 92. Rarely does a gap persist after birth. If your muscles are parallel after the first week—only one to two fingers fit in the gap—you need check no more.
- **Postpone any exercises that cause you to feel strain on your pelvic floor**. Work more on PF exercises until the pressure of stronger abdominal action can be withstood.
- **Your knees should be bent**. This puts you into a pelvic tilt, a mechanical advantage to protect your lower back and for your muscles to work in middle range. (Outstretched legs can be very uncomfortable in pregnancy for the lower back)
- **Half-way is enough**. The abdominal muscles raise the trunk from the horizontal to an angle less than 45 degrees, after which the hip flexors take over and complete the movement. Just curling up seven or eight inches, keeping your waist on the surface, is sufficient to exercise your abdominal muscles. Both shoulder blades clear the floor but your waist stays down.[58]
- **Your feet should be unrestrained. Holding the feet down encourages**

the hip flexors and may obscure weakness of your abdominal muscles. The increasing weight of your trunk during pregnancy may tempt you to stabilize your feet, but remember that the hip flexors will pull on your spine with its softened ligaments, against the diminishing power of your stretched abdominal muscles which struggle to stabilize your pelvis.

- **Both straight and diagonal movements should be performed.** This ensures that all portions of your muscular corset are exercised.[16]
- **The movement must be a smooth roll**, pulling your lower abdominals to stabilize your pelvis. Tuck under your chin before you begin. The use of momentum (jerking) must be avoided. Your back should rounded at all times to diminish hip flexor action.
- **Arm positions increase the leverage as described below.**

Exercise 6. Straight Curl-up

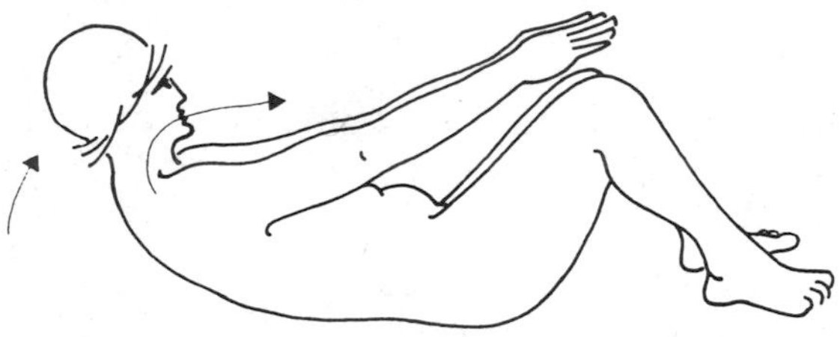

Figure 51. Curl up just halfway to your knees.

Action: Bring your chin toward your chest. As you breathe out, roll forward smoothly with your arms outstretched, reaching to your knees. Come up just as far as your upper back naturally bends, keeping your waist on the floor. Slowly uncurl to the starting position and inhale.

Exercise 7. Diagonal Curl-up

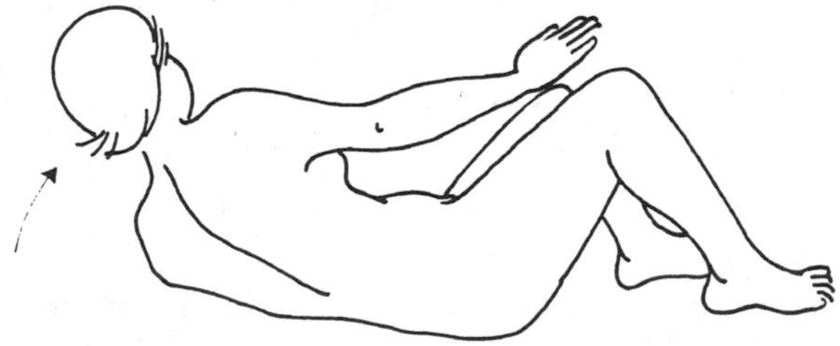

Figure 52. Move diagonally with outstretched arms to the opposite knee: to the left and rest back...to the right and back.

Action: Bring your chin toward your chest. As you breathe out, curl forward reaching with your outstretched arms toward to the outside of your left knee. Slowly return to the starting position, inhale and repeat, bringing your left shoulder toward your right knee.

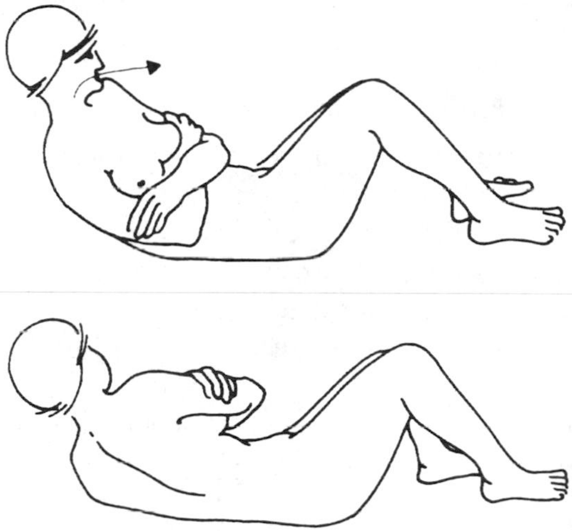

Figure 53. Folding your arms across your chest is a way to progress curl-ups.

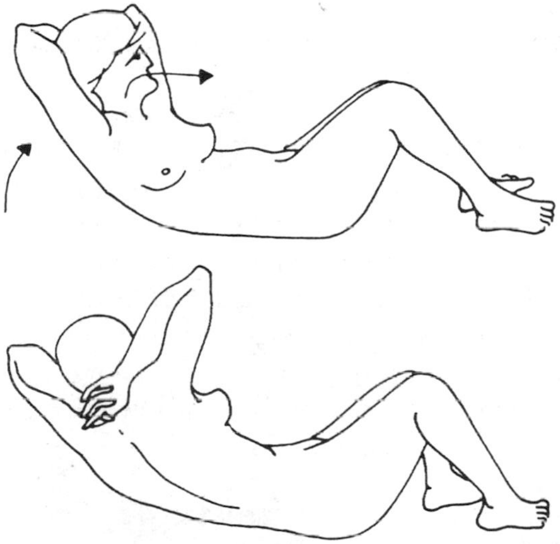

Figure 54. Hands behind head is the most challenging position for curl-ups.

Normal strength is present in your upper abdomen when you can execute a smooth curl-up and roll-back with your hands behind your head.

Few women have normal strength in both upper and lower abdominal areas before pregnancy, and even fewer at the end. However, after birth you must gradually progress to these challenging abdominal exercises for your future health and fitness.

Important Points About Performing Pelvic Stabilization/Lower Abdominal Exercises

Pelvic stability improves with the challenge of leg movements.

- ✦ **Hands should be behind the head**. This encourages you to press with your upper back into the floor.[60]
- ✦ You have **complete control of your pelvic tilt** because you are lowering your **bent** knees, gradually straightening them (controlling the leverage). The action is a **combination of lowering and straightening**.
- ✦ You must **exhale and draw in your abdominal muscles** toward your backbone.
- ✦ The limit is **no less than a 45 degree angle.** (Any lower and your pelvis will tilt like a see-saw.)

Exercise 8. Leg Lowering with Bent Knees

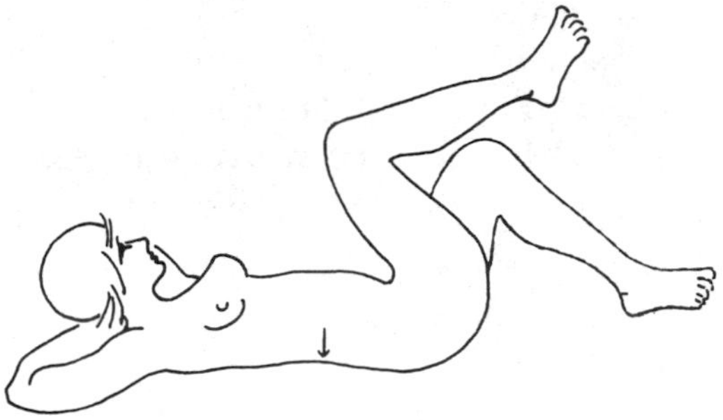

Figure 55. Control your pelvic tilt as you lower one leg.

Position: On your back, knees bent.

Action: Lift one leg in the air and gradually straighten it, bending it back before you lose your pelvic tilt. Keep your other knee bent with the foot on the floor or, if you cannot keep your pelvis in the neutral position, bring that knee over your waist. Alternate legs. Continue as before; now both feet stay off the floor. Move your legs as if riding a bicycle. Low and slow is more challenging. Change direction—pedal backward. To modify, do smaller movements with your knees well bent. Watch for bulging; your abdomen must move **in**.

The cardinal test every time:

Can you control your pelvic tilt?

Lowering both legs involves strong work from your abdominal corset to hold your pelvis stable. You control the **descent** of your legs within the limits of your muscle power, therefore lowering is always preferable to raising both legs.[61] You start with your knees bent, from the easiest part of the range, where the weight of your legs and the force of gravity match your abdominal strength. At any point, you can bend your knees further to reduce the leverage or simply allow your heels to rest on the floor.

Warning: A common error is to straighten both legs and lower them together. (See page 41.) This is far too much leverage. The correct exercise is a **combination of gradual straightening and lowering.** The knees become straight **only** at the final 45 degree angle.

Exercise 9. Double Leg Lowering with Bent Knees.

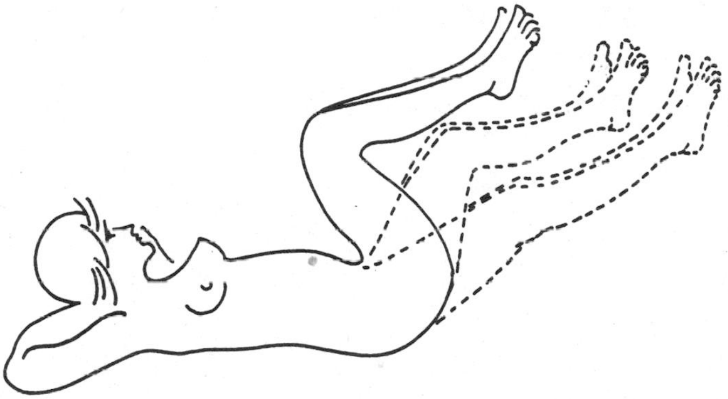

Figure 56. Keep your pelvis in a neutral position as you lower and gradually straighten both legs.

Normal strength has been achieved in your lower abdominal muscles when you can hold your legs straight at an angle of 45 degrees for a few seconds. You can progress the exercise by holding the position longer—but keep breathing! Spreading and closing your legs, or doing "scissors" at whatever angle of descent you reach, will increase duration as well as exercise other leg muscles.

5

Posture, Positions, and Comfort

Posture has to do with feeling and looking well—whether you are male, female, young, old, pregnant or postpartum. Our bodies are report cards on our consciousness. A negative emotional state will be expressed in a slumped, droopy posture. If you feel great, you'll stand tall and walk with a spring in your step. During pregnancy, you want to carry your body and baby so that you feel aligned and graceful, like a tree in bloom.

Body Image

Improvement of body image is a special benefit of prenatal exercise class. I have always encouraged the wearing of cotton stretch clothing; it is much easier for the instructor to observe posture and specific joint alignment. However, most pregnant women choose loose clothes that conceal, like voluminous swimsuits that are made for pregnancy! Art in North America rarely glorifies expectant fullness, nor are pregnant bellies often revealed by bikinis. The absence of role models who are not ashamed of their pregnant body extends through the postpartum period, a time when mothers are rarely seen breast-feeding in public.[62] (An exception, of course, was pregnant Demi Moore on the cover of *Vanity Fair.*) Although we have come a long way since the days of **confinement** during pregnancy, we have not reached unconditional celebration of this magnificent transition. Exercise, yoga and dance classes during the childbearing year are helping this trend.

Hazards of Poor Posture

Naturally, posture varies with different body types. Regardless, certain guidelines determine good alignment and enhance balance.

Your pregnant body needs efficiency and endurance—that is, minimal effort and fatigue in all your resting and working positions. This efficiency is gained by correct body alignment, which results from adequate support and easy coordination of the various body segments. Good posture in all activities avoids unnecessary tension and stress on muscles and ligaments. Crowded internal organs have more space as a result.

Your posture may have been faulty before you became pregnant and sometimes considerable muscle and ligament adaptation have developed. This means that re-education requires more time and effort.

Postural reflexes enable the brain to communicate with certain signal stations in the body—the ears, eyes and muscles being the most important. We can appreciate this by watching the uncoordinated actions of someone who is blindfolded. Because our postural adjustments occur at an automatic level, we are often unaware of bad habits we may have developed. Attention to a few details can help you to cultivate good posture and increase your comfort during changing bodily states.

Posture involves adjustments to the force of gravity, which is why reclining is more restful than being upright. Likewise, postural defects are seen most clearly in the standing position. Ideally, a state of muscular equilibrium maintains the body segments around the line of gravity passing through your ear, shoulder, hip, knee and just behind your ankle.

Once humans stood up on two legs, the vertebral column became subject to compression. The natural curves formed in the spine are a compromise between flexibility and stability. During pregnancy these curves often become accentuated as your center of gravity moves forward. As this shift in the center of gravity increases the load on your spine, you tend to stand further back on your heels. Further compensation may occur. Your head and shoulders poke forward, increasing your lumbar curve, or your upper body sways back from your waist. Backache commonly results from this incorrect weight distribution because the back muscles must do extra work.

Shoes

Together with emotions, habits, muscles and connective tissue, shoes also affect posture. Comfortable and supportive shoes help both your disposition and your appearance! High heels throw your pelvis and body weight forward, hollow your lower back, and strain ligaments in your hips and knees. In this unstable position many muscles work much harder, and the extra weight on the arches and balls of your feet may cause them to protest. If you are accustomed to wearing high heels, adjustment to low heels or flats takes time because your calf muscles will have shortened. They need to stretch gradually. (Fortunately, these unphysiological ornaments are now often carried in shoe bags by women who stride to work in sneakers.)

While it is excellent exercise to walk barefoot in sand, the usual hard surface beneath us needs a buffer. The sole of your shoe should be thick and resilient and the shoe's shank underneath your inner arch should provide support when you stand. If you can press the arch down just with your hand, it is inadequate, and an extra arch support may be necessary as you gain weight during the pregnancy. (See Resources.) The ideal shoe does not change the shape of your foot in any way; your toes are not squeezed and the heel should fit firmly, slanting neither to one side nor the other.

Exercises for the arches of the feet are also important. In fact, foot pain is often experienced by pregnant women who do not do these specific exercises to help maintain their arches. Once you do these exercises regularly, foot pain is most unlikely. Painful pressure under the ball of the foot can also be relieved by a metatarsal foot pad (available in drugstores), deep massage, and mobilizing of the individual bones that form the arch.

Posture While Standing

Improvement follows an ongoing process of regular rather than occasional exercise. You may have been told many times in your life to stand up straight for esthetic reasons, but in pregnancy you need to do so for physiological reasons. As your tight muscles get looser and your weak ones get stronger, you will naturally demonstrate better posture.

Ligaments play a major supportive role when standing at ease. During the childbearing year, supporting muscles must share the stresses of pregnancy and take the load off the softened ligaments. The spinal column forms a subtle **S** curve around the line of gravity; the more pronounced the curve beyond normal, the more muscle work is necessary. The position of your pelvis, which supports your spinal column, is always important; in pregnancy you need a keener sense of pelvic tilt. This pelvic angle determines the prominence of both your abdomen and your buttocks, and affects your appearance as well as your comfort. Naturally, the pelvis tends to angle forward because of the increasing weight of its contents and the stretching of the abdominal wall. You need to keep your pelvis in a neutral position—pulling it up at the front with your abdominal muscles and down behind with your buttock muscles. It is exactly the action described on pages 96, which can be done in every position but squatting, when the pelvis is as far back as it can go (posterior pelvic tilt).

Your Correct Pelvic Tilt

To find the correct position for your pelvis, place the heel of each hand on the edge of each hip bone,[63] just below your waist on each side of your abdomen. You can still feel these bony prominences, even at the end of pregnancy. Then place both hands flat, alongside and underneath your uterus so that your fingertips reach each pubic bone. When both these points of each hand are in the same plane, your pelvis is aligned to the correct neutral angle.[64] For almost everyone this is a backward movement.

A chronic forward tilt of the pelvis causes the muscles in front to weaken and the muscles behind to shorten; consequently, the curve in the lower back increases. The fulcrum of all these forces of stress is where the spinal column joins the pelvis—the most common region of backache. See page 28 for the drawing of this bowstring effect.

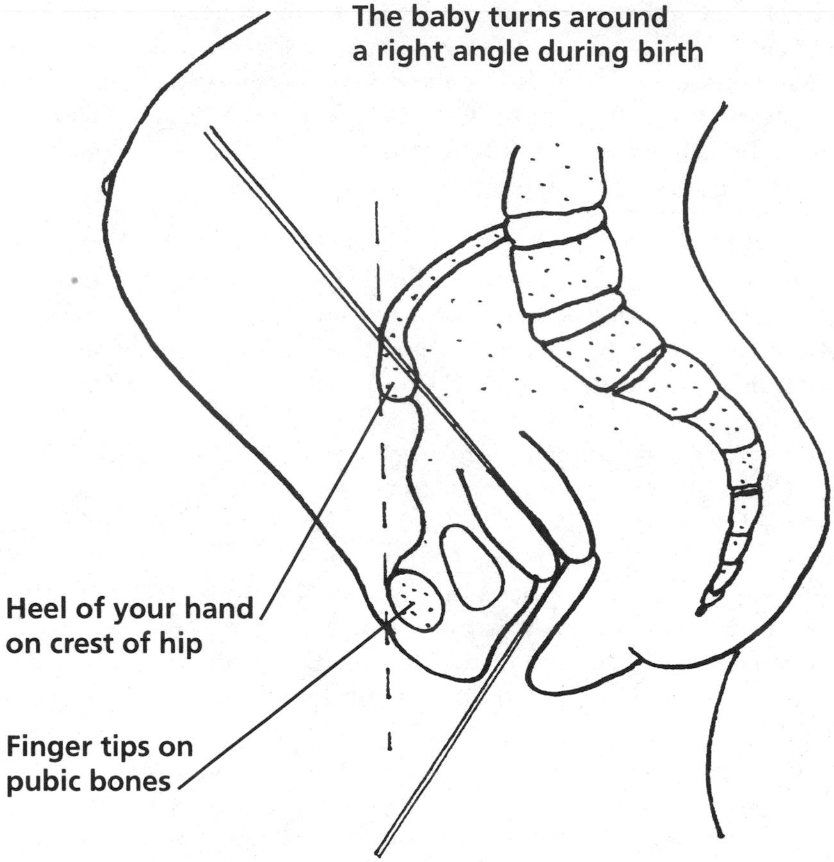

Figure 57. Find your correct pelvic tilt with your hands.

The position of your head is the other important influence on your posture. If you let your head slump and look at the ground, your body will sag too. Just drawing up the back of your neck and tucking your chin in above the notch between your collarbones helps to bring all your body segments into line. Think "tall" and hold your head high, as if an invisible thread were pulling up your head toward the ceiling. Both shoulders and hips should be level; if you wear a belt it should be parallel to the ground. Since in pregnancy it makes no sense to think about pulling in your belly, concentrate instead on tucking under your buttocks. Lift up your breastbone to correct any hunchback tendency.

Postural adjustments are gradual during pregnancy, but after the major weight loss on the day of birth, changes are rapid. Consciously brace your abdominal and buttock muscles when walking around for the first few days after birth.

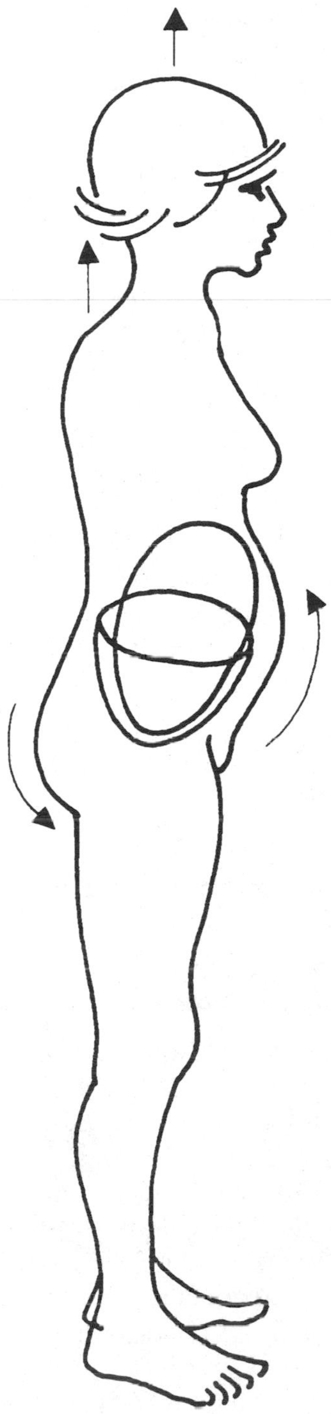

Figure 58. Stand tall and align your pelvis to your spine.

Posture Check

Observe the different features of the two postures shown in the drawing on page 225. Stand comfortably and ask a friend whether you exhibit any of the common defects: chin poked forward, "collapsed" neck, shoulders rounded, pelvis tilted to the front, one or both legs pressed back at the knee, or feet rolled in or out. You can check yourself now and then in front of mirrors and store windows; remember that the side view is most revealing.

Practice holding the corrected position and then returning to your former posture. You will develop the sensation of improved body alignment with new messages in your "muscle memory." It may be tempting to throw your shoulders back, but this stance hollows your lumbar spine. Pulling your the elbows too far back moves your head and shoulders forward. Postural awareness requires that you develop a sense of what **feels** correct and comfortable. Align your body slowly, segment by segment, and notice for how long you can hold the new position. Repeat with your eyes closed; this heightens postural awareness, improves balance and, surprisingly, can be relaxing, too.

Progressions While Standing

Palming

Palming is a relaxation technique for the eyes that facilitates awareness of your posture at the same time.[65] Standing, rub your hands together until they are warm and tingly. Then place them over your closed eyes while you bend your knees as far as you can while keeping your feet flat on the floor. This brings you into an over-corrected position: your pelvis is tilted beyond neutral and all the way back. Soon stress builds in your leg muscles. Allow your thighs to release some tension and trust your feet and lower legs to support you. The strong sensations in your legs are **grounding;** that is, energy and awareness become focused on your feet. Keep breathing in this rather difficult position, feeling your eyes relax with the warmth of your hands. You sense when your eye tension decreases, because the blackness that you see through your closed eyelids becomes blacker.

When your legs start to tire, **slowly** straighten up, but keep your knees at ease. With your eyes still covered, tune into your postural reflexes now as you sway from left to right and front to back. When your arms tire, let them drop down by your sides and gradually open your eyes. Give a good stretch to your jaw (drag it down) your shoulders (pull them down from your ears) and your hands (stretch your fingers long). You may feel taller and lighter. This exercise allows your body to find the most efficient way to stand upright, and it does better unconsciously than under purposeful direction.

Relaxation of the eye muscles is especially recommended for those who wear refractive lenses, or stare at a computer screen for long periods. Studies have shown that computer users blink less often than they do when reading a book, and much less so than in normal viewing.

Wall Presses

Stand with your back against a wall, but your feet a few inches away from it, with your arms at your sides, palms facing forward. Make contact with your head, shoulders, and buttocks. Press back your shoulders and trunk (knees stay at ease) to lessen the curves in your neck and lower back. Next, raise your arms sideways (while keeping them in contact with the wall at all times) and bend your elbows. You are now in a "hold-up" position. Press the back of your **wrists** against the wall—pressing the fingers is easy! Then bring your arms back to shoulder level, and finally down again to rest. Shake out any muscle tension.

Keep breathing...

Pressing against the wall increases the endurance of the muscles that maintain correct alignment. This corrective stretching of tired or tight muscles relieves backache, especially between the shoulder blades. During tedious desk or household jobs, while riding in an elevator or when standing in line near a wall, "iron out" like this to reduce the ache or stiffness in your back.

Keep Mobile While Standing

Standing still for long periods of time is fatiguing. Your muscles work statically to hold your body position stable against gravity, but uncomfortable strain develops as a result of circulatory effects. For your heart, this is the worst position of all; blood must take an uphill path unaided by muscles. Half of your blood is below heart level in the upright position and movement keeps your blood circulating. This is particularly important in pregnancy, because your blood volume is increased by about fifty percent.

Blood is returned from the legs to the heart passively by a "venous pump," which is provided by your leg muscles, because veins, unlike arteries, do not have muscular walls to maintain pressure. Too much pooling of venous blood in your legs can make you feel faint. This is the body's way of protecting itself when no muscles are pumping the blood back uphill to the heart, and blood pressure drops. Then you may feel the need to recline or may be forced eventually to fall to the ground. Thus blood can be returned to the heart more easily; this is why some people faint watching parades and why soldiers "fall out" when standing at attention waiting to be reviewed by a visiting dignitary.

If you have to wait for public transport or if you work mostly standing, there are ways to keep your muscles active. Shift your weight from one foot to the other—side to side or diagonally back and forth; go up on your toes and back on the heels, perhaps resting your hand on some support for balance. Press your toes into your shoes and raise the arches of your feet.

Frequent Position Changes

No one position is comfortable for long, especially in pregnancy. Even if you are blissfully supported on a pile of pillows, after about twenty minutes or so, a feeling of stiffness will prompt you to move.

On the following pages we will consider various postural modifications and how they can be used more effectively to increase comfort and improve body function. The sense of poise and well-being achieved with good posture makes these small efforts worthwhile. In pregnancy and after birth, you look as well as you feel. Many times, looking better makes you feel better.[66]

Posture While Sitting

Posture and comfort in sitting are important because we sit so frequently. Excessive sitting compounds pelvic pressure and congestion during pregnancy. Slumping forward with rounded shoulders increases pressure on your abdomen and can cause indigestion as well. Sitting with your knees crossed interferes with your circulation; it also predisposes to varicose veins, and tightens the hip muscles deep in your groin. Slouched posture increases the tension on ligaments that support your back and neck. Ultimately bad posture becomes disfiguring.

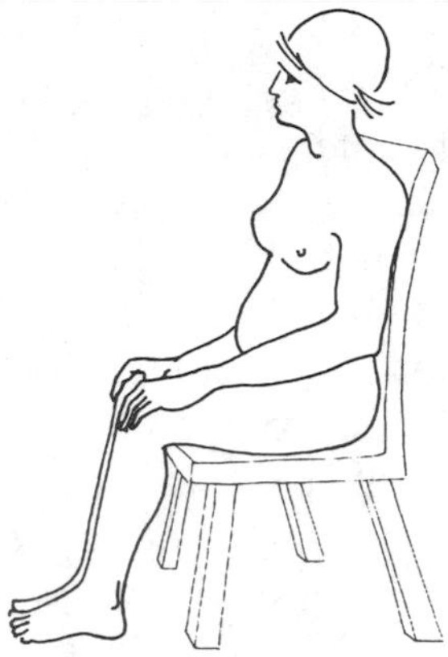

Figure 59. Good posture while sitting.

Sitting also increases disc pressure, especially when you relax without arm or back supports. Good posture while sitting requires active muscular equilibrium. To rest, it is better to lie down. The increasing incidence of back pain, neck pain and carpal tunnel syndrome associated with sedentary work posture give witness to the prevalence of poor sitting habits.

From a holistic rather than a segmental perspective, sitting posture depends considerably on the position of your arms and head. The most common problems are a slight forward bending of the head, together with forward movement of the upper arms from their normal position above the hips. Both of these postural deviations cause increased flexion of the upper back and lower neck, which strains the back muscles in that area. In other words, neck and back posture are closely related, and slight reaching forward of the head is the beginning of postural collapse. For every centimeter that your head moves forward on your neck, strain on your lower back muscles is tripled.

Figure 60. Gradually the shoulders and spine follow a forward-poking head.[67]

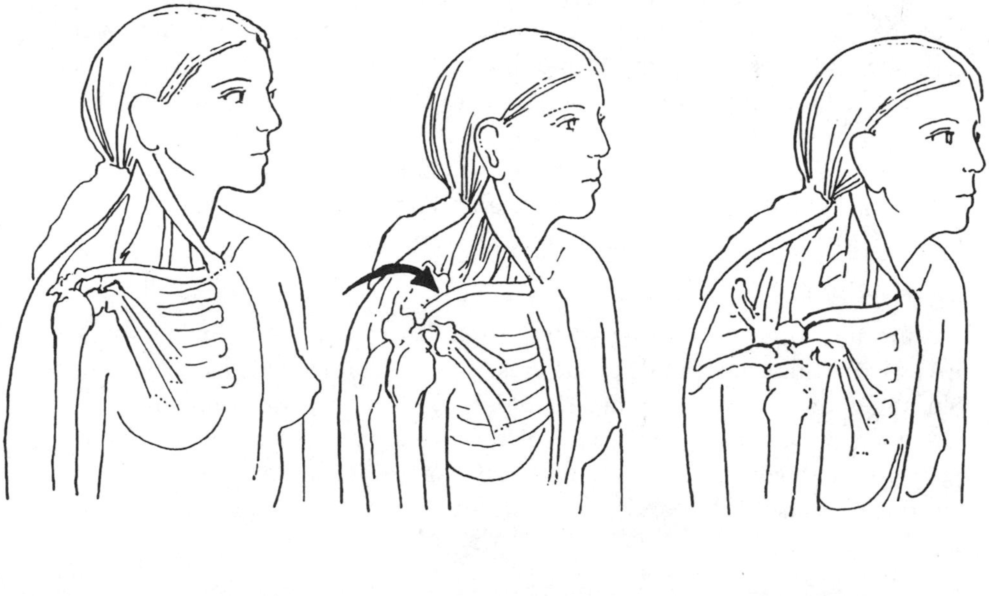

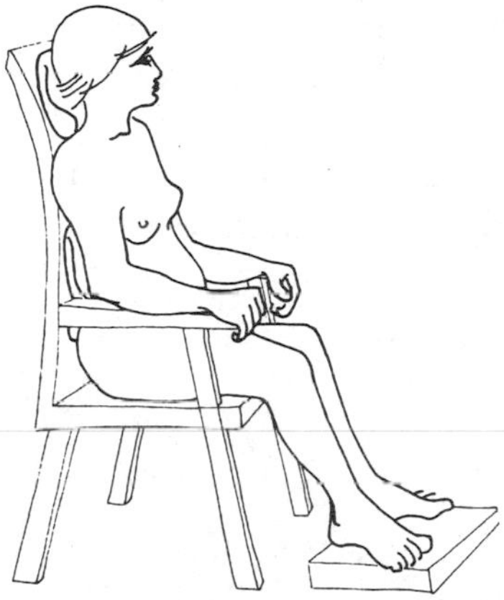

By the same token, sitting in a slumped posture allows your head and shoulder blades to move forward. A lumbar support is often too low to correct this faulty posture. The breastbone needs elevation (often by a higher back support) to raise your ribs, chest and diaphragm to their optimal positions. This automatically improves the position of your head and neck.

Figure 61. Comfort is increased with pillows and a footrest.

The role of vision is also significant. The eyes at rest naturally assume a downward gaze at an angle of about 15 degrees—the normal line of sight. When working, people typically prefer to lower their eyes another 15 degrees. Computer screens are usually too high. For comfortable viewing, the top of the computer screen should be level with your eyes. If the computer screen is too high, the hollow in the back of your neck increases which puts stress on the structures at the base of your skull. The ideal focal distance is between twelve and twenty-eight inches to avoid having to slouch forward and squint. A comfortable viewing distance also reduces the strain on the eye muscles. Other considerations include using an **inclined work surface** (an angle of just fifteen degrees helps relieve shoulder tension) and organizing your desk so that frequently used items are in convenient proximity.

Choice of Chair

Good support while sitting is essential if you spend much time at a desk. The chair seat should support the length of your thigh. Ideally, the chair should be far enough from the floor so that your knee is no higher than your hips. In pregnancy the muscles in front of the hip joints (the hip flexors) tend to become tight. Your legs may be most comfortable when spread apart to make room for your abdomen. Support your feet on the floor or a footrest. An arm rest should be slightly higher than your bent elbow to avoid traction on your shoulders. Support your lumbar spine with a thin cushion in the small of your back—the design of many chairs and car seats is deficient here. A regular pillow will be too bulky. However, today you can find many ready-made lumbar and lower thoracic supports (See Resources.) Press your sacrum from time to time against the back of the chair. This will activate the muscles of your lower abdomen and stimulate the reflexes governing your diaphragm and your back muscles to assist in holding your spine erect.

When you sit in a chair with a high back to support your head and shoulders, add a small cushion at the back of your neck for extra comfort. Take every opportunity to elevate your feet, preferably with your knees supported, when you are sitting. This is also a good opportunity to do foot-stretching and rotating exercises (see page 120) which stimulate the circulation in your legs, ease the aching of varicose veins, and reduce any swelling in your ankles.

Figure 62. Elevate and rotate your feet when resting.

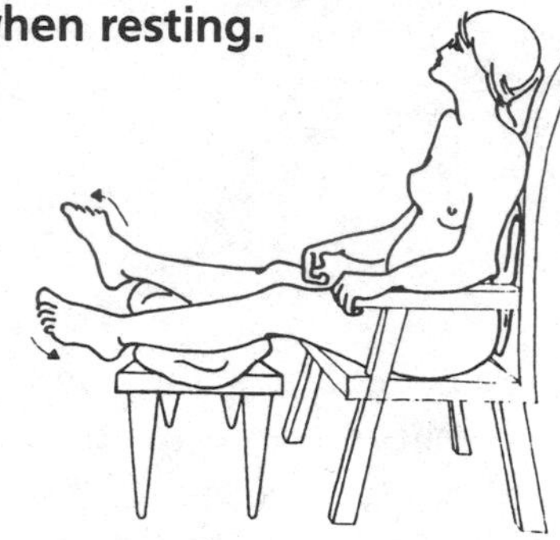

When you stand up, use your legs to raise your body. Slide forward to the edge of the chair and bend your knees for maximum leverage before you rise. Push down with your hands on the chair arms or the seat, rather than pulling yourself up with your arms.

Figure 63. Sit straight instead of slumping on the edge of a chair!

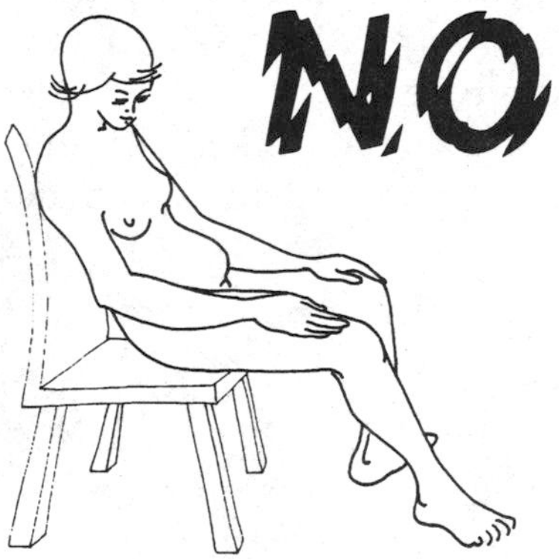

When your feet rest on the floor, "walk" them up and down from your toes. Either sit on the center of the chair on your sit-bones, with your back independently erect, or move further back against the back support. Sitting on your sit-bones puts you in the neutral (correct) pelvic tilt—you can check with your hands as described on page 109.

Figure 64. Lean forward to rest occasionally when at a desk or table. In labor this allows the uterus to tip forward with contractions.

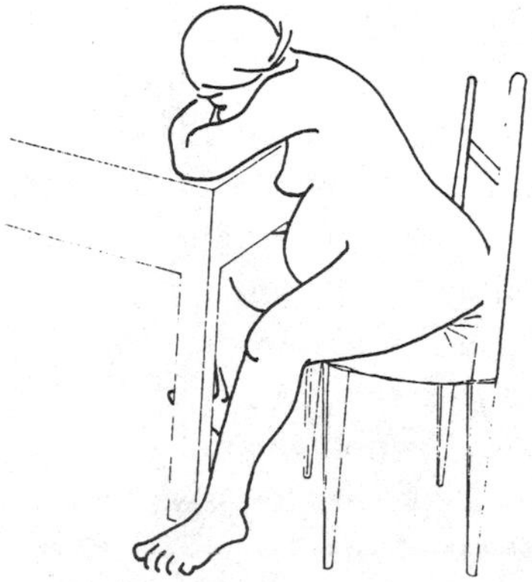

While sitting at a desk, rest your head on your hands occasionally to relieve tension in your neck and shoulders. If you're typing, make sure that you are seated high enough to avoid pain between your shoulder blades from

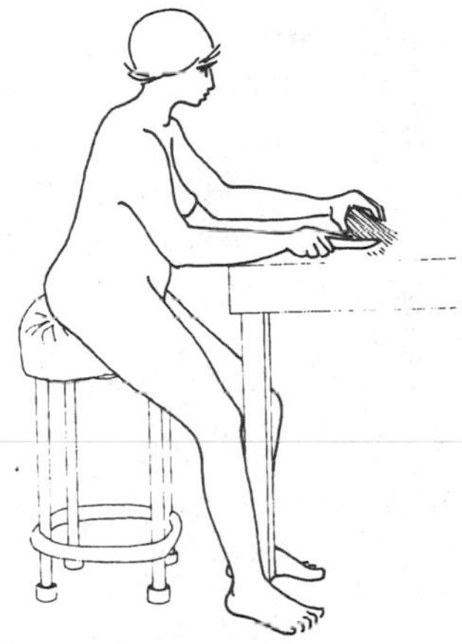

excess muscle bracing while your hands work. Your elbows should be at about a thirty degree angle from the surface at which you work. Nowadays, keyboards are detached from computers and can be at a lower level. I bought a sliding shelf to attach under my desk. Consider buying a high stool so that you can take the weight off your feet if you spend much time at kitchen counters or high surfaces such as an ironing board.

Figure 65. Perch on a stool when working at high surfaces.

Bring Your Baby to Your Breast

I have watched countless new mothers bring their breast to their baby—no wonder they get a backache! When Baby is held low, he or she also drags down on your breast. Support both Baby and your arm on a pillow, or raise your thigh by putting your foot on a stool or the rung of a chair. This way you can keep your back straight, resting against the chair while bringing Baby to your breast. If you obtain a large gymnastic ball (see Resources) you can sit like a tailor on the floor, your baby resting on a pillow, while you lean against the ball. The ball is between you and wall, and being compressible, it accommodates your spine most comfortably.

Figure 66. Sit with maximum support and comfort for feeding your baby.

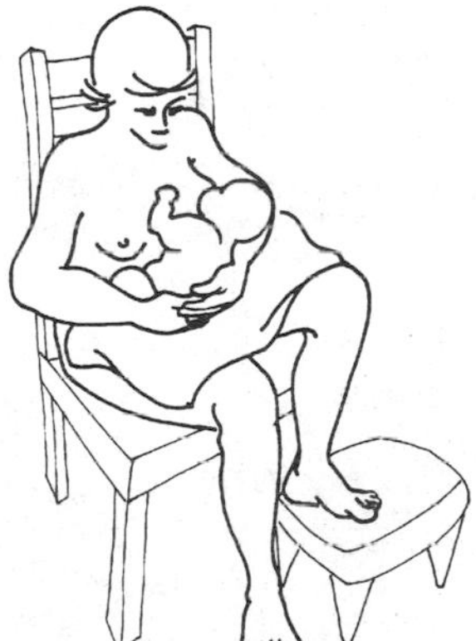

Since nursing your baby usually becomes one of your main activities, these little details make a big difference in preventing discomfort in your shoulder region and enhancing your emotional and physical response to this interaction. Shoulder-rotating exercises relieve upper backache.

Learn to nurse lying down, positioning your underneath arm so it doesn't fall asleep. Whether you plan on a "family bed" or not, you will inevitably have one, and quite often, too! I like plenty of sleep and I never considered a bassinet, crib, or even a room for my children (until school age) because the family bed means more rest for everyone.[68]

Driving

Support for your lower back is often necessary, especially during long distances. Your neck, shoulder blades and right leg are affected, along with your lower back. If your seats are uncomfortably low, sit on a cushion to bring your knees level with your hips. Frequent breaks allay fatigue and discomfort for both the driver and passenger.

Seat belts must be worn by law almost everywhere now. Research on expectant mothers who were involved in automobile accidents[69] revealed that belts really do reduce injury. The abdominal strap should be below your bulge, and a small cushion between you and the strap may make you more comfortable. This cushion also provides more protection for the baby, who is less restrained in a fluid environment.

An infant car seat is necessary for your new baby's safety. Purchase one now and learn how to install it properly. Carrying your newborn home from the hospital in your arms is not safe and is against the law. Consumer organizations and the American Academy of Pediatrics review and make recommendations from the brands available on the market. Some seats stay fixed in the car, and others can be lifted in and out so that you carry your baby in a portable chair. Regardless, the proper use of these seats has saved countless lives.

Posture While Long Sitting (Legs out straight)

Sitting with your legs extended and apart on the bed or floor is another position to use when reading or watching TV. If it's difficult to rest on your sit-bones with your back straight, then put a telephone directory under your buttocks.

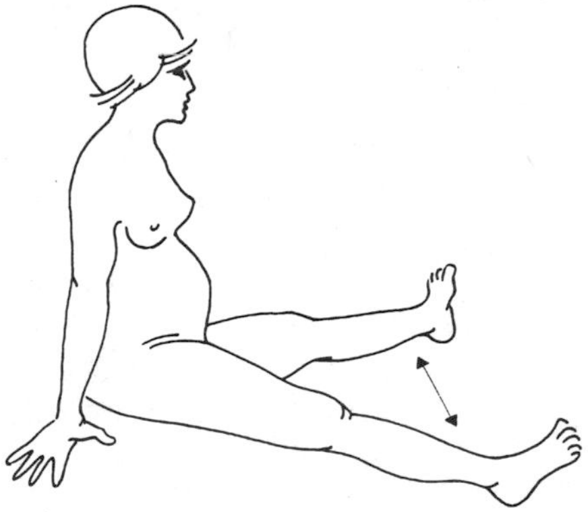

Figure 67. Sit with your back straight and stretch your legs. Bend forward at your waist to stretch your back.

When sitting with your legs extended, your hamstrings are on stretch—which you will feel if your knees aren't comfortably straight. Use your thigh muscles to gently press your knees down until you are flexible enough to allow your joints to extend fully. Tight hamstrings increase the hollow in the lower back; practice sitting like this to lengthen these muscles. Ease out any stiffness in your lower back as you gently lean forward and back, spine erect, bending at your waist (rather than reaching for your toes and rounding your upper back).

This safe way of actively stretching the hamstrings is preferable to bending over in a standing position and forcing yourself toward the floor. After touching the floor you must raise your the trunk upward against gravity, using your back muscles in their most inefficient role. In pregnancy this is even more undesirable because of the increased weight for your back muscles to lift. In any case, your back should never be worked like a derrick; instead use your legs to raise and lower your trunk, as explained below in the section on lifting.

Posture While Tailor-Sitting

From the time they are small, women are usually taught to sit with their legs together or crossed. The muscles and ligaments of the inner thighs, especially the inward rotators of the hip, are commonly shortened as a result. It is a psychological as well as physical change for some women to open up their legs and sit with them wide apart.

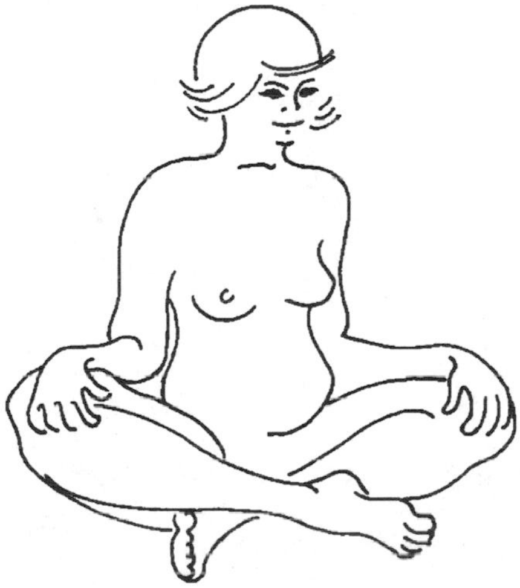

Figure 68. Sit like a tailor whenever you can.

It's unhealthy that we take chairs so much for granted, and rarely sit like a tailor. Cross your ankles and keep your spine erect to provide more room for your uterus and internal organs. The weight of your trunk must be on your "sit-bones." If you find it difficult then sit on a book or two. Most cushions are too soft—a telephone directory (usually the yellow pages!) is about the right size and firmness. You may find that with your ankles crossed your knees are a long way from the ground. In contrast, some women are so limber that they can even place the soles of their feet together (the butterfly position, see figures 69 and 70) and allow their thighs to reach the floor. People's joints vary and must never be forced. Pushing your knees toward the floor in either tailor-sitting or the butterfly position can hurt and be harmful. You will invoke the muscles' stretch reflex and they will contract and shorten. Microtears can occur. Bouncing your knees toward the floor also activates this counter-productive reflex, and can cause pain in your pubic region.

You can more effectively increase your flexibility by actively pressing both your knees toward the floor while **providing resistance with your hands underneath your knees.** Then as your thigh muscles tire and relax, they will allow your knees to drop down further. The resistance from your hands also strengthens your arm and chest muscles. You can also **work your outer thigh muscles actively** to bring your knees nearer to the floor, which, according to the same reciprocal relationship of muscle physiology, relaxes your inner thighs.

Figure 69. Resist the downward movement of your knees to gain relaxation of your inner thigh muscles.

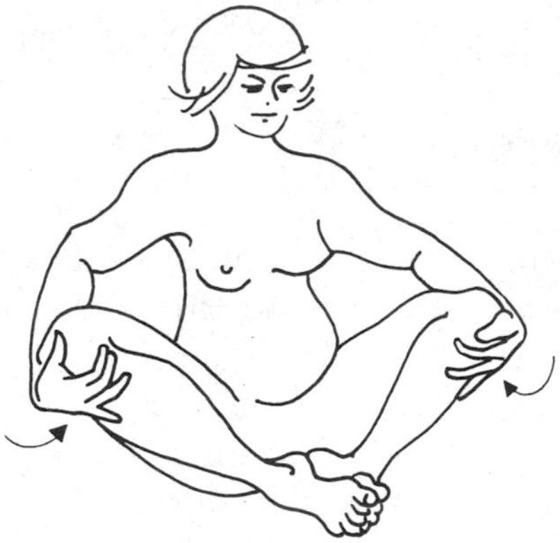

Figure 70. Exercise your outer thigh muscles to bring your knees closer to the floor.

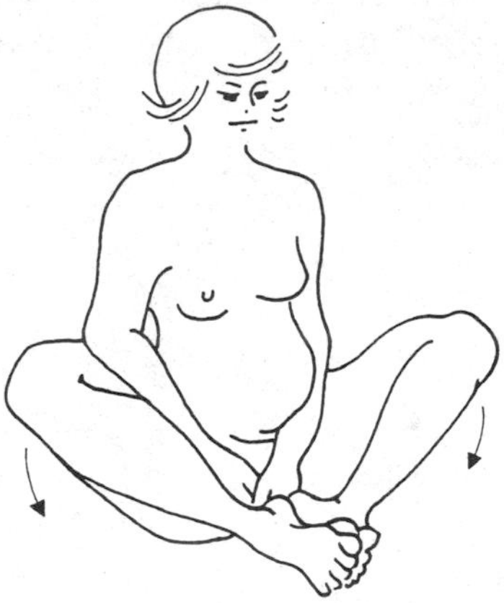

Figure 71. Shoulder rotating relieves upper backache from poor posture or heavy breasts.

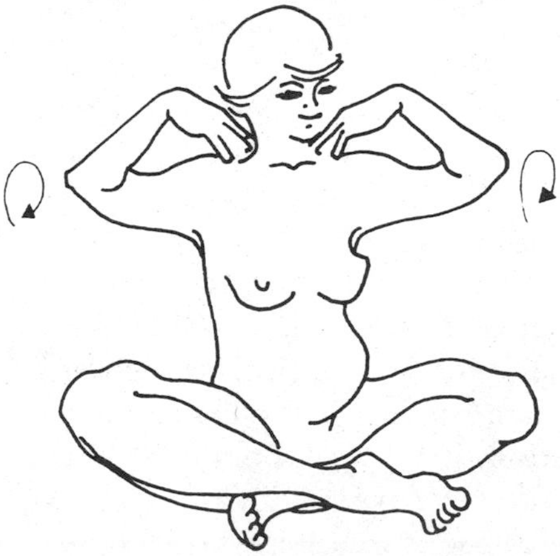

Posture While Prone Lying (On Your Front)

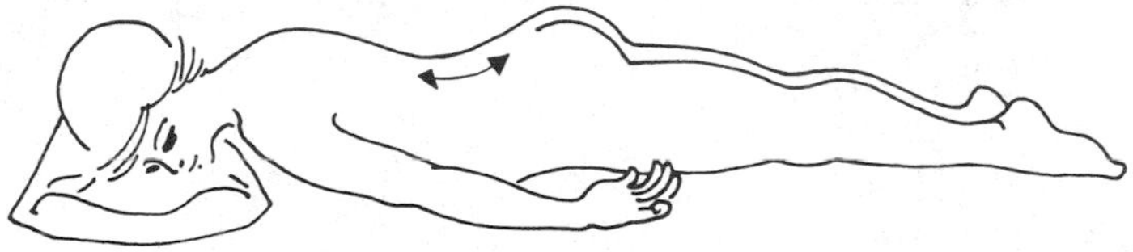

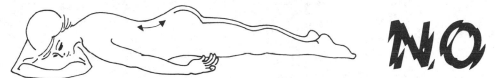

Figure 72. Lying prone without a pillow under the hips, especially with a sag in the mattress, causes the back to hollow.

It is usually with great regret that women give up lying comfortably on their abdomens as their pregnancies advance. Then, because we sit so much, the muscles in front of our hip joints may become shortened, and affect our pelvic tilt and posture. Rest and sleep in the prone position for as long as you can, using pillows for comfort. A bodyCushion™ is a wonderful (but expensive) concave support that accommodates prone lying through pregnancy. See Appendix and Resources.

If your breasts are tender, place two pillows under your hips and one beneath your chin and shoulders. This avoids pressure on your breasts, and the angle of your pelvis relieves any backache and allows your abdominal muscles to relax. Note in the drawing that the pillow is placed under the **hip** rather than the central abdomen. If it is too high you'll soon feel discomfort in your stomach and your spine. Place the pillow a little lower until you feel your pelvis comfortably positioned. This is particularly necessary if you have a mattress that sags, which will increase the hollow in your lower back in the prone position. If you cannot buy a new mattress, place a sheet of plywood underneath for extra support.

After birth, most mothers are very glad to be able to enjoy this position again; others may need reminding, and a few may feel it is an effort to adjust pillows and roll over on to them—but it's worth it. If it doesn't feel exceptionally comfortable, then you haven't got the pillow quite in the right position.

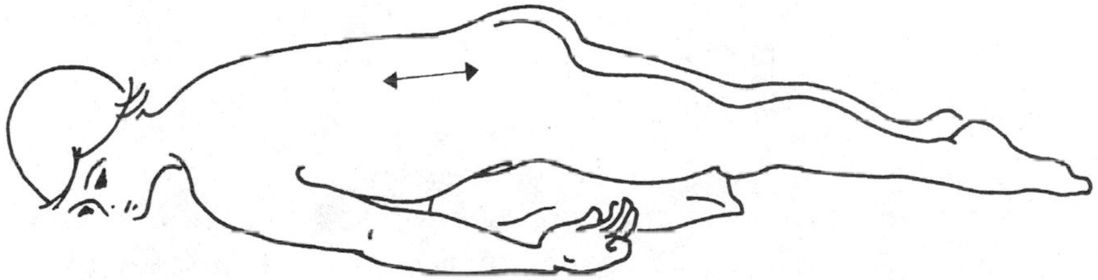

Figure 73. Lying prone with a pillow under the hips: note the raised pelvis, aligned spine and relaxed abdominal wall.

Figure 74. Extra pillows reduce pressure on the breasts: two at the hips and one at the chest to relieve lower back strain.

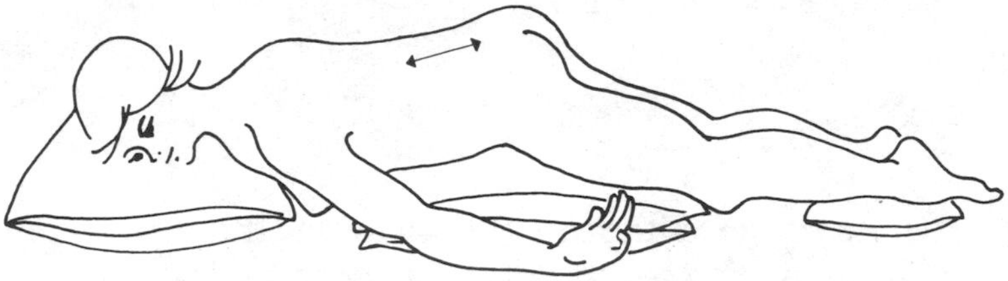

Figure 75. Lying prone on your elbows may cause strain and pain.

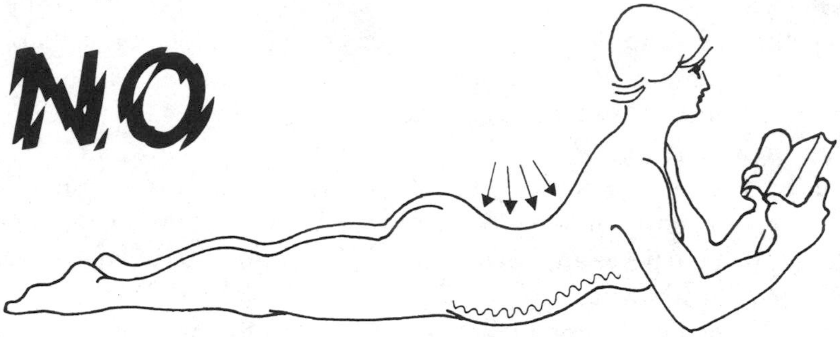

After birth there are many benefits of lying on your front:

- ✦ It feels fantastic!
- ✦ Your stitches won't bother you. You have more awareness of pelvic floor activity. It's an excellent position for practicing PF exercises.
- ✦ Back strain is relieved; the abdominal wall is relaxed because of the tilt of your pelvis.
- ✦ Pelvic organs are encouraged to resume their normal places.

Prolonged prone lying after birth, without suitable support, especially if you prop on your elbows to read or chat, can strain your spinal ligaments. Lying on your front is a resting or sleeping position.

Posture While Supine (On Your Back)

In pregnancy, as the weight of your uterus increases, compression of the major veins in your abdomen can occur when you are in the supine position. This can result in low blood pressure. If lying on your back makes you feel faint or in any other way uncomfortable, move out of it. Fortunately, most women experience no such symptoms and many prefer to lie on their backs for resting and sleeping. Use pillows to support your knees and take any strain off your lower back.

Figure 76. Pillows provide comfort in the supine position.

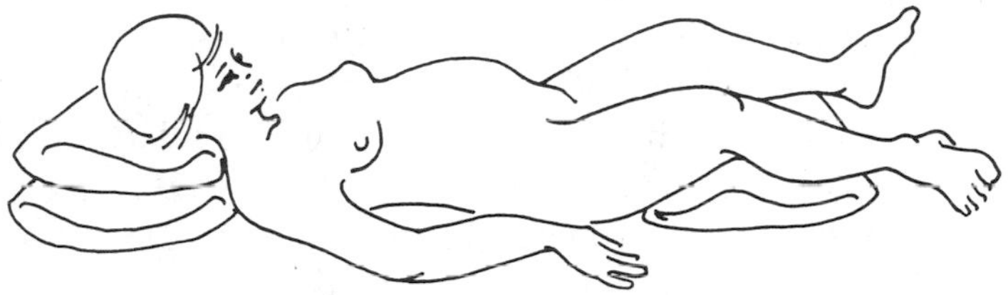

There will be occasions when you will be asked to lie supine: for fetal heart checks and vaginal examinations during labor; for the fetal heart monitor, if used, to be applied to your abdominal wall; and for performing some of the essential prenatal exercises. It is **only** in this position that your adominal wall can be evaluated for *diastasis recti*. (See page 88.)

The following suggestions should increase your comfort.

- ✦ **A folded towel** or **small** cushion provides support to the small of the back if the surface is either too hard or too soft. (A regular pillow is too large.)
- ✦ **Bending your knees,** or supporting them on a pillow, will take the traction off your abdominal area and lessen the hollow in your lower spine. Flat on your back with your legs outstretched is not a recommended position for comfort in pregnancy. (Few non-pregnant people are comfortable like this, either.)
- ✦ **Elevate your feet** to help the circulation in your legs. This reduces leg cramps and discomfort from varicose veins. The foot of your bed can be raised a few inches if you suffer from constant aching in the legs, and this may be recommended as a routine measure to enhance venous return from your legs overnight. Bend and circle your ankles, too, as movement is always more effective than mere elevation.

Figure 77. Take every opportunity to elevate your feet.

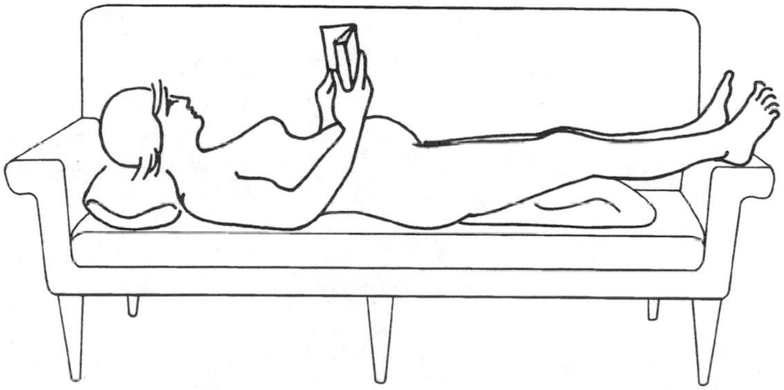

Supine Position During Labor

The practice of placing women on their backs during labor in general, and in the second stage in particular, should be avoided for many compelling reasons:

- ✦ Compression of the major blood vessels between the uterus (especially during contractions) and the spine **interferes with circulation and blood pressure.** (Supine hypotension may result because, unlike a brief session of exercise, laboring women may spend hours on their back.)
- ✦ The **strength of the contractions is diminished** by as much as a third. Staff who are accustomed to women who labor in bed attached to monitors may not realize that more effective contractions occur when laboring mothers walk around.
- ✦ Breathing and **ventilation of the lungs is hampered.** This is known as the "beached whale" sensation!
- ✦ Backache is increased. Many women feel contractions over their sacrum and there is additional pain if the baby's head is posterior.[70]
- ✦ The need for **obstetrical intervention is increased** since your sacro-iliac joints and coccyx are compressed by your body weight and cannot open as wide for your baby as when your pelvis is mobile.
- ✦ Women placed supine invariably arch their backs and necks, straining rather than contracting their abdominal muscles. **This position feels instinctively wrong.** (It's difficult to use a bed pan while lying supine.)
- ✦ You want to watch the birth, not the ceiling!

Research has shown that being supine slows down the progress of labor and is associated with a variety of complications.[71]

Figure 78. Only pancakes should lie flat!

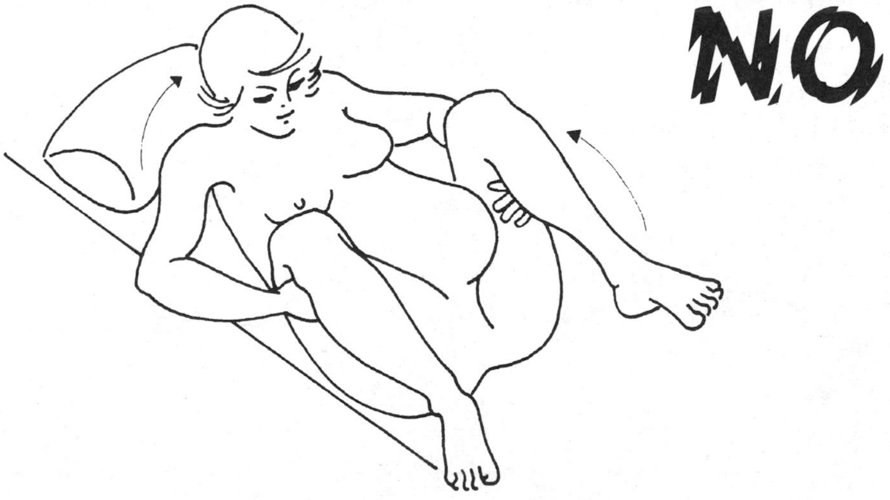

Upright Positions Encourage Freedom and Mobility

When left to choose for themselves, women select a variety of positions for birth that include squatting, kneeling, or supported hanging.

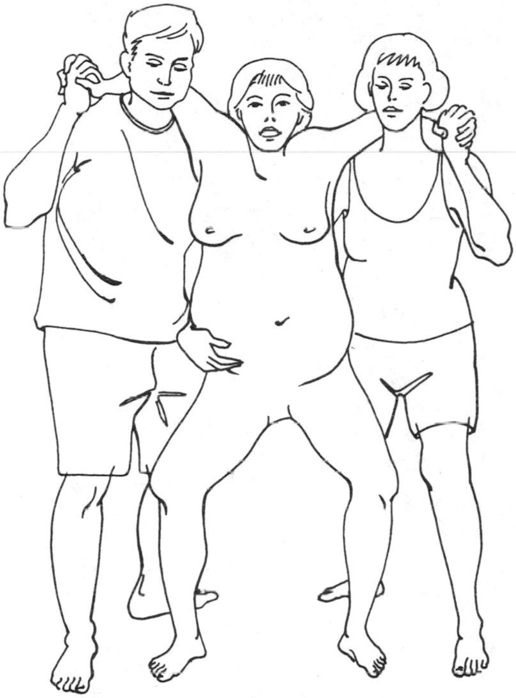

Figure 79. Labor progresses well if you dangle with support on each side.

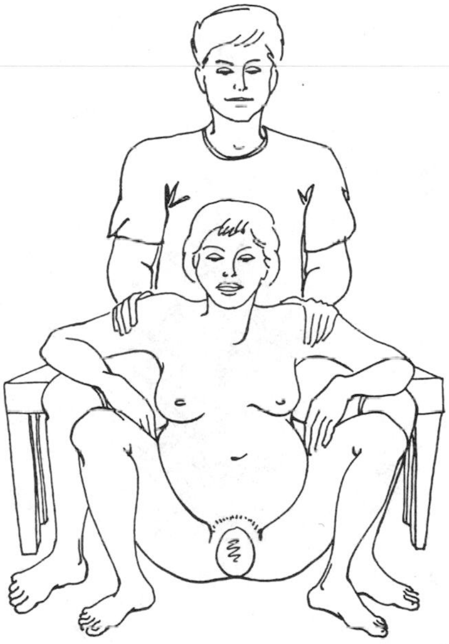

Figure 80. Support for your arms helps you squat during birth.

No animal

selects the supine position for birth.

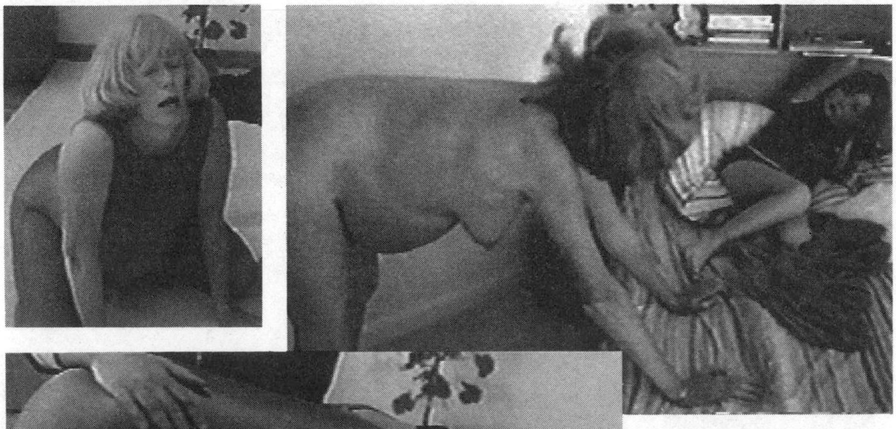

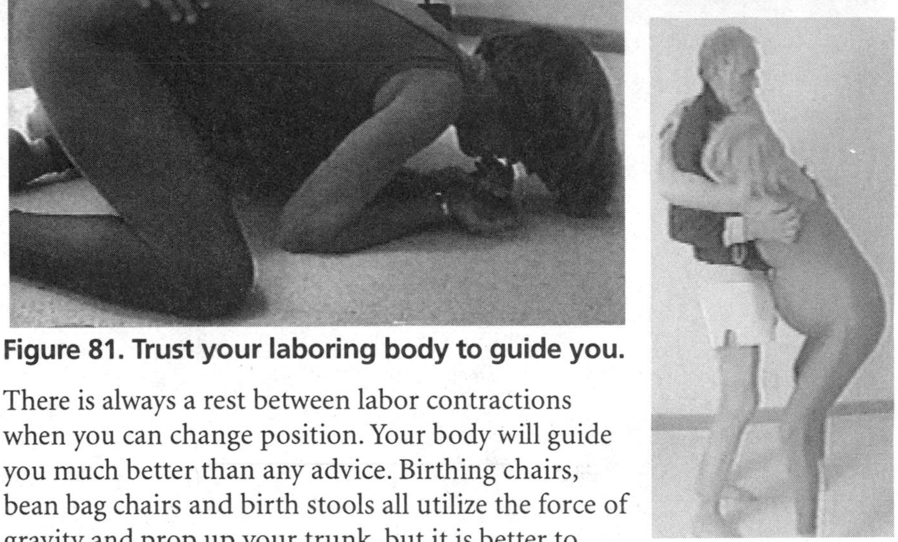

Figure 81. Trust your laboring body to guide you.

There is always a rest between labor contractions when you can change position. Your body will guide you much better than any advice. Birthing chairs, bean bag chairs and birth stools all utilize the force of gravity and prop up your trunk, but it is better to have no weight at all on your pelvis so you can move your body in response to the contractions. We pull a cork from a bottle or a ring from a finger by gentle turns, and women spontaneously make appropriate pelvic motions to facilitate the birth if they are free to do so.

Being upright with your pelvis free to move has many advantages:

- ✦ The most efficient body mechanics for birth; less effort is required.
- ✦ Gravity assists by 15 percent, according to Dr. Michel Odent.
- ✦ Your pelvic outlet is enlarged.
- ✦ Your perineum is stretched equally in all directions and serious tears are less likely.
- ✦ No negative vectors counteract your baby's descent.
- ✦ No compression of your sacrum and coccyx.

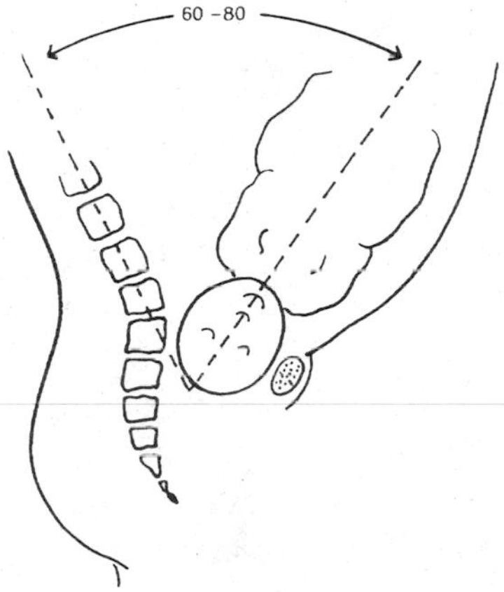

Figure 82. Being upright increases the drive angle of the uterus.

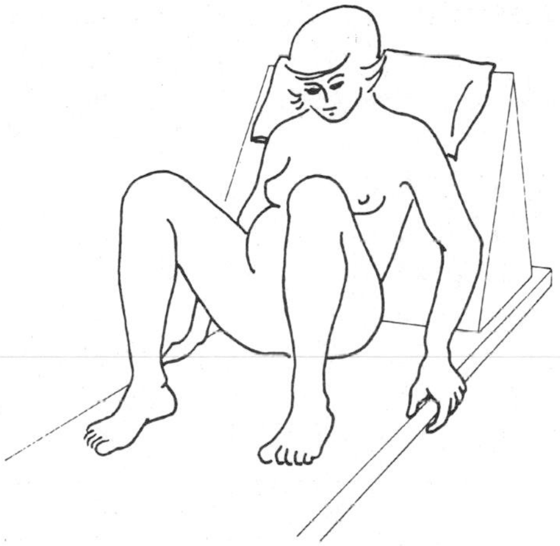

Figure 83. Weight pressed on your pelvis during birth restricts its opening.

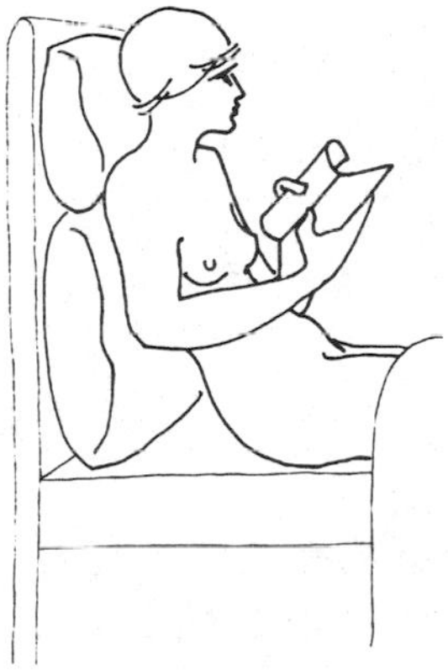

Figure 84. Many people slouch when half-lying, especially in hospital beds.

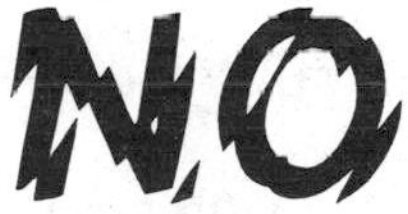

You probably assume this semi-recumbent position when reading in bed, and it is the one in which you will spend most of your days immediately after birth. Usually your knees are a little bent and your legs roll out comfortably from the hips. However, your lower back will ache if you half-lie like this for prolonged periods without support to maintain its normal curve. Stretched ligaments may give rise to joint instability and pain.

An orthopedic specialist, the late Dr. James Cyriax,[72] called this the "nursing mother's position," but it is easy for all of us to slouch in the bed like this, especially after a Cesarean section or other surgery. An extra pillow makes all the difference to support the lower back and keep our shoulders over our hips.

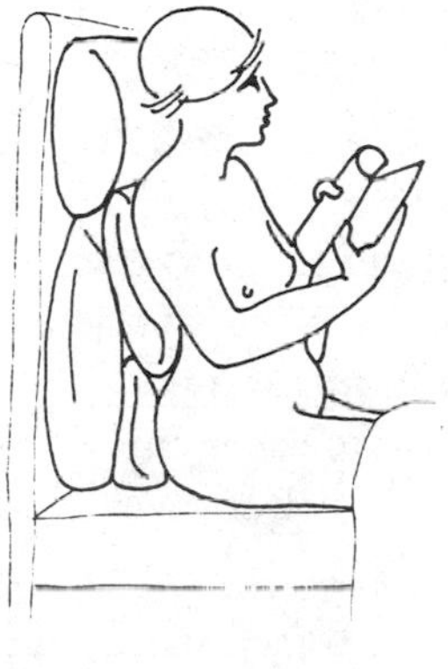

Figure 85.Use pillows to support your spine.

Posture While Side-Lying

Most pregnant women are usually very comfortable lying on their sides. The abdominal weight is off your lower back and groin, compression of major blood vessels is avoided, and your joints are bent to take the stretch off any muscle group. Strain in the upper hip can be prevented by placing **several pillows lengthwise** between your legs to raise your upper foot to the level of the hip. Make sure this foot is also resting on pillows; if it is just dangling, the muscles work in response to gravity.

Lying on your left side (commonly known as left lateral) has two advantages over lying on your right side. Digestion travels through your intestines from right to left, and blood flow back to your heart is a little easier because of the location of the major vein returning blood from the lower part of your body.

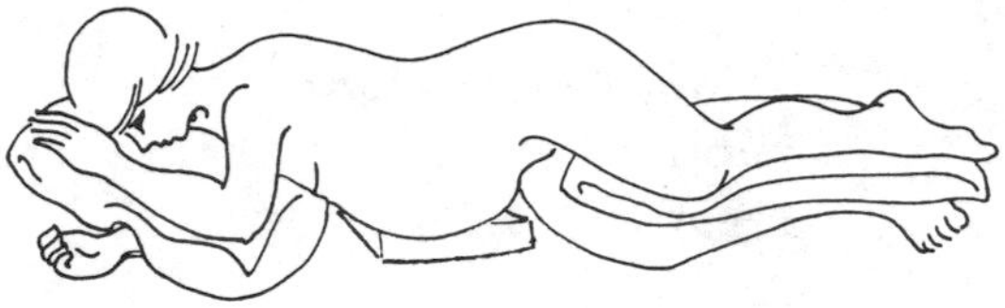

Figure 86. Comfort while side-lying—note pillows between the legs and a wedge supporting the belly.

A **wedge** is perfect to tuck underneath your abdomen to relieve traction on your belly when you lie on your side. You can also use the edge of a pillow or a rolled towel, but the wedge offers a firm incline. Once I discovered the wedge during my last pregnancy, I never went to bed without it. The complete bodyCushion™ provides excellent and extensive support in side-lying. (See Appendix and Resources.) Always bend your knees, one at a time, to turn from side-lying onto your back or to the other side.

Posture While Three-Quarters Over

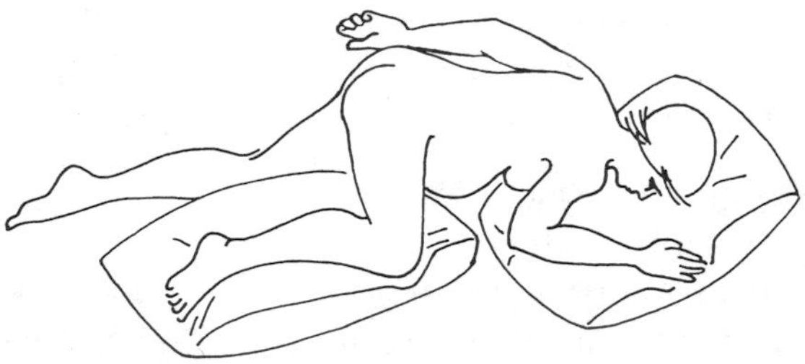

Figure 87. Comfort when lying three-quarters over supported by pillows.

Here you lie more toward your front than in side-lying. Your lower arm is behind your back, which brings your top shoulder further over. The pillow under your head can also be used to rest your upper arm. A second pillow can support the front leg for increased comfort. This position is a favorite for resting and sleeping during pregnancy. In labor, however, the side-lying position is preferable because it prevents your putting any body weight at all on the uterus as it contracts and tips forward.

Posture on Hands and Knees

Take any opportunity to get down on your hands and knees and you can obtain the numerous benefits of the all-fours position, described on pages 98. Being on your hands and knees unweights your spine and relieves the pelvic pressure and congestion that cause hemorrhoids and vaginal swelling. Your circulation improves because the pressure of your uterus is temporarily removed from your back and pelvic floor. This position relieves round ligament spasms, especially when combined with pelvic tilting, and also relieves muscle cramps in the thighs and buttocks. Going on all-fours also helps backache or tired legs that come from continual standing. This position exercises your abdominal muscles against gravity **if you keep your back in neutral alignment.**

A variation on hands and feet, known in yoga as *downward dog*[73] (see the first partner exercise, Chapter 8), is an excellent spinal check for others to see at a glance exactly where you are stiff; segments of your spine will be rounded and prominent instead of in alignment. I do not generally advocate positions and exercises where the head is placed lower than the heart with the extra blood volume in pregnancy. However, like interrupting the urine flow, it is something you can do yourself and it provides immediate feedback of your flexibility. In the postpartum period, however, you can do this exercise as often as you like after your bleeding has stopped. Continue it for the rest of your life to maintain strength in your arms, as well as spinal flexibility.

Posture in Action: Good Body Mechanics

Squatting

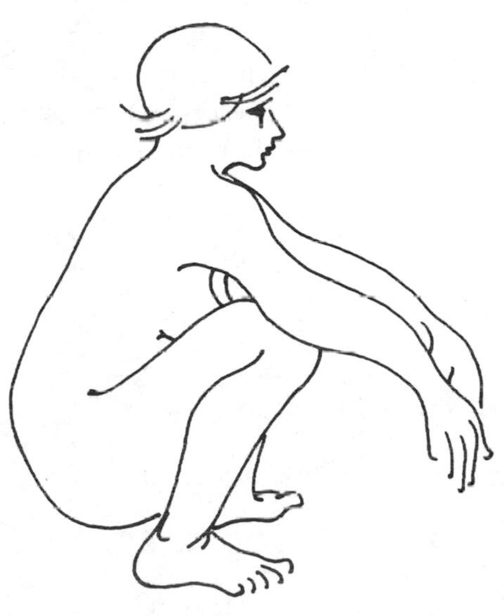

Figure 88. Some can squat with ease and rest elbows on knees.

The squatting position offers many advantages for birth. Moreover, it is necessary for good body mechanics such as lifting (rather than stooping). Lowering your center of gravity increases stability. Your pelvis is tilted backward; in fact you cannot do a pelvic tilt in the squatting position. The small of your back feels most comfortable when squatting, especially if your back muscles are tired and tight. In addition, your calf muscles benefit from a good stretch when you squat.

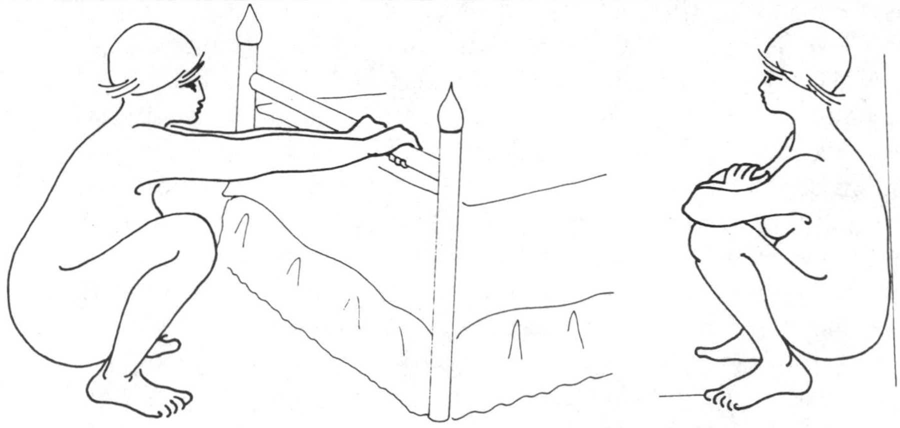

Figure 89. Others need support to squat.

Rest your elbows on your knees when you can balance alone. Use your thigh muscles to stand up. This can be awkward later in pregnancy, so start practicing early. Most people have forgotten how easily they squatted as toddlers. But years of sitting in chairs make it difficult to resume this position again. I have seen 8-year-old children in the U.S. who can no longer squat, whereas in Asia most of the 80-year-olds still squat and rise to standing without using their arms.

Practice while holding hands with a partner (see Chapter 8) or grasping a firm support (bed, chair), or even while leaning with your back against a wall. Make room for your abdomen with your feet flat and wide apart. Keep your weight on the outer borders of your feet and your knees pointing outward. (If the inner borders of your feet roll in, you'll feel an unpleasant twist in your knees.) Those with large calves may find that their legs go to sleep at first, but the circulation improves with practice. Be assured that blood returns to the vital organs via the deep veins.

Tips for Re-Learning How to Squat

- ✦ Wear shoes with heels.
- ✦ Find a sloping terrain outside.
- ✦ Practice on the beach where you sink into the sand.
- ✦ Use a piece of wood or a book under your heels.

Squat a Lot when

- ✦ Picking up objects from the floor.
- ✦ Looking in the oven.
- ✦ Picking up a child.
- ✦ Weeding and planting in the garden.

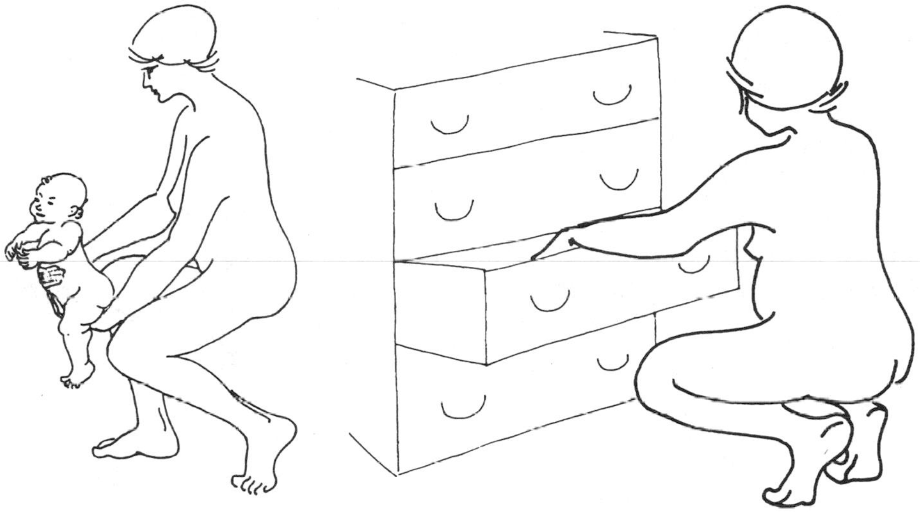

Figure 90. Stoop with ease, bend your knees.

In countries such as France, the Middle East, or Asia, it is common to find toilet facilities that require you to squat: a hole in the floor, sometimes tiled and with flush plumbing. Aim becomes important to spare your feet! This is one reason why women in such countries have better pelvic floor control, and why urinary incontinence is conspicuous by its absence.

Clearly, the human body has the same physical structure everywhere and differences in its use are governed by cultural habits. For example, squatting is the position for delivery in many countries; the pelvis is at its widest and the power of the abdominals and gravity can be well utilized.

Getting Up from the Horizontal Position

As pregnancy advances, you will find it more difficult when arising in the morning, or sitting up when you have been resting or exercising at floor level. Furthermore, your circulation slows down when you recline. Always take care to get up slowly to avoid feeling dizzy or faint.

If you have been on your back, stretch first. Bend one knee and then other. Roll both knees to one side, wait while you take a couple of breaths, then push with your arms to a sitting position. Use your hands to help you stand. Place your legs, one at a time, over the edge and straighten them. Arising with care allows your circulation to adjust and protects your center seam. (This avoids jack-knifing up into a sitting position which strains your abdominal wall and can encourage or increase stretching of your central seam.)

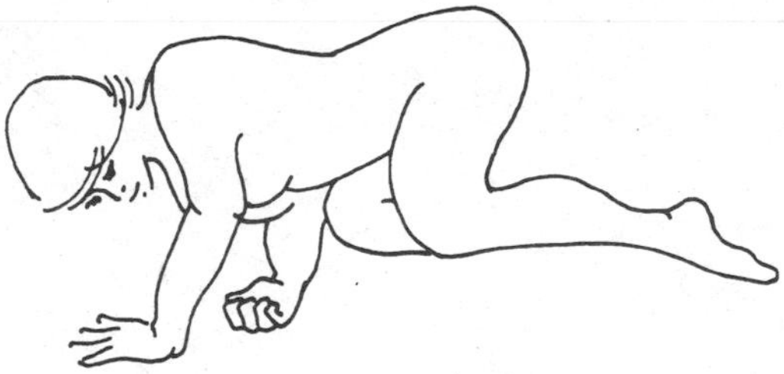
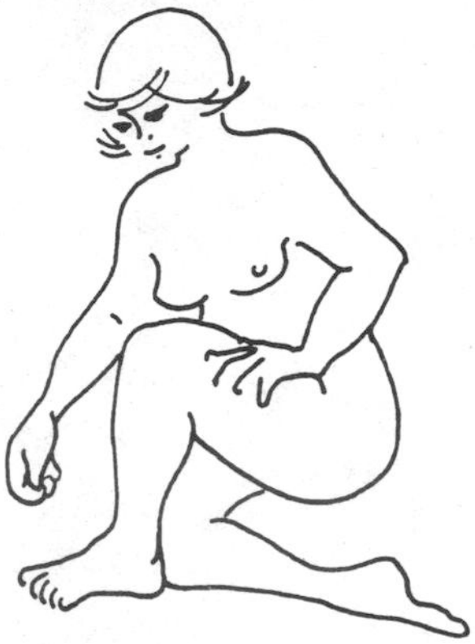

Figure 91. When rising from the floor, push yourself onto one knee, using your arm for support.

Walking

The elements of good erect posture (page 225) should be maintained as you walk. Common faults include: watching your feet, which results in a forward leaning posture; rounded shoulders, with head and neck poked out in front; or a side–to–side waddle, where the legs are swung sideways rather than rotated forward from the hip.

It takes some time and effort to correct bad habits. The easiest way is to concentrate on the key areas—head, pelvis, feet—perhaps just one at a time at first. Tune into your posture during movement; ask those around you to observe. Keep imagining that invisible thread pulling your head up toward the ceiling as you tuck your buttocks under and place your feet, heel first, one in front the other (rather than shifting your legs from side to side.) Beware of the tendency to sway back from your waist with your pelvis forward. Hollowing your lower back to counter your increased weight in front will only emphasize the waddling motion already mentioned, as well as set up a vicious circle of back strain, muscle weakness, and increased forward displacement of your pelvis. The stretching and strengthening exercises recommended in this chapter will improve your muscle control so that better posture follows in all activities.

Climbing Stairs

Use the handrail for balance and make sure that your **legs** are the force that propels your body weight upward. Place each foot firmly and completely on each step, push off from your back foot by straightening your front knee and lifting yourself up with your thigh and buttock muscles. Take one step at a time if necessary. Breathe out as you step up, bracing your abdominals, buttocks and pelvic floor at the same time. Incline your body forward as you go up but keep your body weight over the base of your feet when descending. Hug any packages close to your body and support them from underneath (rather than at the sides or top).

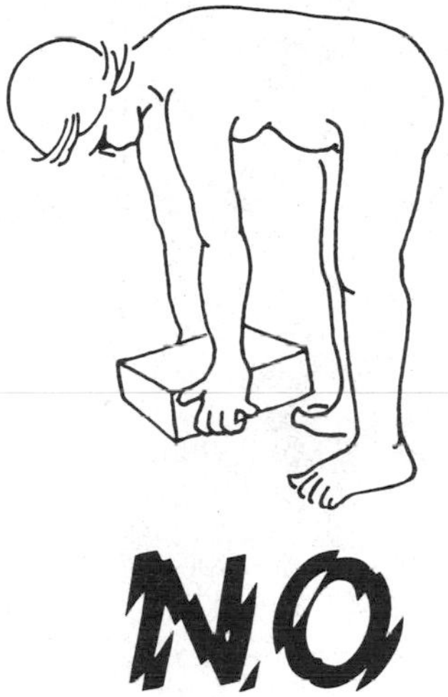

Figure 92. Legs are for lifting.

Your back is not a crane and you risk injury if you lean forward from your waist in order to lift heavy objects. You must lower your center of gravity—to become more stable—so that the weaker back muscles do not lengthen and then shorten again to raise your trunk back up. This action is risky in pregnancy with the increased vulnerability of your spinal joints and extra weight of your torso. We have all watched how weight lifters prepare their muscles and, with a loud grunt, thrust upward by straightening their knees. (Your knees have much stronger muscles than your back.) Watch your family members over the next few days to see how automatically they lean over at the waist to pick up toys, other children, shopping bags, to look in low cupboards, and so on. For light objects, bending forward is fine, although we lose all these opportunities to squat and thus keep our knees and ankles flexible.

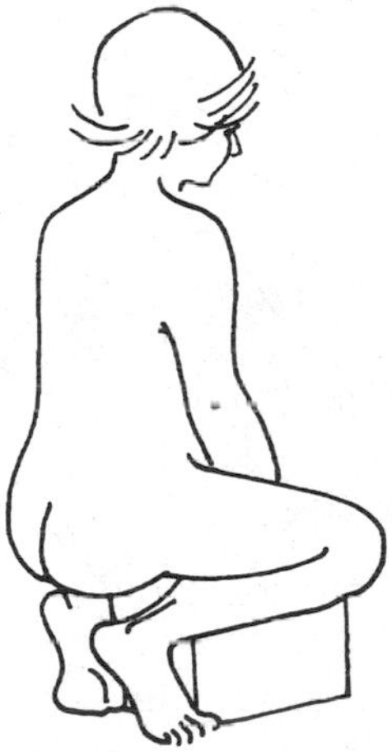

Figure 93. Lift with ease . . . bend your knees.

Most people lift incorrectly—until they get a back problem. In pregnancy, your instability is increased with your forward center of gravity, softening of joints and ligaments, and—if you are wearing them—shoes with high heels. The pelvic floor also registers strain from lifting, as you may well feel. Get into the right lifting habits now if you have not done so before, and make sure your family reinforces them by reminding you and setting an example themselves.

Heavy lifting should be passed on to someone else during the childbearing year. Divide up bulky supplies and place them on lower shelves. Reaching high for moderate or heavy objects can strain your back. If you **must** lift a heavy object, protect your balance by placing your feet apart in a lunge position (See page 137.) When you need to be at floor level, assume a squatting position—it's easier with one foot in front. Remember to stand up **from the knees**—the quadriceps muscles on the front of the thighs are the strongest in the human body. Encourage children who want to be picked up to climb on to a stool or chair so that you lift them a shorter distance.

When you do have to lift heavy objects, remember:

- ✦ Stand close to the load and carry it close to your body.
- ✦ Divide up loads so that you carry them equally on each side.
- ✦ Have a firm footing; one foot in front of the other in a lunge position is easier when you are lifting with the opposite arm. Keep feet parallel for large objects requiring both arms.
- ✦ Bend your knees, keeping back straight.
- ✦ Take a steady grip.
- ✦ Move smoothly.
- ✦ Brace your abdomen and pull up your pelvic floor, as you exhale. Rise up, straightening the knees.
- ✦ Face the direction of movement.
- ✦ Shift feet if the object turns out to be heavier than you thought.
- ✦ Move the object with a sideways lunge rather than an upward lift.

Carrying Your Baby

Supporting your baby on one hip causes your spine to twist in compensation. Similarly, carrying your baby over one shoulder increases the hollow in your lower back. Avoid using these positions on a regular basis.

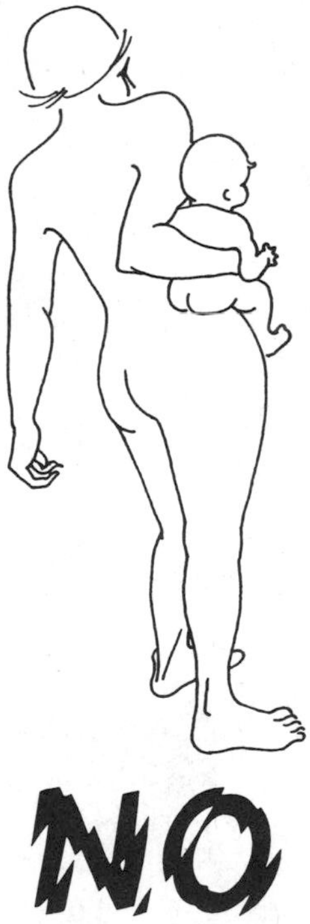

Figure 94. If you carry a baby on one hip, change from side to side. A back pack is better and leaves both hands free.

In recent years, many infant carrying devices have appeared on the market, so now we can enjoy the advantages that most women always have had in other cultures. The mother's hands are liberated and the baby feels the reassurance of her body motion. Baby is upright, which aids digestion, especially after feedings, and allows him or her to face the world. Babies carried this way rarely cry.

Carriers on the back are the most comfortable for the parent. However, for the first couple of months, before your baby gains head control, you may prefer him or her in a front pack. In reality, most infants can go on the back if they sink right down in the carrier, as they typically do. Put your baby on your **back** as soon as you can, to avoid muscle strain from a front load equivalent to being fifteen months or more pregnant! Let out the straps so that the baby sits around your waist, taking his or her weight near your center of gravity. Most people place the back pack too high. (The only advantage of this otherwise undesirable position is that you must bend your knees while lifting or stooping forward, otherwise the baby may fall out over your head!) It is much better to have the baby ride you as you would ride a horse.

When lifting Baby out of the back seat of a two-door car, climb in and sit beside the infant seat. Lift your baby on to your lap and emerge as a unit, supporting Baby from his or her base.

The side rails of a crib drop only so far and you must reach over the top. Take a wide stance and raise your back leg with your knee straight to keep your spinal alignment. Better still, consider enjoying a family bed.

The Haptonomic Circle

Figure 95. Cradle your baby in a circle of support.

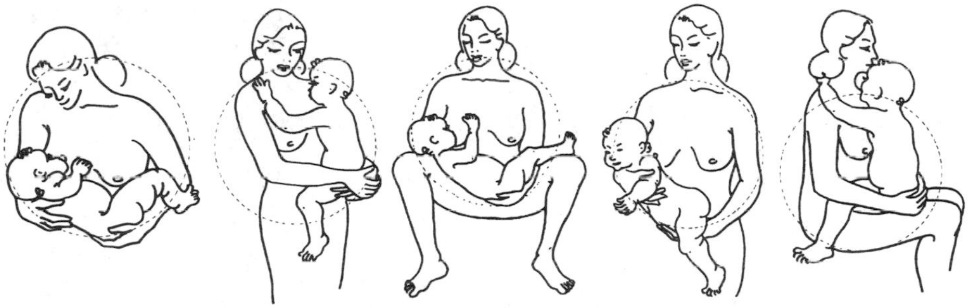

A child who through infancy is lifted, supported and thus affirmed from his or her base, illustrated above, develops an expanded sense of his or her self through the body. That is, the child *is* her or his body rather than *having* a body. Amazingly a baby held at his or her base can and will hold the spine and head erect—from the moment of birth. (It may take a few minutes. Be assured that a head has never fallen off!) Most people will not believe this because they are afraid to try it. By "protecting" the baby in a crumpled position, caretakers actually fulfill their own limited prophesy of a baby's postural abilities.

Lifting a baby from his or her base spares the new mother from wrist and thumb pain, which is treated commonly by physical therapists. When the baby is supported under the buttocks, postural reflexes keep him or her upright. When lifted conventionally, the baby is a dead weight dangling from the armpits, with the ribcage squeezed and no possibility of using either the trunk or limbs. Frans Veldman, the founder of Haptonomy (see Resources) observed that "this leaves the child in control only from the neck up—the cerebral personality of modern western society." Veldman further points out that in the "circle of affectivity," the mother's arms entirely enfold and hold the child; breast-feeding naturally accomplishes this. In contrast, the circle is broken when one arm and hand must separate from the embrace for bottle feeding.

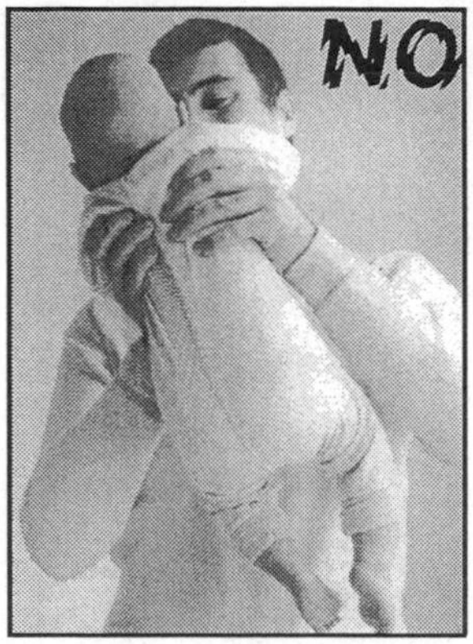

Figure 96. Baby's center of gravity is unsupported.

The baby on the right is ten days old and feels safe after just a few minutes of being held by his base for the first time. After a few more opportunities, his head will be quite erect.

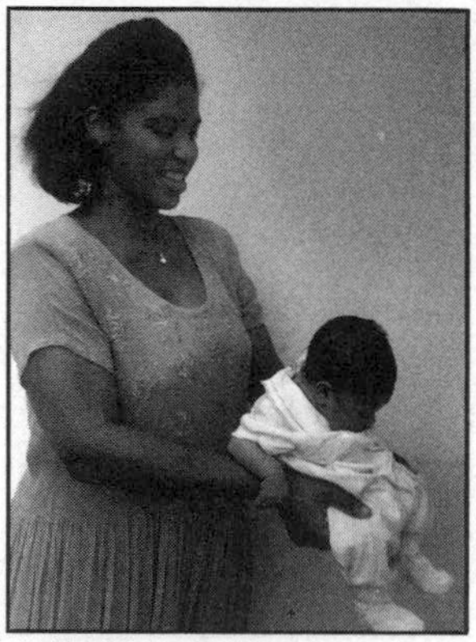

Figure 97. Baby holds up his head when held from

Wheeling Strollers, Utility Carts, Supermarket Carriages

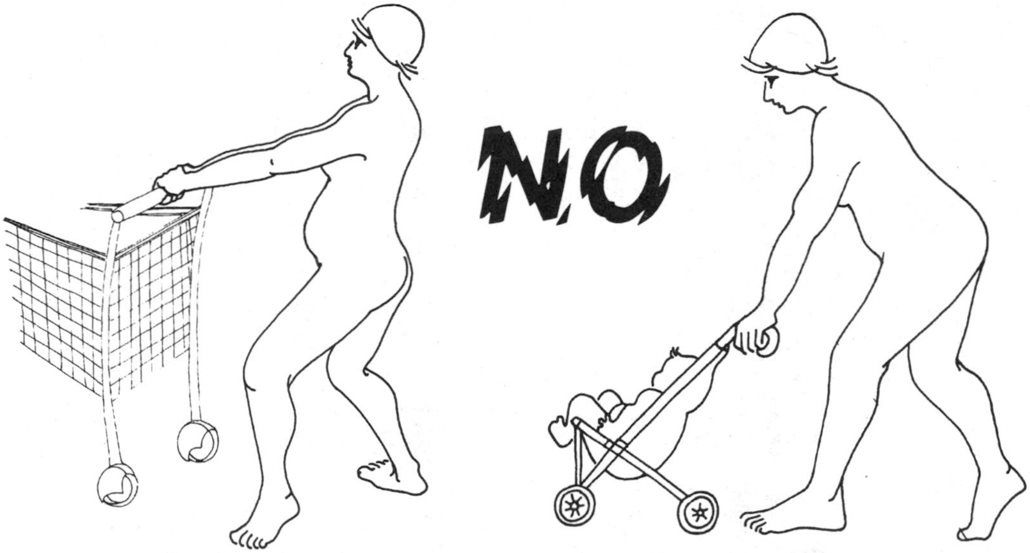

Figure 98. Equipment you wheel should be high and close.

Take care to buy a stroller or baby carriage with the handle at the proper height. If the handle is too low, you will have to lean toward it. Push grocery carts held close to you—not as in the sketches above.

Vacuuming, Mopping, Sweeping, Raking Leaves, Shoveling Snow

These activities involve long-levered tools, which can be tiring for your arms. Turn these tasks into a beneficial exercise for your abdominal and back muscles: work diagonally in a lunge position. Footwork is the key to performing these movements with ease, comfort, and grace. As a tennis player puts the left foot forward to serve with the right arm, you should use the same principle with household equipment. (Reverse if you are left-handed.) It is a good idea to change sides anyway, as most of us are asymmetrically developed. Bend your forward knee a little, as you thrust from your straightened back leg. This makes the work easier because you swing your weight back and forth into the movement instead of standing alongside the tool with one arm doing all the work and your trunk muscles in prolonged and tiring contraction.

Figure 99. Exercise while you work. Use the lunge position.

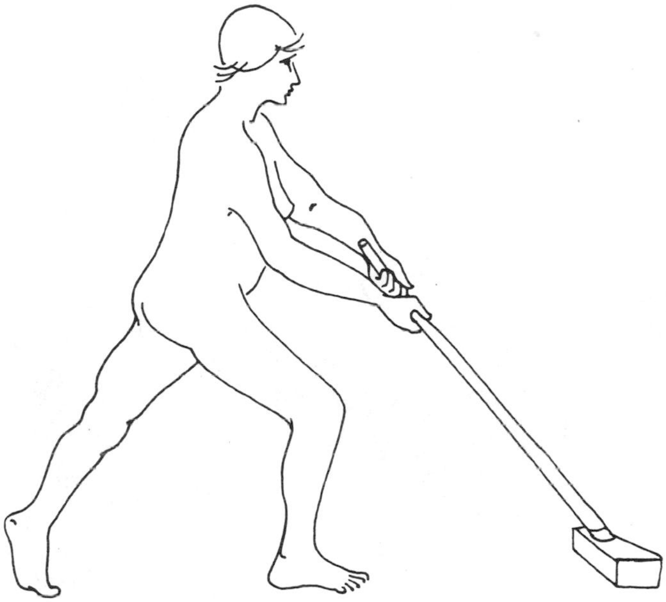

When moving furniture, use the same position, and bend your knees and hips a little to line up with the object. Lean close with your back straight, bend your elbows and push with both hands. The force is provided by your body weight as you thrust forward from the back foot. Pushing and pivoting movements are easier than pulling and lifting ones. If you bend your knees and lower your trunk, you economize on effort and objects are less likely to topple over.

Working on High Surfaces

Make sure that the height of a counter, desk, ironing board, table, or similar flat surface is appropriate. The surface should be near the level of your hip bone—so that you work with elbows bent at an angle of about 30 to 40 degrees. A sink is always lower than these surfaces; you can wash in a basin supported on another basin that is turned upside down. This will prevent your having to lean over when doing dishes and laundry.

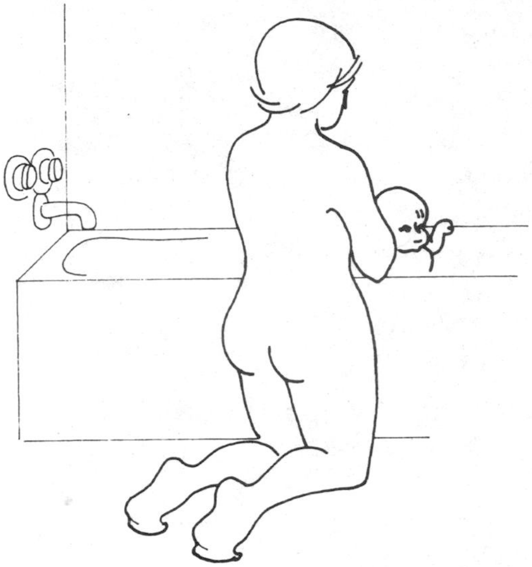

Figure 100. Kneel by the bathtub.

Figure 101. Move back and forth with your feet apart while ironing.

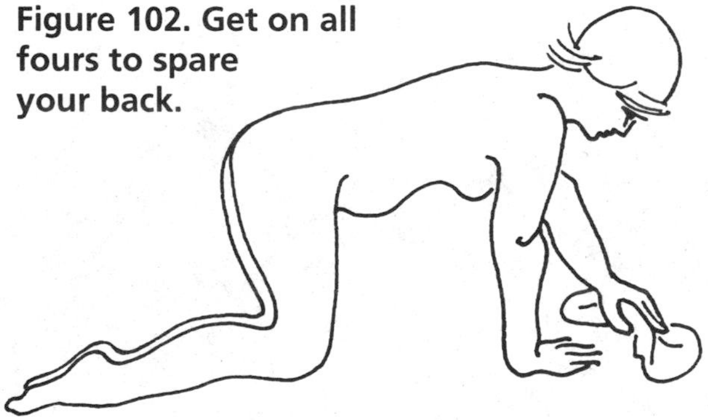

Figure 102. Get on all fours to spare your back.

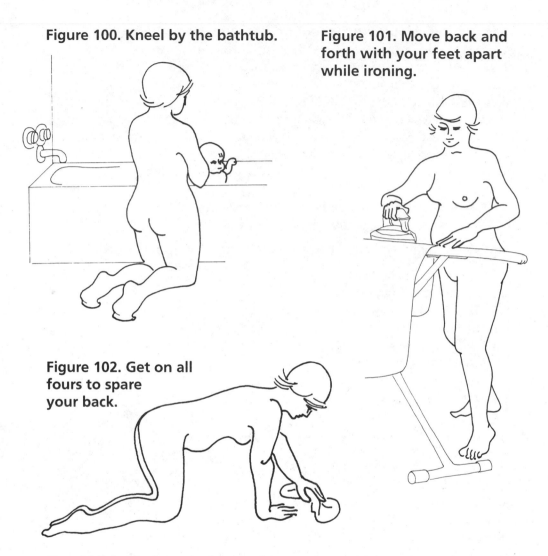

Use a high stool where possible, perching on the seat if you are moving back and forth, when standing at the ironing board or when cleaning furniture, for example. Place your feet so that you have both a firm base and the freedom to move backward and forward in the direction of your arms and trunk. An alternative that prevents backache when standing is to rest one foot on a low stool, chair rung, or an open drawer.

Bending over a bed to fold clothes is a fast way to get a backache! Instead, sit like a tailor on the bed or move the clothes to a counter top. Kneel or squat when you wash the floor, clean the bath tub, wash a child or work in the garden. Squatting is preferable to putting your body weight on your knee caps.

The easiest way to wash your baby is to take him or her into the bathtub with you. I rarely took on the daunting task of washing a slippery baby in a sink or baby bath. Besides, it's much more fun to get in the tub together. Baby can feel your skin, float and move, and nursing is instant! It takes a baby four to five months of postpartum development to move as he or she did in the fluid-filled uterus. Therefore, introduce Baby to water right away and make bath-time fun for the family. (The cord stump can get wet.)

Artificial Supports

Girdles

Only on rare occasions do I recommend a corset in pregnancy, or a binder after birth, because artificial supports give your natural muscular corset—the abdominal muscles—a vacation. Allowing muscles to remain passive retards their return to normal function.

In some cases, however, a support may be needed in pregnancy if obesity, multiple pregnancy, *diastasis recti* or spinal curvature cause back pain. Maternity support garments can also help pelvic floor pressure and varicosities by taking some weight off the pelvic floor. (Various products are listed in Resources.)Likewise, after birth an abdominal binder may be necessary when there is severe muscle weakness. Its use in the postpartum period should be temporary; it is a splint to assist in restoring the muscles to their normal strength. Such garments should be removed during exercise sessions.

Bras

During pregnancy and nursing, a supportive bra can increase your comfort, especially if you jog or play sports during which your breasts bounce. There are **no** muscles in the breast, although exercises for the muscles lying beneath the breasts are often given to improve circulation and lactation. During pregnancy, the familiar factors of increasing weight and gravity apply to your breasts in the same way as to your uterus and pelvic floor. A well-fitting bra can improve your posture and minimize upper backache from the increased weight of your breasts.[74]

Make sure that the bra you select has broad straps and provides stability and support. Check also to make sure that it allows proper circulation and you should never see any red or indented areas on your skin when you remove it. Numerous styles of nursing bras are available for breast-feeding mothers, but buy these after birth so that you get the best fit and support. Some people like front closures, but I preferred the trap-door style. When the flaps are down, there is still a supporting contour of fabric underneath and this is handy if you need to air sore nipples.

Support Hose for Varicose Veins

Venous blood must be returned against the force of gravity when your body is upright. Valves placed in the thin-walled veins direct the blood back to heart. If blood becomes backed up, some veins may become distended and prominent. Both your increased blood volume and growing pressure within your abdomen challenge your circulatory system. Socks or knee-highs with tight elastic tops interfere with the blood circulation in the legs. Regular exercise is a help in preventing varicose veins; if you do develop them, support hose provides relief.

For best results, elevate your legs while you put the support hose on **before** arising in the morning. Your legs have been horizontal all night, and swelling and venous congestion is less than after you stand. All these external supports, however, treat the symptoms—not the cause. Exercise, changes in position, and massage will minimize these pregnancy-related problems. Walking backward in knee-deep water is very good for varicose veins.

Leg Cramps

Calf cramps are common in pregnancy and can often be brought on simply by pointing your feet. Stretching usually works as a preventive measure and it is certainly the cure if you experience a cramp. **Calf-stretching** in the lunge position is best. Stand with one foot well in front of the other. Keep your back leg straight and heel on floor. Align your second toe with your knee which keeps the inner border of your foot straight. (If your toe is turned out slightly you will not stretch the **inner** calf muscle, which is the one that cramps.) Gradually bend your front knee and lean your weight forward, keeping your back heel on the floor. Take a wider stance to increase the stretch. A variation is to stretch both heel cords while doing wall push-offs to strengthen your arms and shoulders. Squatting also exerts a stretch on part of your calf muscles.

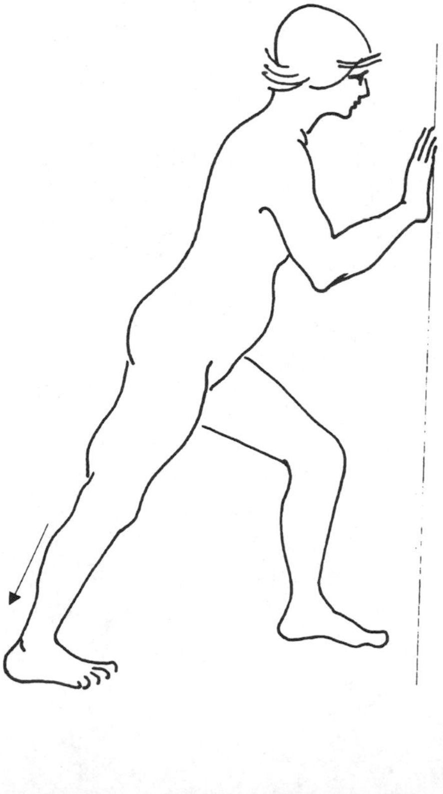

Figure 103. Lean against the wall and stretch your back leg.

Round Ligament Spasm

Exercise, together with frequent changes of position, relieves common twinges of pain in usually felt in one groin. These sudden stabbing sensations result from spasm of the muscle fibers in the round ligament of your uterus.[75]

Discomfort and pressure in the groin can be relieved by your partner raising and lowering your hips while you are lying down. This activity is similar to lifting a wheelbarrow. You relax completely with your legs loose and bent so that your thighs can be grasped. Stay quite passive as your buttocks are raised a few inches from the floor; your weight provides counter-traction. Relief is usually immediate after your uterus has been tipped off the cramped structures a few times in this manner. (Make sure your helper's knees are bent to protect his or her back.)

If you are by yourself, lie on your back and do some bridging, or else go on all fours and tilt your pelvis back and forth a few times.

Symptomatic Relief for Nerve Compression Syndromes

Sometimes postural changes cause pressure on nerves, and tingling, numbness and even pain in the fingers may result. *Thoracic outlet syndrome* occurs when there is pressure on the cluster of nerves lying between your collarbones and armpits. This is usually from a combination of postural changes and increased fluid in your tissues. *Carpal tunnel syndrome* may develop when there is pressure from fluid accumulating in your wrist on the median nerve which supplies your thumb and first two fingers. (It is a common problem for anyone who works long hours at a keyboard.) Finger symptoms can also arise from nerve compression in the neck and shoulders. (See page 114, Figure 60.) A night splint may be helpful so that you don't sleep with your wrist bent backward. Many individuals have both carpal tunnel and thoracic outlet syndromes.

Some women develop swollen fingers while pregnant and have to remove their rings. After birth you will lose your extra fluid very quickly; it is amazing how much urine is voided in the first day or two. But until then, exercises help to pump fluid along. Ice can also be tried on your wrists, along with squeezing a soft ball or Silly Putty® from a toy store. Occasionally similar symptoms develop in the feet and toes from fluid accumulation in the nerve tunnel at the back of the ankle. Ice and movement can help here, too.

Decreasing your fluid intake will not affect these conditions; on the contrary, you must be sure to drink at least twelve to sixteen glasses of water, juice, herbal tea, or soup a day. Beverages that contain caffeine—coffee, sodas such as Coke and Pepsi, black tea—are diuretics and by increasing the excretion of fluid, they also increase your need for it. The amount of sugar (usually several teaspoons!) in sodas also makes your thirstier. You are adequately hydrated when your urine is a pale yellow color. Conversely, when you are dehydrated your urine is darker.

Compression of intercostal nerves between your ribs can give rise to localized discomfort. (This can also happen when the baby persists in kicking in a certain spot.) Friction massage can bring relief, as do the side-bending exercises with partner. (See pages 186.)

Placing your fingers on your shoulders and making circles with your elbows, **backward only,** will help these symptoms as well as relieve upper backache from heavy breasts and bending over the baby, counters, and appliances. (Forward shoulder circles only make round-shouldered people more so. I always advise women and men to do **double-time in the backward direction,** opening the chest and straightening any hunch-back posture.)

Toward the very end of pregnancy, pressure on vaginal nerves can give rise to tingling, even minor "electric-shock" sensations in your vagina. Bridging helps relieve this discomfort, but usually it is time to give birth!

Exercises to Improve Posture

Exercise 1. Stretch Out the Kinks

This exercise has its greatest use in late pregnancy and during the immediate postpartum period when you want your back and abdominal muscles to work **isometrically,** with minimal leverage on your joints. After birth, your body has to readjust suddenly to its loss of weight. It's easier to retrain your posture in the horizontal position, before you take on the force of gravity.

Position: Lying on back, arms at sides, **palms up**, legs out straight.

Action: Bend your feet toward you to stretch your calves as you press your knees into the bed. Pull in your abdominals to reduce the hollow in your lower spine and press down the back of your neck. (Spinal curves are normal; you will never get your back completely flat, but it is a helpful image during exercise.) Squeeze your shoulder blades together. Press the **back of your hands and thumbs** onto the floor. Hold this stretched position for a few seconds—keep breathing—and then rest.

Progression: Standing or sitting against the wall. See pages 144.

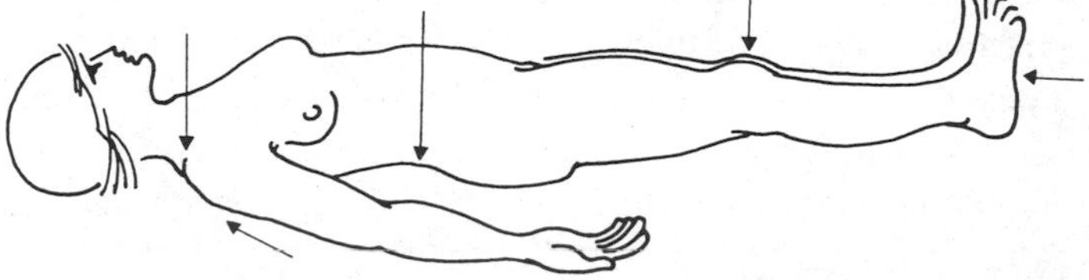

Figure 104. Perfect posture lying on your back.

Exercise 2. Pelvic Tilting
This essential exercise for good posture in pregnancy and after birth was discussed in the last chapter, pages 95-101.

Exercise 3. Bridging
Bridging, or raising your hips from the floor, exercises your buttocks muscles, which control your pelvic tilt together with your abdominal muscles. In pregnancy and after birth, as your abdominal muscles become stretched and less able to do their share, your buttocks have more work to do. We sit on these muscles, and they work strongly in running, jumping and climbing stairs, although not in ordinary walking. Known as the glutei, they extend the hips when we get up from chairs or the floor, providing an anti-gravity thrust. The buttock muscles also contribute to erect posture in standing.

When you make a bridge with your hips, your buttocks work strongly to lift your body weight against gravity. Bridging exercises benefit the circulation in your legs because the glutei exert a pumping effect on the veins and an elevated position assists the return of blood to the heart. Furthermore, strengthening this muscle provides additional support for the back of the pelvis where the muscles attach and blend with ligaments.

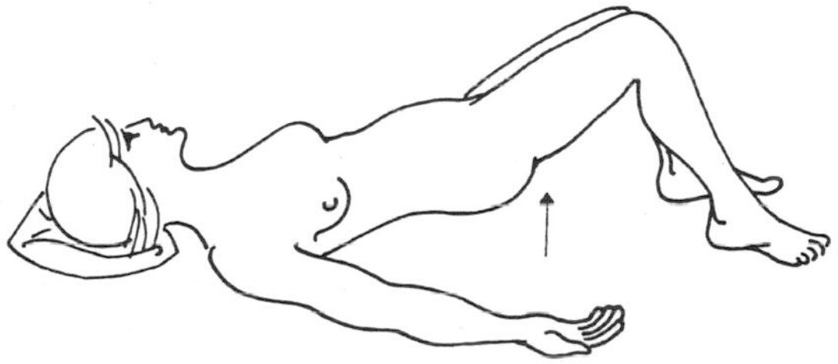

Figure 105. Your hamstrings help bridging when your knees are bent.

Position: Lying on your back, knees bent.
Action: Contract your abdominal wall and buttocks and slowly raise hips off the floor until trunk and legs are in a straight line. Hold for a few seconds while breathing, then slowly lower. Contract your pelvic floor during this exercise because gravity is now a help rather than a liability. After birth, close your sphincters as tightly as possible and clench your buttocks to protect your perineum from gaping.
Action: The closer your feet are to your buttocks, the more leverage you use from your hamstrings. This exercise also maintains the normal length of the muscles at the front of your hips which are often tight.
Progressions:

- Move your feet farther away from your buttocks. Squeeze your buttocks together as tightly as you can, so that you lift with these muscles rather than the hamstrings in the back of your thighs.
- Raise your buttocks with one knee bent and the other straightened. Keep both thighs parallel.

- Remain in a bridge position and move the straight leg to the side and back to the center for additional strengthening of your hips and thighs.
- As well as opening and closing the straight leg, circle it to challenge your balance.
- Increase the duration by bending and stretching your ankles or doing two or three pelvic floor exercises.

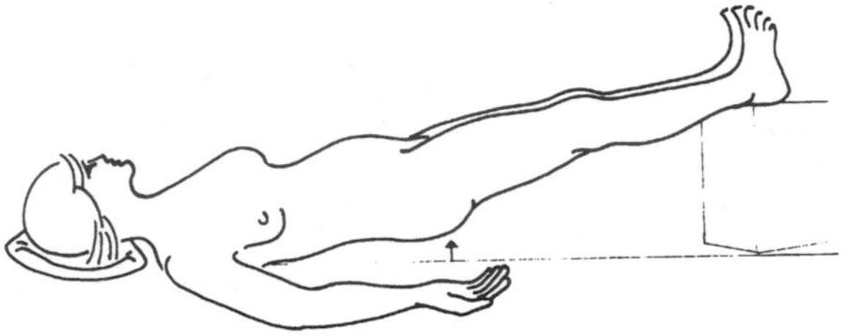

Figure 106. Bridge with straight legs to increase the challenge.

Position: Lying on your back, feet elevated on low stool, end of bed or coffee table. A gymnastic ball can be used if you want to challenge your balance.

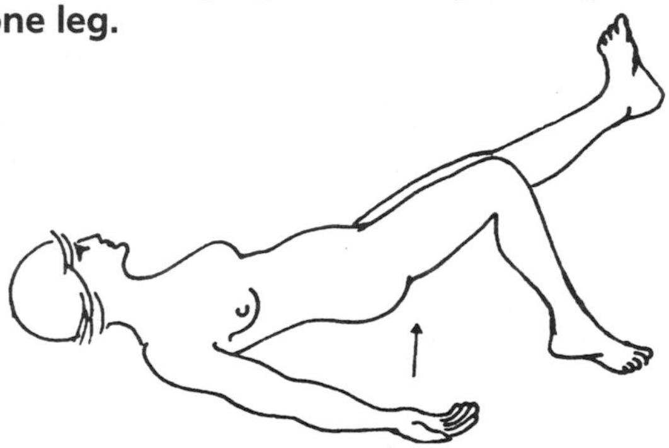

Figure 107. Progress the bridging exercise by raising your body with one leg.

Exercise 4. Lift Your Ribcage Off Your Uterus

Raise your ribcage off your uterus to relieve pressure that gives rise to heartburn and breathlessness. Overhead stretching smoothes out tightness in your shoulders and upper back.

Position: Sit like a tailor against a wall, with your hands above your shoulders, pressing against the wall.
Action: Stretch tall with your arms over your head—reaching higher with your right hand, then higher still with the your left hand. An added lift is gained if you bend to opposite side while stretching. Keep your pelvic tilt during these movements.

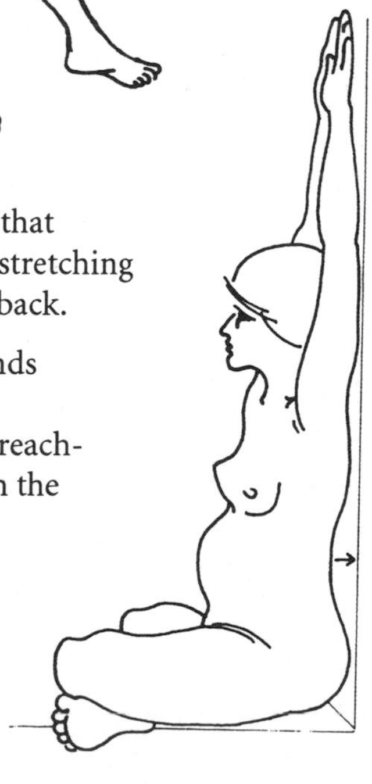

Figure 108. Stretch and press your arms and back against the wall.

Variation: Do this while standing and allow your hips to shift away in the opposite direction to which you bend. This will keep your ribcage expanded on both sides.

Foot Exercises

Note: Exercises that bend, stretch and rotate your ankles keep things moving if you are confined to bed for any reason. These movements are very important postpartum to prevent thrombosis if you've had general anesthesia for a Cesarean section or other complications—but they can be discontinued once you are walking around again.

Exercise 5. Foot-bending and Foot-stretching

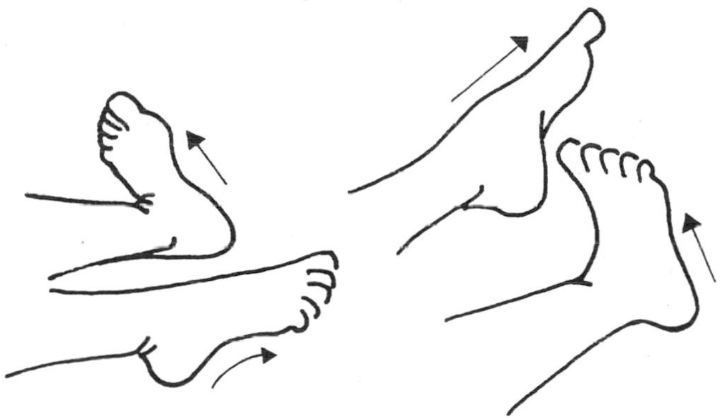

Foot exercises prevent discomfort and deformities from the increasing weight incurred during pregnancy. The feet often increase in size during pregnancy and may remain larger afterward.

Figure 109. Bend and stretch your feet, one at a time, and together.

Frequent bending, stretching, and rotating of your ankles assist the return of blood from the lower legs and minimizes swelling of your ankles and varicosities. Cramps, which often occur from lack of exercise, may be relieved by stretching your calves, pointing your **heels**. (Pointing your toes commonly results in cramp.) When moving your feet, use your thigh muscles to stabilize each knee; this localizes the movement to your feet and ankles.

Raise up the arch underneath the ball of your foot while keeping your toes **straight.** This can be tricky to learn. Stand with one foot unweighted and placed out in front—a necessary adjustment in late pregnancy for viewing your feet. It is the same action as holding a book between your thumb and fingers—your fingers remain straight. Curling the toes uses long muscles in your calves, which need stretching instead. You may experience cramps in your arch as you begin exercising these muscles.

Position: Sitting or lying. In either position, your legs can be relaxed over a pillow or your feet can be elevated. At other times, rest your foot on your oppo-

site knee. (This also makes it easier to see your feet in advanced pregnancy!) It's also a good way to put on socks or pantyhose. Sitting with your legs out straight provides an additional stretch of your hamstring muscles.
Action: Bend your ankle as far as you can, pulling your toes up toward you, stretching your calf muscles. Do this several times throughout the day whenever you are sitting. It can also be done when you stand on one leg, which is another way to improve your balance.

Exercise 6. Ankle Circles

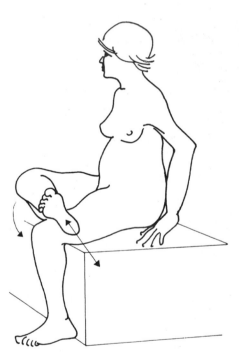

Position: Any time you're off your feet.

Action: Make large slow circles with each foot, first in a clockwise, then in a counterclockwise direction. You can do both feet together or move them in opposite directions, or rotate one at a time. Some people have difficulty coordinating their feet, so start off rotating one foot at a time if that's easier. If you have swollen feet and hands, for added challenge, circle your feet while you make figure-eights with your wrists!

Figure 110. Rotate your feet at every opportunity.

6

Breathing

Breathing is both a voluntary and an involuntary function. Unlike other inner metabolic activities, we can choose to become aware of our breathing at any time. This normal activity is fundamental to improving body performance whether through yoga, athletics, meditation, relaxation training, pelvic floor control or prenatal exercise classes. Breathing indicates our degree of physical exertion and the way we use our energy. Blocking the breath holds back energy, whereas breathing freely and fully lets it flow through the body. Research by the International Society for Research and Development in Haptonomy discovered that there are consistent respiratory patterns for different psychological states, such as aggression and inner- or outer-directed activity. Interesting graphs have been made documenting spontaneous changes in breathing of people doing exams, in arguments, and listening to music.

All our lives we have been effortlessly experiencing the expansion and relaxation of the chest, as the lungs inflate and deflate with our natural rhythm. Yet it is possible to emphasize breathing activity in different areas, although not completely isolate it because the chest functions as a coordinated whole in normal breathing.

Some people find it quite difficult to localize diaphragmatic movement. Instead, they breathe more using a sideways expansion of the rib cage or the top of their chest. It is important to take a **complete,** deep, refreshing breath. Deep breathing is important during pregnancy and labor, before and after operations, and for lung and chest problems.

The actual exchange of oxygen and carbon dioxide takes place in the farthest recesses of lung tissue. Shallow breathing does not permit this exchange of gases, and if done habitually, can lead to breathlessness on mild exertion. During shallow upper chest breathing, partial air intake is shuffled at the tops of the lungs.

Tense, anxious people breathe with their chests and shoulders, instead of with their diaphragms. Likewise, chest breathing leads to feelings of anxiety and tension, which interferes with our ability to relax and remain aware of our feelings. Rapid, shallow breathing, through over-oxygenation and increased muscular activity, further diminishes body awareness. Mostly, we are unaware of our lungs. However, we have all experienced how breathing changes with our emotions. When angry, excited or afraid, we become aware of a racing heartbeat and feel tight in the chest. Messages from the gut reach our mind, and we hold or accelerate our breathing.

Breathing is thus both a mirror of the emotions and a way of modifying them. It is intimately involved with relaxation, since neither of them can be achieved without the other. Easy breathing means a relaxed body and greater comfort. Holding one's breath leads to tension. Attending to one's breathing, then, is a way to stay calm.

Exhalation is the natural relaxation phase of the respiratory cycle. No one can exhale too much air. The subsequent breath is physiologically regulated to replace the amount of exhaled air. Emphasizing exhalation is a way to increase inhalation without getting dizzy, as often happens when inhalation is stressed.

Breathing During Pregnancy

Efficient breathing is essential in pregnancy because your body is coping with an increased load. Your blood volume expands to supply your growing baby with oxygen and nutrients, and to remove his or her carbon dioxide. While these natural adjustments provide adequate oxygen for you both, the decreased movement of your respiratory muscles, together with the increasing pressure within your abdomen, can cause discomfort and limit breathing.

In early pregnancy, intermittent breathlessness results from hormonal shifts; in late pregnancy, mechanical factors such as climbing stairs put you out of breath. Good breathing habits bring many benefits: circulation will be improved, breathlessness avoided, and your heart and lungs will function better.

Expectant mothers who suffer from chronic bronchitis, asthma or even a cold during the last trimester need to improve lung function with breathing exercises. Complete breathing can and must be combined with activities and exercise. **It is *never* necessary to hold your breath.** Exercises involving elevation of your shoulders and rib cage combine well with conscious breathing. They help relieve indigestion, heartburn, and improve your posture.

The general rule is: **exhale as you exert.** The abdominal muscles and pelvic floor can only contract when the diaphragm is ascending on outward breath.

Functions of the Diaphragm

The *diaphragm* is a broad sheet of muscle separating the chest region (with lungs and heart) from the abdominal and pelvic cavity (including the uterus). You feel this muscle when you have the hiccoughs. In addition to being the major muscle of respiration, it plays a key role in singing, crying, coughing, sneezing, vomiting and elimination. The diaphragm also assists the expulsive contractions of the uterus in the second stage of labor. In all these activities, the diaphragm is an agent of pressure control. Power is provided by your abdominal muscles, which can actively contract and shorten **only** if a balance of air is released by the ascent of your diaphragm. This is the most efficient way of increasing the pressure—by decreasing volume—in the abdominal–pelvic cavity.

As you push during birth, your abdominal wall is drawn in, with the slow upward movement of your diaphragm, as air is exhaled against the resistance of your lips or throat. It is commonly taught that the diaphragm must be forced down like a piston and "fixed." This puts undue pressure on the pelvic floor, but fortunately the diaphragm poorly maintains a prolonged contraction. Fatigue occurs in the actual muscle fibers, as well as the central nervous system according to a 1993 article in *Lancet.*[76] The author concluded that if expectant mothers practiced a few maximum expulsive efforts a day, the increased muscle strength of both the diaphragm and abdominal muscles would reduce the second stage of labor. Singing or playing a wind instrument offer pleasant opportunities for such training.

You can well imagine how advancing pregnancy limits the action of the diaphragm. Around the eighth month, the uterus reaches its highest position abdominally, with the uppermost surface *(fundus)* at the level of the breastbone. The increasing resistance from the abdominal contents restricts the downward diaphragmatic movement by several centimeters—until the baby descends into the pelvic cavity *(engagement),* usually by the end of the following month. This makes breathing much easier—although relief of these symptoms is traded for the onset of others, such as pressure on pelvic organs and blood congestion.

Learn diaphragmatic breathing for the following reasons:

- Efficient **expansion of your lungs** and complete exchange of gases.
- The pumping action of the diaphragm will **improve blood circulation** because the main vein from your lower limbs, abdomen and pelvis passes through it.
- Slow, deep rhythmical breathing helps general **relaxation** and requires specific relaxation of the abdominal and chest muscles.
- A complete fulfilling breath feels good and does good as a refueling breath at the start and end each labor contraction. It adds a psychological benefit: **signing on and off** that lets you relax between contractions.
- Postpartum, diaphragmatic breathing helps **to rid the body of waste products,** and the effects of **medication and anesthesia.**
- Combined with tightening of your abdominal wall, breathing with your diaphragm improves lung capacity and **tones your abdominal muscles.**
- If you are confined to bed for any reason before or after delivery, a few complete breaths every hour are essential to help **prevent complications.**

Diaphragmatic Breathing

During *inhalation,* your diaphragm moves downward, allowing your lungs to fill with air. As your abdominal contents are displaced outwards, your abdominal wall rises like a balloon. This differentiates a deep breath involving your diaphragm from a shallow gasp, where just your collarbones and upper ribs move. On *exhalation,* your diaphragm moves back up into the chest, emptying your lungs of air.[77] This is important for pelvic floor function, too.

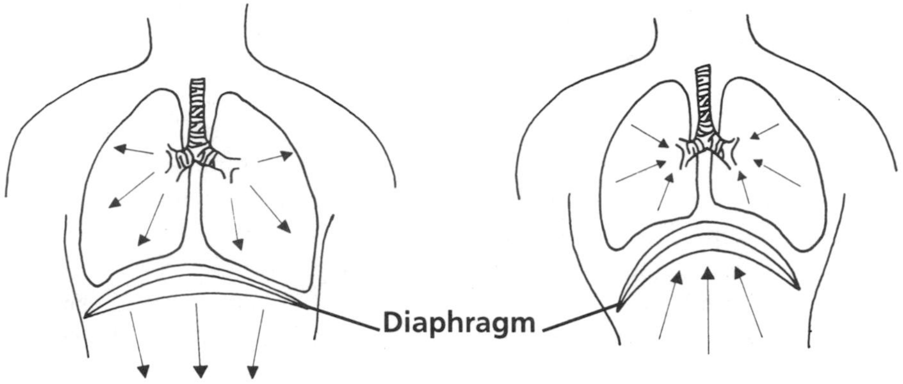

Figure 111. The lungs fill with air as the diaphragm descends.

Figure 112. As the diaphragm ascends, air is exhaled.

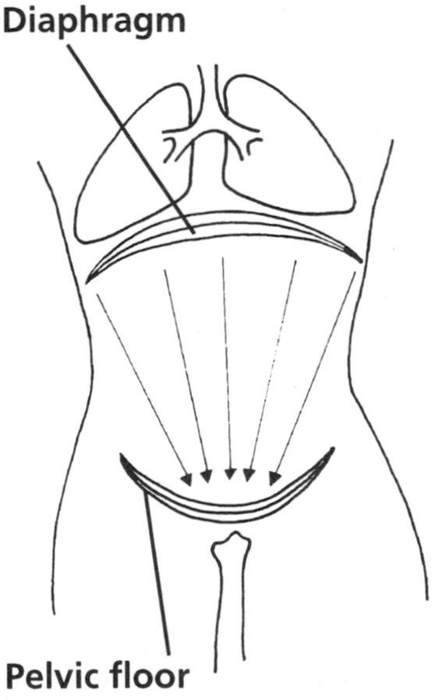

Figure 113. When pressure is increased from above, strain is felt below.

The misnomer *abdominal breathing* is common, but we cannot breathe with the abdomen! Respiration at rest is performed most significantly by the diaphragm, and movement in the abdominal area is secondary. In fact, if the muscles of the abdomen are not relaxed and passive, breathing is forced up into the chest. This phenomenon has consequences for the first stage of labor, where diaphragmatic breathing and relaxation of the abdominal wall complement each other and allow the uterus to tip forward during contractions.

Exercise 1. Diaphragmatic Breathing

Position: Any position. It is easier to learn while semi-recumbent, with your knees bent to relax your abdominal wall. Place your hands on your waist.
Action: Blow all the air out of your lungs, pulling your bellybutton toward your spine. Now, allow your relaxed abdominal wall to rise as it "fills up with air." Next, exhale, noticing how your abdominal wall "deflates" and flattens again.

Note: It is easy to reverse this action, so take care that you do it correctly: like a balloon, fill up as you breathe **in;** flatten back down as you breathe **out, emptying your lungs.** Practice often throughout the day to improve your breathing capacity.
Warning: Breathe with moderation. Too many deep breaths in succession can cause dizziness. Deep breathing must always be slow, according to your own natural rhythm.

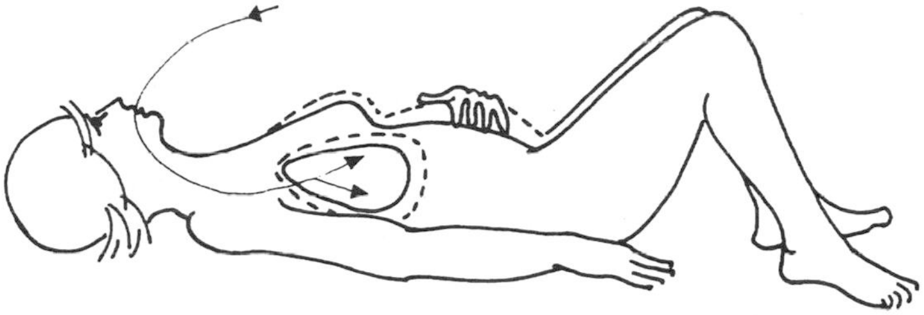

Figure 114. Diaphragmatic breathing can be felt with your hand on your waist.

Breathing for Labor—First Stage

Ideally, breathing is easy and comfortable. I encourage women to "flow with the contractions," and allow their breathing to adjust spontaneously to the changing intensity of the labor. This way you conserve energy and avoid a dry mouth. Nevertheless, patterns of controlled breathing are the foundation of most prepared childbirth programs. Taught with the best of intentions, paced respiration usually prevents relaxation, and increases effort and performance anxiety.

> *Formulae are for those who sidestep the challenge of new experience.* —*Alan Watts*

Dr. Fernand Lamaze stated several decades ago[78] that "respiratory exercises must be directed and controlled carefully and none should be done without medical direction." However, childbirth education evolved into a paramedical activity, and breathing techniques in labor are of no interest to obstetricians, especially in the age of epidurals. The woman's partner became the coach, who supposedly recognizes the phases of labor and supervises the different breathing patterns—such as *choo–choo, hoo–ha,* panting and blowing combinations, "spiral staircase" breathing, or "sheep's or butterfly breaths." (One can't help but ask what is wrong with normal human breathing!) All these breathing techniques emphasize use of the chest to limit the "downstroke" of the diaphragm, as Lamaze put it, claiming that pregnant women feel pain on deep inspiration. Yet proponents of shallow breathing who believe that the diaphragm irritates the uterus during the first stage of labor also believe that it acts as a piston to push out the baby in the second stage of labor! Mammals have a diaphragm precisely so that breathing, which occurs in the chest, can continue during activity of the abdominal and other muscles.

The term *coach* evokes images of organized sports, teams and captains. It reflects an underlying belief that the natural event of birth is a game to be played, with rules to be followed, behavior to be modified and appropriate rewards to be received. In the space of just a few weeks, the partner is supposed to become expert and confident in his or her ability to evaluate, prompt, or direct a laboring woman. Training is based on discipline, concentration, conditioning and dissociation. The use of such "tools" requires a good deal of effort, both mental and physical, to "stay on top" of the contractions with both acceleration and variation of breathing. As contractions become more intense, the mother is encouraged to do more elaborate breathing patterns for distraction, which naturally causes fatigue. Couples are greatly relieved when I explain why I consider all of this is completely unnecessary, as well as unphysiological. When the conscious mind attempts to regulate ventilation, disturbances result such as hypo- or hyper-ventilation.

Hypoventilation

Under-breathing may occur if respiration is artificially paced. When there is inadequate intake of carbon dioxide, the major regulator of respiration, there is less stimulus for oxygen intake. Breathing must be sufficiently deep to traverse the space between the nostrils and the air sacs of lung tissue where gaseous change occurs.

Hyperventilation

Over-breathing results in surplus oxygen being circulated in the body. This disturbance occurs when excessive oxygen is inhaled (during "cleansing" breaths or with the use of an oxygen mask). Hyperventilation also results if there is normal oxygen intake, but carbon dioxide levels are lowered (such as during forceful blowing in labor, or inflating an air mattress). Carbon dioxide, a waste product, dilates blood vessels to facilitate its own removal. During hyperventilation, the relative amount of carbon dioxide is decreased and, as a result, blood vessels become constricted. The surplus oxygen causes the blood to become more alkaline, impairing the release of oxygen from the hemoglobin in the red blood cells that transport it.

The paradoxical result of hyperventilation is that although the mother is taking in surplus oxygen, the combination of these two effects means less blood flow carrying less oxygen to the tissues. If circulation to the uterus and placenta is decreased, then the baby can suffer from a lack of oxygen. This situation is more likely if there is a fall in your cardiac output from other causes, such as supine hypotension or epidural anesthesia. Clinical symptoms associated with hyperventilation include slowing of the baby's heart rate and a build-up of waste products, causing fetal circulation to be more acid. Fetal distress leads to intervention in labor, often Cesarean delivery.

Typically, hyperventilation occurs with rapid, deep breathing that accelerates at the peak of a contraction's intensity. Accelerated breathing patterns sound like a train passing, as the breath follows the waxing and waning of the contraction. Of course, it is normal for respiration to adapt to any physical exertion, whether in labor or jogging. However, if women are taught to accelerate their breathing in prenatal classes, then they will do so even more during the actual labor. At rest, the frequency of normal breathing ranges from about five to twenty-two breaths per minute, the average being twelve to sixteen. Researchers at the Bristol Maternity Hospital in England found that many mothers trained in psychoprophylactic[79] breathing patterns took **over one hundred breaths per minute** during labor!

Side effects of diminished blood flow include: visual clouding, dizziness, tingling in the fingers or lips, even muscle spasms in the hands and feet. Carried to extremes, or combined with breath-holding, hyperventilation can lead to fainting. Usually the mother just decides to breathe normally, or someone hands her a paper bag so she can inhale her exhaled carbon dioxide.

Moaning, groaning or chanting may help women center themselves during contractions. Often women invent their own techniques. It is best to be directed from within rather than by those around you. Of course, your partner and other attendants of your choosing lend support and encouragement, as well as providing comfort measures. Practice the surrender stretch (page 187) for a realistic preparation for labor. While doing this stretch, experiment with different ways of breathing to determine for yourself what helps or hinders your ability to surrender.

The first stage of labor usually has three phases. *Early labor* is when the cervix is thinning out and dilation is getting started. This is followed by the *active phase,* when your uterus works hard and consistently, gaining momentum, until the last final burst of effort *(transition).* When dilation is completed (ten centimeters or five fingers), the first stage is over.

The sequence of events is always the same, but the nature and timing of their progression, as well as women's experience of each phase, vary greatly. Some labors start slowly, allowing the mother to adjust gradually to the nature of events. Others are heralded by immediate strong activity which tends to rush the mother along through the whole process. Given the wide differences that are possible, guiding principles are more valuable than a rigid set of rules.

As you near the end of the first stage, you may feel the (perhaps premature) urge to push, which begins as an involuntary grunt or gasp in the throat. Often this is due to rectal pressure stimulating the proprioceptors, especially if you are lying on your back. Brisk panting is helpful in overcoming the desire to push before full dilation is achieved. Blow briefly with your cheeks, to avoid using your abdominal muscles. However, if Baby's head is pressing on your pelvic floor, the urge will be irresistible and then it really is the right time to bear down.

Breathing is a tool that you always carry around with you. It's not something you can leave at home by mistake! The slow, deep breathing already discussed will stand you in good stead for any situations of stress, including labor.

You do not control your labor. It is a normal physiological process during which you need to be emotionally aligned with your baby. In order to flow with the process, let go of resistance in your mind as well as your body. This obviously requires considerable self-confidence as well as total trust in the birth process. The best preparation is prenatal exercise in general, and partner stretches (see Chapter 8) in particular.

Remember, every birth is different, even for the same woman. You cannot know in advance how you will react to the demands of your labor. Normal breathing is clearly the most physiological. The respiratory system is very sensitive to the oxygen requirements of the body. Adjustments happen automatically.

Breathing for Labor—Second Stage

Coordination of pushing with exhaling is essential to avoid exhausting straining with prolonged breath-holding.

The Hazards of Breath-Holding

To hold your breath is to hold yourself back. People with good body mechanics or intuitive physical awareness keep breathing during exercise or physical exertion. A baby manages all kinds of feats without interrupting his or her breathing, or bracing unnecessary muscles. Children, as they grow up, commonly develop the habit of tensing the diaphragm to control their emotions and "gut" feelings, by holding their breath and tightening their abdominal walls. Children also learn breath-holding and the use of accessory muscles when premature toilet training is enforced. Breath-holding thus becomes associated with tension, discomfort and an inability to let go. While elimination should involve only the physical act of letting wastes pass from the body, habits of strain and effort easily become deeply entrenched. Children on toilets strain to please their parents. Women in labor strain to please their attendants. Whatever the result, the obvious effort reassures parents and birth attendants and encourages their exhortations.

Most of us have grown up forcing ourselves to compensate for movements that no longer happen naturally. We are so accustomed to control that the idea of spontaneity is often frightening. It is no surprise, then, that expectant couples latch on to the ideas of control and effort to avoid coming to terms with their intense emotions, fears, and the unpredictable nature of birth.

When respiration is interrupted, there is no oxygenation. Straining with the breath held is known as the *Valsalva maneuver*[80] and can cause marked cardiovascular effects. Old people have died straining on bedpans, and there have been rare reports of strokes and even death in laboring women who were made to strain excessively during birth.

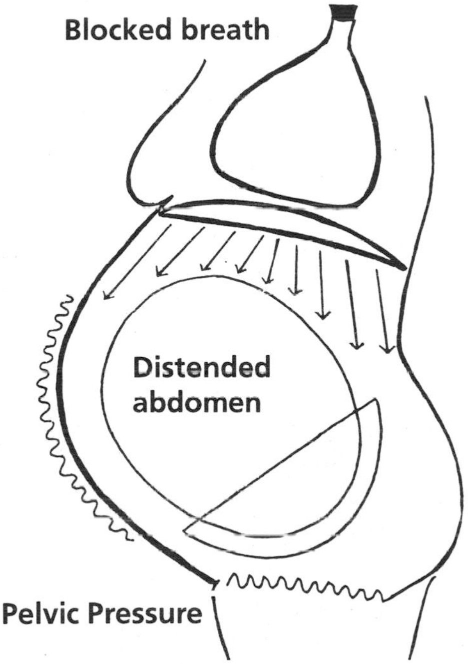

Figure 115. Forced pushing creates a closed pressure system, like a balloon.

"Purple Pushing"

Visible signs of straining include a red face, taut neck muscles, bloodshot eyes and burst capillaries in the cheeks. Exertion with a closed glottis affects your circulation. Blood pools in the veins of the legs and pelvis because its return to your heart is impaired by the increased pressure in your chest. (This pooling is made worse by epidural anesthesia and the back-lying position.) As a result, both your blood pressure and the output from your heart fall. Abnormal changes in brain waves and heart rates have been recorded on research subjects, usually young, healthy men performing hand grip tests for just a few seconds.

Like a balloon, a closed pressure system is formed when straining distends your abdominal wall outward. This strain puts great stress on your abdominal muscles and the vulnerable midline uniting them. Reflex tightening of your pelvic floor is inevitable: pressure goes in equal and opposite directions (Pascal's law). This unnecessary forcing also strains attachments of your pelvic organs, and interferes with your venous return which often causes hemorrhoids.

Blocking the breath during any exertion produces a closed pressure system. Very high pressures created in the chest reduce the blood flow back to the heart. Less blood and less oxygen reach your lungs, the rest of your body and the placenta. After only about five seconds your baby's heart rate may slow down. More serious, however, is the long recovery required for your baby's heart after prolonged breath-holding. Your blood pressure, which is very high at the onset of strain, will fall as a result and there is an increased chance of Cesarean delivery because of fetal distress. A few moments of strain, though giving no advantage to a laboring woman, is usually not harmful.

Prolonged breath-holding also causes you to gasp air suddenly when you reach your breakpoint. At this time, various protective mechanisms are aroused and you gasp with relief. Until your cardiovascular system returns to normal, there is an overshoot phenomenon, which causes imbalance of pressure throughout the various body fluids. After the suddenly release of air, the resulting retraction of your abdominal muscles creates a suction pull, which tends to negate your effort. Unless you are in an upright position, your baby's head (which slips back and forth a little as it works its way through the flexible vaginal passage) will regress even further. Jerking head movements often go along with this pattern of pushing.

Dr. Roberto Caldeyro–Barcia investigated[81] the effects of pushing in the late Seventies. He found that bearing-down efforts are always longer and more forceful when the mother is made to push than if she responds spontaneously to the contractions. Forced pushing is also associated with the need for an episiotomy. If there is insufficient time and relaxation, then the perineum is not able to distend adequately. The central seam of the abdominal wall, where the recti muscles unite (and sometimes spread) is also strained. Pelvic floor dysfunction may follow a forceful second stage labor, with prolapse of the bladder, bowel or uterus. The mechanism by which this occurs was pointed out in 1957 by a British obstetrician, Dr. Constance Beynon.[82] She used the analogy of the lining in a coat sleeve being dragged down, to describe how pelvic structural supports are weakened when forced downward from pressure above. A considerable amount of blood pools in the pelvis during the Valsalva maneuver, because blood flows with difficulty up to the heart against the high pressure in the chest. Veins in pregnancy are dilated more easily due to hormonal softening, thus the Valsalva maneuver may cause varicosities such as hemorrhoids. While brief straining tends to raise blood pressure, when straining is prolonged (and women in labor are usually told to hold their breath for at least twenty seconds), low blood pressure results.

I've noticed that women in labor rarely hold their breath for as long as they are taught or told to do, which is fortunate. Conducted in such a manner, the second stage of labor has been limited to one and a half to two hours, with good reason. Could mother and baby stand much of this stress and strain?

As in all stages of labor, normal breathing is the goal although respiration fluctuates in response to contractions. This enables experienced birth attendants to recognize progress in normal labor without needing to do vaginal exams. Grunts and groans are primal sounds echoed by women in all cultures. Feel free to make these sounds. If your attendants object, remind them that they are not laboring. I recall one woman who said, "I'm paying the bill, it's my birth, and I'll make as much noise as I like!" Remember, the alternative is breath-holding. This increases tension and retards the process.

Figure 116. Sound is energy and energy flows.

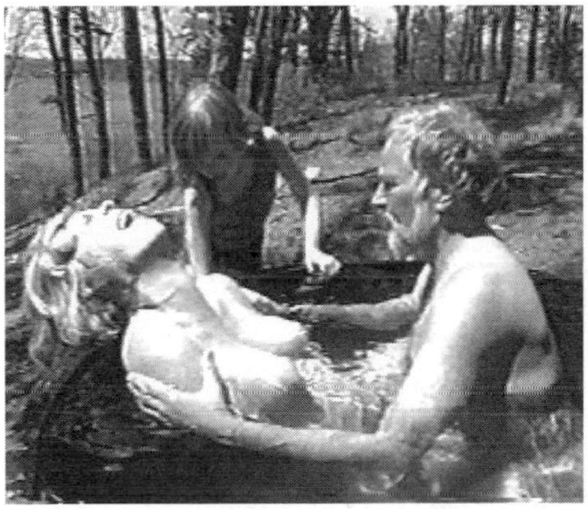

The coordination of breathing with your abdominal muscles to bring your baby down to your pelvic floor was described in Chapter 4, page 81-84. Toward the end of second stage of labor you may be asked to refrain from pushing so that your baby can be born gently through your intact perineum. The strength of contractions at this time, however, is more intense than at the beginning. Gasping or moaning is a natural response to allow your uterus to ease your baby out of your vagina. Birth was a sensual experience long before it became a medical event; some women who are particularly in tune with their sexuality experience orgasm at this point.

Feel for Yourself: Examples to Experience

A way to understand these principles is to hold your breath while you increase the pressure inside your abdomen. Notice that your bellybutton moves **away** from your backbone, bulging your abdomen like a balloon. Feel how your pelvic floor is part of this closed pressure system, reflexively tightening to contain the tension. This is purple pushing, the *Valsalva maneuver.*

Now make a fist and blow into it so that your breath slowly escapes against resistance. Feel how your bellybutton moves **toward** your backbone. Note the absence of pressure on your pelvic floor because air is leaving your body. This is *physiological pushing.* Your abdominal muscles shorten and move inward as air is forcefully exhaled. Exhaling during birth makes sense for the same reasons as during elimination, exercise or any form of exertion. Oxygen levels and blood pressure remain steady. There is no strain on your pelvic floor or abdominal wall. Letting your air out encourages the physiological flow of energy in your body. The pressure within the abdomen is increased by decreasing volume, like squeezing toothpaste out of a tube. The rib cage, diaphragm and abdominal muscles all interact as a unit.

The uterus contracts radially, like making a fist.[83] The walls move inward from all directions. When you exhale slowly and forcibly, with some resistance in your glottis, your abdominals shorten and contract, moving inward in the **same direction**, unlike breath-holding, during which the abdominals move **away** from the uterus.

Figure 117. Pushing as you exhale maintains normal physiology.

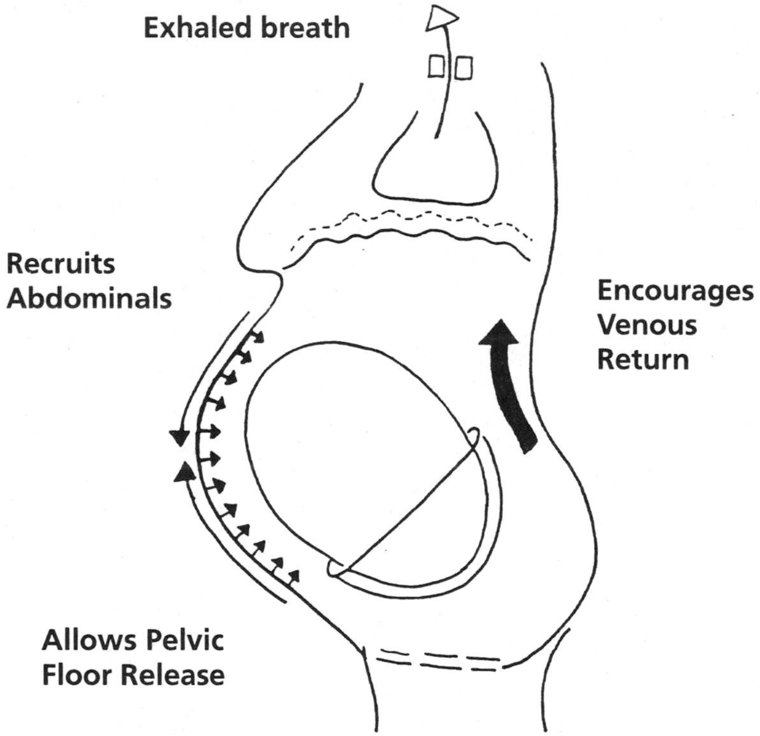

Spontaneous Participation

In contrast to the unnatural and grim picture I have just painted, with spontaneous pushing your breath is audibly exhaled, just like you hear when the tennis players serve at Wimbledon! Traditionally, hospital staff have discouraged vocalization during labor. But sound is normal expression of emotion and effort. Exhalation during exertion in sport is accepted—why is effort during birth considered different?

Your breath escapes slowly and noisily because your glottis is partly open. Braking the breath in this way allows your rib cage to stay firm, and your diaphragm to ascend slowly **as the abdominal muscles are drawn in around your uterus.** Indeed, if you make no sound, then you are holding your breath.

If you practise this your throat will become sore—that's why I recommend that you blow into a fist instead. However, in labor, the increased circulation to your vocal cords permit the most amazing gutteral sounds without any subsequent discomfort.

You may feel the urge to give one or several pushes during a contraction. It is a little like swimming breaststroke or treading water: there is a time for the abdominals to retract and a time for air to be exchanged. Consciously allowing your body to respond like this, instead of relentless pushing, allows time for your vagina to fully distend around your baby's head, and prevents undue fatigue. Spontaneous pushes also are of much shorter duration.

Breathing Postpartum

After birth you need to help remove the waste products that accumulated during the hard work of labor, plus any medication or anesthesia. Diaphragmatic breathing hastens this process, through its pumping effect on the blood returning from the legs and pelvis.

Breathing to expand the three key regions of the chest is described on pages 197-198; the same routine is used after a Cesarean section.

The usual type of coughing is replaced by **huffing**—a sudden retraction of the abdominal muscles on **outward** breath. Exhaling is mechanically more effective and less tiring. Remember to pull up your pelvic floor muscles as you pull in your abdominals to avoid the sometimes alarming sensations of strain and pressure that are often felt during a regular cough. **Everyone** should huff, not cough, to clear the lungs of any secretions. Remember this advice for the rest of your life.

7

Relaxation

Any exercise program, like one's daily life, should include periods of rest and relaxation. Even your heart, which beats rhythmically for the whole of your life, rests more than it works. Rest and recuperation occur when your heart beats at half its maximum rate, and this is important for fitness. During strenuous exercise muscle tissue breaks down, resting muscles replace glycogen, and growth takes place.

Fatigue not only interferes with the ability of muscles to contract, but also to relax and even to grow. Cramps may appear if certain muscles are worked overtime and waste products accumulate. Just as significant, however, is the tension that results from stress and anxiety, especially in the absence of physical activity.

The Importance of Relaxation

Tension within the body can become habitual without our being aware of it. It can be localized to certain areas, such as the neck or lower back, or the effects can become more pervasive and cumulative, causing changes in posture, habits of elimination, eating, reading or even personality. Effective relaxation, which reverses these detrimental effects, is clearly essential for good health.

The tension that all relaxation techniques aim to alleviate concerns the state of readiness of the muscles for a sudden action or emotion **when such a state does not exist.** Tension serves a useful purpose only if the body needs to mount a "fight, freeze or flight" response. If tension persists when the need is no longer there, it may become habitual and interfere with rest and sleep. We have all seen the tense types: face set, shoulders hunched, arms folded, knees crossed. Irregular breathing, a tapping foot and drumming fingers are other nervous responses. People displaying this kind of body language often make those around them tense, too!

Relaxation is more than doing nothing, napping, or sitting back and being entertained. Genuine relaxation requires that we gain insight into our muscular system, with which we make all purposeful actions in life and express our emotions. We can learn to recognize and release excess tension, which is still present even when muscles are not in use. Biofeedback has proven that we can become aware of muscular tension and learn to decrease it. Even monkeys have been successfully trained to control their muscle tension precisely.

Levels of resting tension vary tremendously between individuals. Unnecessary "bracing" of voluntary muscles causes a simultaneous alerting of the nervous system and vice versa. This vicious circle of stress is one of the dangerous threats of Western life. Bookstores are full of advice on how to cope with it. Over half of the deaths in the United States are from strokes—high blood pressure—and heart disease is the number one killer of women after menopause. Diet and lack of exercise are influences too, of course.

Techniques of Relaxation

There are countless ways to achieve a state of repose—listening to music, having a massage, rocking in a hammock. Water, especially the ocean, can be a powerful agent for relaxation. Yoga and meditation have been practiced in various parts of the world for centuries. Using these techniques, you gain the skill and benefits of relaxation through self-direction. No pill, prescription or other external agent is required. Such relaxation is free, always available, and is far more effective than any mood-altering substance for regeneration.

Biofeedback produces rapid and scientifically verifiable results. Sensitive monitoring equipment makes degrees of tension audible and visible, so that you learn to reduce muscle tension consciously. Because you are accurately and continuously informed of your progress, it takes a very short time—sometimes just one session—to gain impressive control of muscle activity. Unlike meditation, the activity is direct, specific and purposeful. However, biofeedback and meditation both achieve on-going measurable results. Equipment that records muscle activity or skin temperature as an index of relaxation is becoming cheaper and more available. (See Resources.) Pulse readings can also be taken for biofeedback.

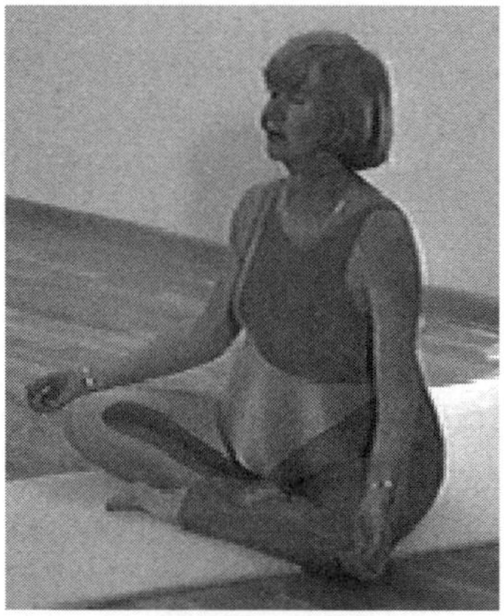

Figure 118. Meditation is a time for inner bonding with your baby.

Meditation and its modification, the *relaxation response*, require no equipment; any quiet place will do. It may take several weeks for you to let go of the "chattering monkey" in your mind and surrender into this process. Release occurs indirectly since you remain passive in a state of "restful alertness," which is quite different from sleep. The many benefits reach beyond relieving muscle tension to improving internal bodily functions.

Passive relaxation occurs when you temporarily withdraw into your private world. Release can pervade your entire body because your mind is neither reflecting nor analyzing. Instead of forcing your mind to remain blank, you enter a state of low arousal. This process may be enhanced by repeating a simple word or a meaningless sound (such as a mantra), listening to music, visualizing a peaceful rural scene or focusing on your breathing rhythm. Thoughts pass in and out of your mind, but your mental attitude remains detached from any idea or emotion. Another technique is simply to concentrate on all the experiences in the present, such as sounds, smells, pressure on parts of your body, the breeze against your face, your breathing and so on.

Initially, it may be difficult for a goal-oriented person accustomed to "purposeful" activity to feel comfortable being alone with her or his self, doing "nothing." The process is similar to attaining orgasm; you must stay in present time. In both states you release both the mind and the body; if you continue as a spectator, evaluating how you are getting along, participation is blocked. In other words, trying to relax makes you tense! The very phrase "try to relax" is an oxymoron, a contradiction in terms. As self-consciousness diminishes, self-confidence increases so that it becomes easier to let go.

Sessions last ideally about twenty minutes but five-minute sessions in a traffic jam or a break from the computer screen work well, too. A quick release of body tensions with your head dropped forward is an instant refresher. At first the muscles and ligaments at the back of your neck may protest if they are tight from maintaining the head constantly in an erect position. They will lengthen with practice, and discomfort in this area, commonly felt by commuters and desk workers, will be relieved.

Visualization is a powerful and self-regulatory tool. Cassette tapes are available with all kinds of guided imagery with appropriate sounds. Individuals are primarily visual, auditory or kinesthetic; a good tape combines all three elements. Some people choose to spend time by a waterfall in the mountains, others may prefer the warm sun and a light breeze at the ocean, and yet others may enjoy listening to birds chirping in a meadow. Individual visualization sessions can encompass the personal situation—the client's back pain, pre-term labor contractions, or experiences of birth and before.[84] All kinds of therapeutic breakthroughs have been documented by such researchers as Carl and Stephanie Simonton[85] and Dr. Bernie Siegel.[86]

Active relaxation differs from passive because you now interact with your environment but without undue tension or muscle expenditure. You need to cultivate the ability to be mentally attentive while at the same time relaxing the parts of the body that are extraneous to the task at hand. All of us have experienced occasions when our nervous system seems more excitable than usual, and a telephone or honking horn causes us to jump abruptly. Clues are provided by posture, work habits and parts of the body that feel tired and stiff.

Movements, such as stretching or shaking (never tensing), help you to recognize the contrasting states of tension and relaxation. Reversing habitual patterns of muscle contraction results in lengthening and relaxation of tight muscle groups. These physical approaches, however, are limited to the nervous system that communicates with *voluntary* muscles. The deeper tensions of the *involuntary* muscles, and those of the gut (the *psychotonus)* are a greater challenge. It is my experience that **anxiety is the number one human problem.** It underlies a host of symptoms, dysfunctions and diseases as well as social ills and political crises. Addressing the particulars of a person's anxiety[87] is the central issue, especially as people only learn relaxation when they feel safe.

Reciprocal relaxation is based on a physiological law, namely that muscle work involves two actions.[88] A muscle contracts and shortens or it relaxes and lengthens. In this way muscles also work together—but in an opposite and reciprocal relationship. For example, when we bend an elbow the biceps muscle contracts and the triceps muscle behind lengthens to allow the movement. Sometimes this interaction may be disturbed, as when your foot goes into cramp. The muscle remains in a state of prolonged and fatiguing contraction, which becomes painful. Furthermore, you may be temporarily unable to work the opposite group of muscles, which bend your foot upward, without applying some extra force to stretch out passively the cramped muscle. Normally, however, you can freely move your foot up, shortening those muscles while the neighbors relax.

Relaxation at its most basic is the physiological state that follows muscle contraction. Even the simple act of breathing in and out is a natural way to experience mild tension and relaxation. Muscles contract as air is taken in and their release allows the air to be exhaled. As you become skilled at observing your breathing, you will notice another state—the pause between the inhalation and the exhalation.

British physical therapist Laura Mitchell, in her excellent book, *Simple Relaxation,*[89] selected a few photographs that show the characteristic body language of tension. Anxiety, whatever the cause, results in a typical pattern of muscle contraction and shortening. The difficulty with relaxation, as she rightly points out, is that information about muscle tension is not conveyed to the conscious brain. A simple experiment verifies this experience. Even with our eyes closed, we know exactly the angle of our bent elbow, but we cannot know the state of the muscles above and below the joint. Proprioceptors give us information about joint position, but the mind knows movements, not individual muscles.

Mitchell's approach is based on the physiological principle of reciprocal contraction of one group causing relaxation of the opposing muscle group. She refined a series of specific orders to reverse classic muscle tension patterns. For example, pull your shoulders down from your ears and the tight muscles that hunch your shoulders will lengthen, releasing their tension. This clear and concise method of relaxation can be learned by anyone. Sessions may involve any or all of the significant movements. For example, stretch your fingers "long" to achieve relaxation of the tense flexor muscles. Dragging down the jaw is also an important action.

In **yoga**, relaxation is achieved through a combination of physical and mental techniques. The mental discipline in yoga also involves meditation, a key to which is listening to the breath. However, concentrating on *asanas* or other activities that quiet the conscious mind in itself produces a meditative state that leads to calm and well-being.

The *asanas* are positions that involve the body in a series of stretches. Most of these extend areas of the body which in sedentary people usually are tight. (Certain positions are not advisable during the childbearing year; see pages 40-43.) The challenge and rewards of yoga lie in the confrontation and surrender of your physical and mental limitations. Forcing, however, only increases the resistance; yielding is the key. If a difficult posture is painful, "become" the pain, focus deeply and **exhale** "into" it. You will find that as you reflect on the sensations (What color is it? Is it hot or cold, sharp or dull?) that acceptance of the pain actually eases it. (This contrasts with the Lamaze approach of dissociating and blocking out discomfort.) Yoga thus provides excellent training for childbirth, as you learn to associate ever more deeply and amaze yourself with your ability to extend your limits further and further.

Tensing Leads to More Tension!

A common technique actually uses muscle contraction to make tension more obvious—making a fist or raising your shoulders. In theory, this is supposed to provide a sense of relaxation through a contrasting experience. However, the problem is that you are undoubtedly making tense muscles more tense. It has never been shown that this approach lowers your initial tension level; in contrast, biofeedback readily demonstrates that returning to a former resting level is often difficult after contraction of the same muscle. Sometimes it is helpful for your partner to see and feel a tense muscle. It makes much more sense, however, to contract the opposite muscle group so that the tight muscles are obliged to relax and lengthen according to natural laws of reciprocal relaxation described above. Test this with a simple "organic experience." Make a fist with your left hand, and "relax" (which is meaningless to the brain). Now, stretch your right hand, open wide, fingers long. Then stop (that's how the nervous system works). I have never met anyone who felt the tensed hand to be more relaxed than the stretched one. This is why yoga and stretching classes, with more extension than flexion activities, leave you feeling relaxed. Yet the old way of progressively tensing muscle groups is still described in just about every book on health and exercise! If you find yourself in one of these tension sessions, simply reverse the instructions and **s t r e t c h** each muscle group.

Benefits of Relaxation

As we become more aware of our mind–body connection, we can modify our psychosomatic processes. Gaining relaxation skills pays off with greater poise and emotional serenity as well as such physiological benefits as reduced blood pressure (since better circulation is allowed when the muscles are free from undue tension). With bodily tensions reduced, there are fewer cramped muscles, headaches, backaches and insomnia. A 1995 report from the University of Pittsburgh found that pregnant women could often relieve their headaches through learning how to relax.

Learning to unwind is of value for the rest of our lives, whatever our age, sex or occupation. Life today is ever more stressful. Anxiety about the unknown is raging on a global scale, and I believe that women desire epidurals for birth, not primarily for pain, but for a measure of control, predictability and shoring-up assistance.

Preparation for Relaxation

Relaxation is best practiced after an exercise session, when your muscles are slightly fatigued. It is important to slow down gradually—from activity to rest to relaxation. Without this gradual slowing down, waste products accumulate in the body, and muscles ache or feel stiff later.

Lie or sit in a completely supported position of total comfort. (See Chapter 5 for various options.) Gravity has the least stimulating effect on the body when you are lying down, on your back, front, side or three-quarters over. Check that all your joints are slightly bent. This prevents the stretch reflex that readies the muscles for action. All parts of your body must be supported, otherwise gravity will stimulate any dangling extremity to do muscle work. For example, check that your hands and feet are resting on pillows, rather than hanging over the edge. In sitting or half-lying positions there is less resistance under the diaphragm from the abdominal contents, so you may prefer these positions in later pregnancy and particularly if lying on your back makes you light-headed. We spend so much of our time sitting; if we can relax only when lying down, then our opportunities are truly limited.

You need to be adequately warm, your clothing loose and shoes off, and in an atmosphere that is conducive to relaxation. The supporting surface should be firm. If it sags, then support will be lost and strain may occur. Use as many cushions and pillows as you need to accommodate your body completely and relieve all pressure points. Large bean bag chairs and hammocks are comfortable for a short period, but you may need assistance to get out of them. Resilient foam or rubber pillows interfere with relaxation; they often cause or aggravate neck tension. A feather pillow does not require continual adjustment of the joints, as does a springy surface. Instead, you just let your head sink right down into the down or feathers.

People vary greatly in their ability to relax. Rare are those individuals who are regularly in a state of repose; others always have a self-defeating battle with the process. The large majority of individuals lie between the two ends of this spectrum and can improve their relaxation skills with regular practice.

Conventional Childbirth Preparation

The foundation of childbirth education has traditionally been the instructor's concern for psychological control. The expectant mother's mind is the chief weapon in the struggle. Indeed, the term for the best-known type of preparation is *psychoprophylaxis,* which means "mind prevention." Rehearsed response to commands, concentration, focal points for the eyes, and complex breathing patterns occupy what Dr. Lamaze called the "cerebral machinery." In this way a laboring woman will attempt to dissociate her mind from her body to gain control over painful contractions. Lamaze's disciple, Dr. Pierre Vellay, author of *Childbirth Without Pain,*[90] wrote, "Like expert engineers with perfect machines and carefully presented information [women] control, direct and regulate their bodies." To these male physicians, giving birth is not like learning to walk, which is preprogrammed and happens without instruction when the individual is physiologically ready. Dr. Lamaze wrote, "A woman must learn how to give birth in the same way that she learns how to swim or write or read." Dr. Vellay advised that a mother "must insist on being trained in the proper way." Because these prominent obstetricians held typically mechanistic views, pregnant women are commonly seen as machines that can be regulated. Dr. Lamaze actually stated that "as the obstetrician is the only one conversant with the nature of the uterus, he (sic) alone can decide how such a labor is progressing."

Lamaze believed that "speech is the best means we have to prepare women for childbirth" and Vellay echoed this with "words by their direct meaning enable the human being to have precise and complex stereotypes, far superior to those formed by the animal through direct signals." The key words are *without pain.* Experts promised pain relief through words *(verbal analgesia)* following psychoprophylactic instruction for dissociation and distraction.

Conditioned Response

Psychoprophylaxis is based on classical conditioning (Pavlovian reflexes) and conditioning in the behavioral school of psychology popularized by B. F. Skinner. Training is accomplished with an expectant couple's repetition of the proper words and techniques. These skills supposedly become so automatic to the pregnant woman that in labor the real contraction can be easily displaced, like Pavlov's dog who learned to salivate at the sound of a bell. The promise of an easy, painless or brief labor is a strong incentive for a woman to practice breathing patterns and other control mechanisms taught in class. Her behavior is thus conditioned to operate for an anticipated reward. Negative reinforcement also operates. If a woman does not follow the method, her labor will surely be painful and the attending medical staff will disapprove of her lack of commitment to her birth method. As Dr. Lamaze[91] wrote, "[A mother's] mind carefully educated, steadfast and alert, will know how to abolish pain. In the same way, it can magnify pain if misfortune and negligence decree that she should fail in her task."

The mother concentrates on breathing patterns and a visual focal point to distract her from her bodily sensations. But the law of reversed effort dictates that no one manages to concentrate intently by sheer willpower. When one is interested, concentration occurs naturally.

With regard to a focal point, it is more relaxing to let the eye make natural random movements, such as scanning and blinking, than to stare fixedly at one point. In his classic *The Art of Seeing*,[92] Aldous Huxley describes how forcing the eyes to fix on a point interferes with body relaxation and respiration. Eyestrain leads to shallow, suspended breathing and it is tiring to repress natural bodily movement, however small. While eye contact between a laboring woman and her attendant or partner is helpful for communication, if it is maintained for prolonged periods, it can become forced and mechanical.

> *Sexuality and anxiety are functions of living organisms operating in opposite directions: pleasurable expansion and anxious contraction.* —*Wilhelm Reich*

Methods of childbirth preparation based on the work of male obstetricians Grantly Dick–Read[93] and Robert Bradley[94] allow the laboring woman more association her body and feelings than other methods, but they are much smaller and less influential than the Lamaze organizations. I personally find it hubristic for any individual or organization to declare a method of childbirth and I have successfully resisted attempts by colleagues to create the *Noble Method!* Birth is *birth.* As Dr. Moyses Paciornik said, "It is magical, but not mysterious."[95]

Relaxation During Pregnancy

Your body's changing condition affects you psychologically. Discomfort, bizarre dreams, ambivalence about being pregnant, fear about the well-being of the baby, concern for your relationship with your partner, or feelings of inadequacy regarding your ability to be a parent—these are all commonly experienced. Superstitions and performance anxiety about labor are also frequent. Some women think (mistakenly) that no one else would have such thoughts and feelings, and thus they repress them instead of expressing them to others. The baby's father is probably experiencing his own worries. In fact, since fatherhood has no outward visible signs, in our culture a father tends to be overlooked until the arrival of the child. Regular relaxation helps to reduce the emotional stress that accumulates with focusing too much on *D-Day.*

Read widely and attend various classes on the subject of childbearing. Knowledge is the first step in gaining gain self-assurance and faith in one's body during this natural process. You will also be more committed to taking care of yourself postpartum when meeting the demands of a new life.

The mind must be at ease for the body to relax—if one can use dualistic language that belies the unity of mind and body. Although the mind is the dominant center of control, relaxation in the voluntary muscles influences relaxation in the involuntary muscles and elsewhere in the body, too.

During pregnancy you can relax passively, like a rag doll. You recognize the state of blissful rest with a calm mind and body, usually in a recumbent position of complete comfort. When you lie still, your baby usually becomes more active because the rocking motion, which soothes your baby when you move around, has ceased. Also your baby finds it easier to turn when your uterus relaxes. Uterine tension is not under your conscious control. It happens indirectly when you are in an altered state of consciousness. Many women admire their taut abdomen and firm uterus, and some feel very hard. But I identify with the baby inside—would he or she rather grow in a soft stretchy surround or a rigid one? Babies in a difficult position, facing forward instead of backward, or with their buttocks instead of the head in their mother's pelvis, may be unable to change unless the mother is guided to allow her uterus to relax.

You may feel the customary, painless, intermittent tightening of your uterus (*Braxton–Hicks contractions*) when you lie still. A change of position usually causes these transient contractions to pass, although they provide a useful opportunity for practice. (When labor is established, contractions increase in duration, intensity and frequency, and they will not substantially diminish whenever you lie down.) Practicing relaxation in pregnancy helps your comfort level during those months. Furthermore, it prepares you for labor and birth, a time of stressful, physical, involuntary events when your intellect must allow the body to follow its own wisdom. Although the muscles of your uterus, like those in your heart, will perform without your conscious control, you can ensure relaxation in the muscles that you can effect.

Human feedback may be provided by a partner who also becomes more personally involved as a result. This person assists by evaluating the state of tension in various muscles when checking limpness of your limbs and your response to touching, stroking, massage and such. Practice this on each other so that you become trusting and adept in the gentle handling and can let your partner know what pleases you.

Readers who have been accustomed to regular yoga, meditation or other forms of relaxation will, of course, continue to experience benefits during the maternity year. Yoga and meditation help develop trust in your body so you can release both mental and physical resistance. In my personal and professional experience, releasing resistance is of key importance during the birth process. As a result, I have developed a surrender–stretch exercise to be done with a partner, to prepare you for labor contractions. (See Chapter 8.)

Relaxation with a Partner

All your joints must be slightly flexed and supported in one of the positions described in Chapter 5. Your partner starts with observing your outward signs. Your face should be expressionless and your breathing quiet and effortless. Next, your partner should gently check the weight of the limbs. Neuromuscular principles determine that release spreads out from the center. Therefore, when checking levels of relaxation, work in reverse order from the periphery. Below are some guidelines for your partner to follow.

Begin by gently raising her hand a little. If relaxed it will feel loose and heavy; this means it **is** relaxed. If it is stiff and light, it is not relaxed. (Often a person helps with the movement; it takes trust to become a dead weight in another's hands.) Next, go to the joint above. Ease her elbow up and down; if you feel resistance, take her whole arm next. Support it above and below the elbow and "work it loose" with a gentle slow circling motion from the shoulder joint. Let it drop back, softly checking that the muscles have released and the limb is heavy. Raising a leg may be too disturbing whereas just rolling the thighs in and out will loosen the hip and knee. Rotating the ankles or stroking the calf may also help. Handling the feet can be ticklish (unless done firmly); downward bending of the toes can cause cramp.[96]

Next, place your hands firmly on a part of your partner's body for deeper relaxation of the underlying muscles. (Both hands must be placed; otherwise you may wonder with some anxiety where and when the other hand will arrive!) This quiescent, nonverbal contact gives you the opportunity to allow more release.[97] Some people are also aided by the repetition of suggestive words, such as *limp, droopy, loose, calm, give, ease, slow, heavy, slack, warm, floating* and so on. These words can be used affirmatively to acknowledge and reinforce your state of repose.

The contact should be smooth and continuous; otherwise muscles respond when the hands are taken on and off all the time. You may prefer firm pressure or light touch. The rhythm of slow deep breathing assists relaxation. Allow a little more residual tension to escape as you sigh gently on each outward breath, since relaxation naturally occurs on exhalation. Become aware of your breathing in this way **without controlling it.** This awareness engages your conscious mind and frees your body from tension in a way that you cannot achieve directly. The more you relax, the quieter your breathing becomes. With practice you become increasingly aware of the pause within the respiratory cycle, knowing that your breathing, like the growth of your baby and its eventual birth, takes care of itself. Your eyes may close naturally during relaxation sessions or you may prefer to keep them loosely open, gazing vaguely at a point. Harmonizing mind and body is a personal and variable experience.

Massage

Massage will increase sensory awareness, improve circulation, reduce swelling, relieve stiffness and discomfort; it feels wonderful. (I have met very few individuals who dislike being touched. Most mammals enjoy body contact—just visit a pet store and see how the kittens or puppies huddle together!) Stroking downward avoids friction against the body hair. Deep massage of the neck and shoulders, light circling with the fingers on the muscles of the face, firm counterpressure on the small of the back and light stroking of the taut abdominal wall are some suggestions.

A thorough massage of the feet feels marvelous and benefits the whole body. Reflexology involves stimulating pressure on points on each foot to improve the function of organs and systems throughout the body. I highly recommend it. During my first pregnancy I had a full body massage on Mondays, and reflexology on Fridays. Some points on my feet were so exquisitely tender (in other words, the pressure felt good despite the pain!) that I saw colors in my mind's eye. I surrendered to these sensations and colors and found this type of a massage a wonderful preparation for labor, which turned out to be no more intense.

Perineal massage may prepare you for the sensations of stretching during birth and perhaps the absorption of Vitamin E oil, or castor oil, makes your tissues more supple. It is certainly worth doing as well for the sexual sensations and to focus your attention on this key area.

Finger-painting induces relaxation in just a few minutes, even when standing. One partner strokes lightly over the entire body surface of the other, as if the fingertips were ten soft paintbrushes [98] and imagines painting with a specific color. The person being painted allows his or her intuitive sense to tune into the color. After switching partners, find out if you guessed the correct color in which your were "painted". There are always individuals who guess the color in my groups, especially pregnant women.

Relaxation During Labor

Understandably, an expectant mother feels apprehension as well as excitement when the inevitable process of labor commences. After all, labor is a process filled with unknown events which the mother cannot control. As Dr. Grantly Dick–Read advised in his 1933 book on natural childbirth, "Cultivate a sense of mystery." Time passes pleasantly with normal activities at home in the early stages of labor; many women arrive far too early at the hospital. Your labor will progress more quickly and more comfortably if you walk around for as long as you can. The mechanical direction of the contractions (known as the drive angle of the uterus[99]) is most efficient if you keep upright. If you are planning a hospital birth, the fetal monitor and/or intravenous may curtail your freedom, although you can walk around if you push the IV drip pole alongside you.

Usually no position is comfortable for long and you will feel the need to make changes. For routine checks and examinations, you may be asked lie on your back, usually a very uncomfortable position at this time. Relaxing under these conditions is demanding. Use different positions and lots of pillows if you lie down. Remember to empty your bladder from time to time.

Birth is as safe as life can ever be.

Hospital Policies

The labor bed is not the place to negotiate hospital procedures. These are best discussed with the medical staff beforehand and documented in your chart. (A Birth Plan can be found in my book *Childbirth with Insight.* See Further Reading.) Much of childbirth preparation is information to acquaint a couple with hospital procedures and interventions, and to provide them with coping mechanisms for this environment. Visit the maternity unit during pregnancy and become aware of the hospital rules and routines. Also, talk to women who chose a midwife and those who gave birth at home.

One would assume that, since every labor and delivery is different, institutions and practitioners should be responsive to the personal needs of each woman. Some certainly are, but, in general, women need still far more input and autonomy with regard to their birthing circumstances. Although four million women give birth each year in the United States, regrettably they share no collective power. As transients in the health care system, they usually are obliged to labor according to the expectations of others. As a result, women frequently experience "unfulfilled transitions" or "missing pieces," and I have spent many hours with such women, helping to put the puzzle together and to process their disappointments. Medical decisions, of course, must be made by qualified professionals, but **we must never forget that birth in at least 90 percent of cases is a physiological rather than a medical event.**

Nevertheless, because childbirth has become medicalized and institutionalized, its experiential value is often overlooked. It is not enough to focus on "healthy mothers and healthy babies." We want a healthy baby and mother **and** a good experience. Health in its broadest sense is much more than the absence of disease; it is a state of well-being. As one empowered pregnant woman once stated in one of my groups, "I vowed, when I entered the palace of technology, that I would not let them separate the dancer from the dance."

Childbirth, like life, is never without some risk, and no culture approaches this life crisis without some foreboding or ritual. Despite this truism, **birth is as safe as life will ever be.** The keys are empowerment and trust in your body, both of which have to be re-learned in this culture. The child trusts that she will learn how to walk, even when she keeps falling down. We have lost that kind of faith, somehow, somewhere.

If a woman has a choice, she will choose a place of birth where she can feel safe. In the Netherlands, for example, where birth was never medicalized, the majority of women give birth naturally at home with a midwife. In the United States, on the other hand, most women feel safer in the hospital and with a physician attending, "just in case anything happens."

Labor and delivery may be the hardest work and greatest challenge that a woman ever experiences. However, it is not an athletic event in the sense of preparing yourself for a marathon. As the saying goes, you cannot push the river. Think of being on a log that's floating down the river. Support and cheering on the sidelines may keep your spirits up, but only **you** are on that log! The greater your ability to go with the flow, the more empowering you will find the process of **giving** birth. After all, it is **your** power, your body, your baby. Feeling this unequivocal energy is thrilling and much easier than say, white water rafting—you don't even need to steer or watch out for rocks!

Understandably, women seek a supportive birth environment, but my advice is for every pregnant woman to entertain the idea, seriously, that she

may give birth **totally alone.** By **may** I mean to stress that nature has prepared for this. Notice that I did not use the word *should.* I am in no way advocating unattended birth—just for you to explore the concept in order to tap your inner resources. Just imagine that there may be a hurricane, an earthquake, whatever . . . your contractions are getting stronger . . . no one is with you. What will happen in this fantasy?[100]

Pain

Women are very suggestible in pregnancy and may readily become afraid. They are particularly vulnerable in labor, not only because of the overwhelming power of the contractions, but also because at this time they may see themselves as dependent on those around them.

Shore up your self-confidence well before your due date with education, physical exercise and the partner surrender-stretch. Positive support and comfort during labor obviously helps; a medical study[101] was even done to prove this! Negative emotions inhibit the activity of the uterus; fear often stops labor. Contractions may slow down or even stop for a while when a laboring woman arrives at the hospital.

During labor the muscles of the uterus open the cervix, contraction by contraction. However, if your "flight or fight" mechanisms are activated, tension will spread to the circular muscles of your cervix and cause them to constrict. This conflicts with the work of the uterus, and antagonistic muscle work causes pain and slows down labor. During the first stage of labor, the cervix is like the pelvic floor during the second stage—ideally yielding to the forces from above without tension or resistance. Relaxation is difficult when you are tired and uncomfortable, with contractions continuing to become stronger and closer together. I prefer the concept of yielding, which may involve powerful sounds and movements.

Figure 119. There is always a rest between contractions.

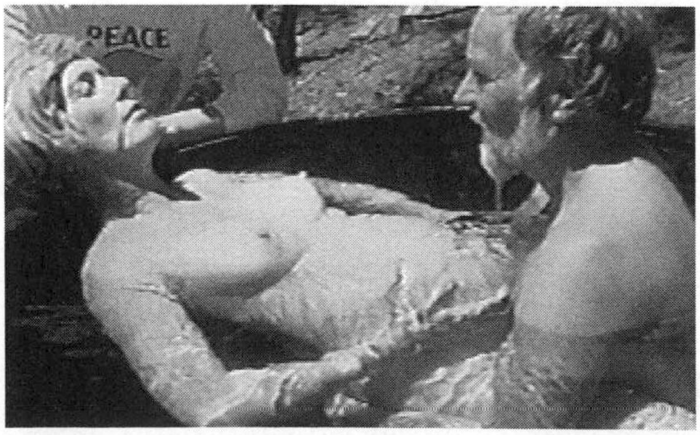

Understanding what is happening and why is essential if you are to trust your body and flow with its natural rhythms. The uterus is simply a muscular nest that contracts when it is ready to open the door and guide your baby into the world. You may feel referred backache from the stretching of the cervix (in first stage) or from the position of your baby. During second stage, there will be increasing pressure in your pelvis, which will turn into an irresistible urge to push when your baby's head reaches your pelvic floor.

Of all the sensations experienced by women, it is possible that perceptions of labor vary the most widely. Pain is felt and interpreted (two different experiences) according to influences from one's culture, ethnic group, religion, past experiences, time, place, mental preoccupation, and suggestibility.

Fear, as we have seen, brings more pain with it than the pain. When combined with fatigue, nausea and tremors, fear can make contractions unbearable. In a similar way, the effectiveness of drugs depends greatly on the circumstances under which they are administered, as research with placebos (dummy drugs) has consistently shown. I am fascinated by the fact that a large percentage of people who take a placebo will have the same response as those who take the real thing. How powerfully our expectations affect our bodies!

Physiological processes generally are not painful. Having a baby is not like having a tooth drilled; normal teeth do not need drilling. Thankfully, Mother Nature did not design the reproductive process with biblical torment in mind. On the contrary, pregnancy and birth, like conception, are primarily sexual events and provide experiences of ecstasy.

Hypnosis, acupuncture, medication, anesthesia and Lamaze techniques for dissociation all share in common the goal of diminishing the painful sensations of labor contractions. Distraction has been the hallmark of conventional childbirth preparation for decades. This concept is based on the theory that you feel less pain by diverting your attention elsewhere—breathing, watching your partner or focusing on something external. If you have difficulty relaxing or if your labor is stormy, you will probably find that breathing patterns make you tense and tired. Paced respiration may be a useful tool for some, but, unlike relaxation, it consumes energy rather than conserving it. In my experience, it is easier, more natural and integrated to *associate* with the intensity of the pain. Cancel any thoughts of control; **the nature of birth means no control** and, sooner or later, **you surrender to the life force**. Entertaining the concept of surrender from the outset makes labor and birth less threatening. For me it was exhilarating. I loved setting my intellect aside to be a channel for the incredible energy bursting through me.

Surrender Your Resistance

I believe pain in labor is just the mother's resistance to opening up—physically, emotionally, mentally and spiritually. We all have resistance at some level which usually results from deep-seated anxiety. During labor and delivery, the cervix is stretched, of course, as are the vagina and pelvic ligaments. Preparation for such powerful physical sensations is essential, and the more sedentary the society, the more frequent the need for birth interventions. The mother's heart and mind must also open to the new life, by aligning herself with her baby so they journey through the process together at the deepest level.

The simulated contractions described in the partner exercises (see Chapter 8) provide a stretch to help you to give in when it hurts, to learn that it is the **not** yielding that hurts. Together, you and your partner learn what relaxation involves while experiencing a strong sensation. Stretching like this during pregnancy gives plenty of opportunities to explore your limits and, at the same time, develop your self-awareness and courage. The word *courage* comes from the French word meaning *heart.* Your heartspace is the place for the wellspring of birth energy, not your head. A partner who experiences stretching to the edge of pain will appreciate that letting go cannot be taught, only learned, and that such changes occur only from within. As Einstein once said, "All experience begins and ends in individual reality." For further information about this approach to birth, consult my book *Childbirth with Insight*, my birth video, *Channel for a New Life*, and *Creating a Joyful Birth Experience* by Lucia Capacchione and Sandra Bardsley.

Keeping alert, staying in the present time and going with the flow gives you a better psychological advantage than distraction and dissociation. If you resist a labor contraction that you "know is going to feel awful," you will prove yourself right. It is more empowering if you tune in to the contraction as just muscle energy, the guiding force that will bring your baby into your arms.

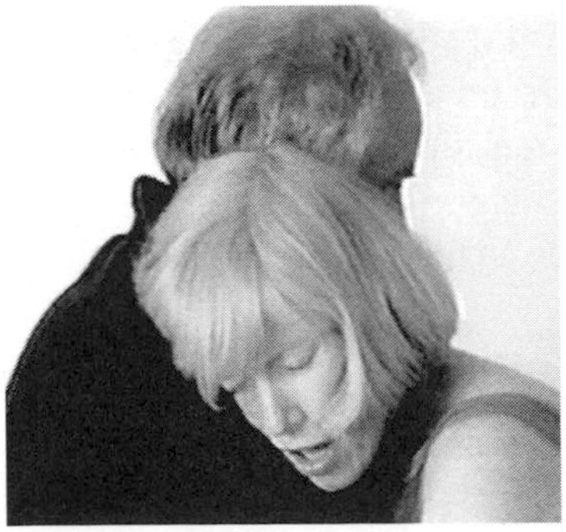

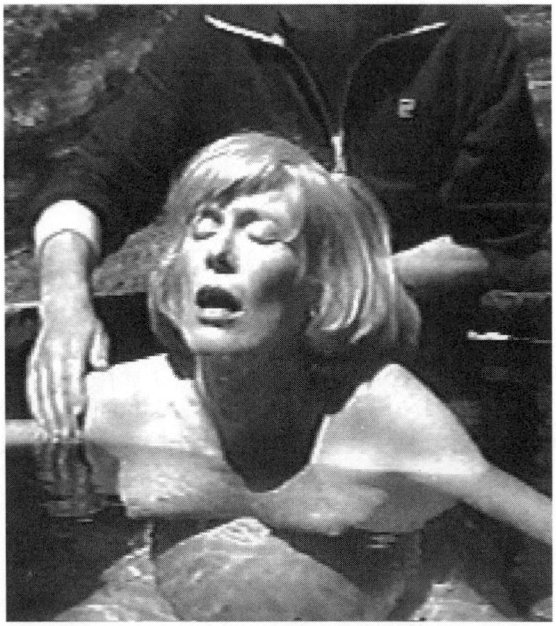

Figure 120. Take each contraction as it comes—allow your body and mind to yield.

Nourishment in Labor

Herbal tea, juice and high carbohydrate food that is light and digestible help allay the exhaustion that makes pain worse. Many hospitals prohibit anything by mouth except ice chips in case the mother should require general anesthesia for a Cesarean section. General anesthesia is rarely used today, and even if it should be required, a tube in the windpipe will prevent aspiration of the stomach contents. Pregnant women feel weak, tired and nauseated if they go a few hours without sustenance. Those feelings are compounded with the exertion of labor, at a time when nourishment may have been withheld for over a day or more! Mashed potatoes with gravy, or soup with pasta or rice go down well in early labor. Obviously, if labor is progressing rapidly you will not feel like eating anything. Antacids may be offered to you as vomiting is not uncommon as labor advances.

Comfort Measures

Interventions in labor can be reduced by making pain *bearable.* Simple physiological methods such as hot or cold packs can relieve discomfort along with hot tubs, and showers, massage and pressure on acupuncture points. Touch involves your partner physically and emotionally. As an experience of human connection, touch needs to convey affection and respect. Often partners complain after the birth that despite all the massage techniques they practiced in pregnancy, during the labor the mother didn't want to be touched at all. I have mulled over this common experience, and decided that it is the *way* she was touched that was the problem. Since making that observation I provide expectant parents with different types of touching among the group so that each person can decide which type of touch is a pleasing, warm, emotional connection rather than mere mechanical contact.

Staying Upright

Studies have demonstrated a decreased need for drugs, anesthetics and uterine stimulants, as well as less heart rate abnormalities in the baby, when women stand and walk during labor. Often, women instinctively "rock and roll" the pelvis during contractions.. If you are upright and mobile you will have a faster, easier birth.

Breathing

Your breathing will take care of itself—just keep breathing. Your sounds lets everyone know that you are not holding your breath or overbreathing. Then your breath flows with the contraction. Any control of breathing works against your body's equilibrium; it limits feeling and impairs relaxation. Vocalization—singing, moaning, chanting—keeps your breathing physiological. Women who have been to prepared childbirth classes often feel pressure to conform and to be "in control." They are reluctant to let go and as a result hold back from noisy or uninhibited behavior. Unfortunately, self-restraint opposes the surrender that is essential for birth.

Maternal Effort

It is odd that physiological principles well understood in sport and exercise are actually reversed in obstetrics. The conventional "management" of the second stage of labor, when the uterine contractions push the baby down the vaginal canal, makes no sense at all. The mother is made to hold her breath, fix her chest, tense her shoulders, stiffen her neck and concentrate her effort on command. Although many people are used to the daily ritual of forcing their bowels, others find straining uncomfortable and self-defeating. (Imagine, as you are reading this, how you would react if you were forced move your bowels within the next five minutes, and perhaps flat on your back!)

Labor is one time when the cues from the body are immediate and powerful. Why isn't support for a laboring woman simple patience and encouragement for her to do what she feels is natural? Perhaps one reason is because the sounds that a laboring woman makes may be the same as she makes approaching orgasm. Let your sounds emerge! I don't know whence the expression "let your hair down" comes, but this is the time to do just that. The best support you can anticipate is affirmation—soft comments such as, "Yes . . . that's it." or "Mm, hm . . . good." Then you relax, knowing that all is going well, instead of striving and straining to force the birth.

Remember: **for the actual birth you must not put weight on any part of your pelvis** in general, and your sacrum in particular, for the reasons given in Chapter 5, see pages 125-127.

Medication and Anesthesia[102]

No anesthetic is totally effective and at the same time entirely safe for use in childbirth. Pain-relieving drugs are always available in a hospital setting, but they should be used as sparingly as possible because of their potential depressant effects on the baby. Some powerful evidence for unmedicated birth can be found in a six-minute videotape[103] showing how babies, right after birth, can crawl to a nipple and attach themselves like any mammal does, **without assistance.** Babies born to mothers who had received narcotics in labor are unable to do this. **Also, taking the baby away from the mother to wash and wrap him or her disorients this instinctive behavior.**

Medication in general, and some epidural anesthetics in particular, slow down the process of labor and block out important feedback. Unfortunately the majority of women have epidurals in the United States. We rarely hear about the side effects of this "Cadillac of anesthesia." However, I have treated women who have had difficulty moving and walking afterward, and some have persistent back pain localized to the area where the epidural catheter was inserted. (I personally find the idea of a needle invading my spine terrifying. I trust my own body in birth much more than any anesthesiologist.) However, if a Cesarean is necessary, regional anesthesia can allow you to be awake and aware and it is safer than general anesthesia. There is generally a use for every piece of technology that has been developed; it's the **overuse** that I protest.

Dr. Eva Reich suspects that epidurals result in decreased sexual feeling; that is, there is never quite full recovery after the sacral nerves were numbed. Indeed, the package insert for Marcaine/Bupivocaine (the anesthetic solutions that are injected) warns against "partial or **complete** loss of sphincteric control or sexual satisfaction." Several women have also confided to me that they have never had an orgasm after the birth with epidural anesthesia. Research needs to be done on this problem. I advise you to read the entire leaflet which is available at your local drugstore, or in the *Physician's Desk Reference (PDR)* at your health care provider's office, or a library.

Although it appears that there may be actual nerve damage in some instances from the anesthetic, my feeling is that psychological issues are just as influential. Birth is the most powerful, creative act that a woman can experience; to block your awareness of it is contrary to Nature. As a result, you meet life and yourself on diminished terms. Women have been subject to misleading promotion by drug manufacturers, physicians and hospitals who benefit financially from our vulnerability and submission. This same medico–industrial complex will continue to profit from hormone replacement therapy that will be recommended to the same women when they reach menopause.[104]

Relaxation During Labor—Second Stage

There will be longer rest intervals between contractions than you experienced at the end of first stage. Some women shiver from heat loss or experience quivering of muscles from the effort of pushing or from pressure on nerves. Wait until your body directs you to push. It makes sense to expend your energy only when the urge to do so is **irresistible**. Your role when pushing is to use your abdominals to assist your uterus in bringing your baby through your birth canal while remaining relaxed in your arms, legs, face, jaw and pelvic floor.

The birth canal consists of your vagina and the bony passage with its yielding ligaments. Your jaw is related to your pelvis, and your mouth to your vagina—let them be slack during birth. If your breath is slowly released (rather than held), your pelvic floor will stay loose.

During the actual birth you will ideally allow your baby to slide out with light pants or groans, your perineum yielding easily. This can be a challenge because the urge to push is now at its strongest.

My son shot out in one contraction because I used my abdominals very strongly. Having seen so many adults relive their births with no help from a knocked-out mother, I was determined that my children would never complain, "She didn't push!" Luckily, he was born underwater, so I had no anxiety about his need to be caught. My second-degree tear healed well without sutures, but I did use ultrasound.

Giving birth is letting go...

Relaxation Postpartum

Natural childbirth creates a feeling of euphoria. Right after birth your baby is very alert and eager to make eye contact with you both, as well as to breastfeed. Rest or sleep is often difficult after such a time of exhilaration. However, you've worked incredibly hard and undergone some very sudden changes, and you will certainly feel tired later.

In the first week, you will experience many profound adjustments. Your uterus, which took nine months to grow to term, begins its six-week shrinking process. Your breasts will start to produce milk around the third day; many of the hormonal changes associated with this may make you feel overwhelmed. Occasionally an anticlimax follows the birth event and the glamour of motherhood seems to evaporate with the demands of being both a wife and mother, and the feeling that all your energy and time is tied to your baby. Though others may disagree, I believe that stress and fatigue, together with inadequate help, not "hormones," is the cause of most postpartum depression.

Continuing relaxation at this time is even more important than before, and breastfeeding is a ready answer. It can serve you as much as your baby in obliging you to rest. You will nurse more often than you would have ever expected. I view this function as a gift, because I took every opportunity to lie down when nursing! Sometimes I would read or talk on the phone, but it was still a peaceful time and a chance to put my feet up. You will be much less tired breastfeeding than bothering with bottles. The intimacy and satisfaction of suckling your appreciative baby is indescribable. I nursed each of my children until they were three years old; on the rare occasions when they were feverish I can't imagine what else I would have done. Breastfeeding serves both of you in more ways than you could fathom in our repressed society. Although we value "the milk of human kindness," we admire breasts for their brassiered appearance instead of their marvelous function.

Discomfort may be experienced during the shrinking contractions of the uterus, mostly by women who have had more than one child. Known as "after-pains," these contractions can be quite intense for the first few days, especially during breast-feeding, which stimulates them.

You must have rest and relaxation to complement any exercise program if you are to renew your strength and vigor. If your rest is inadequate, you may never have the energy or inclination to exercise! Domestic activities and chores are a low priority. If your partner can take over your usual duties or get a few days off work to ease the adjustments, your first week or so at home will be much smoother, especially if there are other children.

Women can help each other enormously if they form an informal support network, donating credits of time that could be used after birth. For example, an expectant mother would help a new mother for a few hours a day during the first week or two. This would be an invaluable experience to learn what life is like with a newborn. In turn, this assistant would receive the same kind of help after she gives birth. Despite the simplicity and clarity of this arrangement, the nuclear family continues to struggle alone. Allow your visitors and well-wishers to perform odd jobs for you. Make sure that you are not concerned with appearances or other unimportant matters at this time. Mothers of twins **have** to make these plans and the sooner the better. Mothers of singletons tend to be less realistic about postpartum life and often suffer for it.

The childbearing year includes at least three months postpartum before the mind and body have reached a state of adjustment. How well you look and feel at the end of it will be the reward for your efforts.

8

Partner Exercises

Exercising with a partner is fun and a great incentive as well. With a partner you will experience additional stretch to improve flexibility, and extra resistance to build strength. All of the exercises in this chapter are beneficial not only in pregnancy but for all men and women. They help to reverse the effects of our modern sedentary lifestyle.

Caution: Warm Up First. Stand and move your joints sequentially from head to foot, and directionally from the center of your body to the periphery, as described in Chapter 2, pages 35–36. Additional exercises can also be done prior to the partner stretches.

Exercise 1. The V-Stretch

Almost everyone can benefit from this upside-down, anti-gravity thrust in a weight-bearing position. The **V**-stretch (a modification of "downward dog" and part of the Sun Salutation in yoga) stretches your spine, hamstrings and heel cords. This exercise can be done alone; an easy way is to rest your heels on the top of a baseboard for secure fixation. However, as with all the partner exercises, the interaction between you both increases your motivation. Importantly, by watching your partner's spine align, you understand better what you need to do.

More than any evaluation tool I know, this stretch exposes the relative flexibility of your spine. Tight areas will be very obvious! In pregnancy, the extra blood volume creates pressure in your head and you may get heartburn; therefore, just do it briefly. However, it is an excellent daily exercise after all bleeding has ceased[105] and **for the rest of your life.**

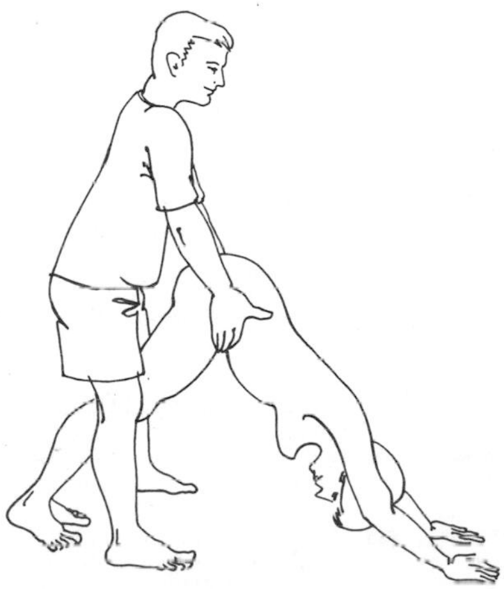

Figure 121. Form a *V* to stretch your spine and strengthen your arms.

Position: You begin on your hands and knees with a lengthened spine. (See page 99.) Your partner stands behind you, ready to give assistance when you are on your hands and feet.

Action: Exhale as you straighten your knees and imagine there is a string from your tail-bone to the ceiling, aligning your spine. Keep your elbows at ease. Unless you do yoga, your heels will not be on the floor. (That may come later and there are other exercises in this book to stretch your heel cords.)

Partner Assistance: Your partner grasps each side of your pelvis, or the top of your thighs at the groin, and with steady traction guides your spine toward normal alignment. Keep your hands in their original place on the floor; often people bring them closer in response to the stretch, losing the point of fixation upon which the stretch depends. However, you may need to place your feet further away from your hands; the space between should be about four feet. A common error is to have the feet almost under the hips, so that the spine is then like a horizontal **C** instead of a **V**.

Now your partner has lengthened your spine to its limit, you should hold the position alone. He or she stands away and you experience new possibilities of alignment and strength, holding the corrected position by yourself.

Exercise 2. Squatting

Please refer to pages 129 for additional hints and precautions about squatting.

Position: Both stand with feet placed wide apart for a steady base. Hold hands with arms outstretched in front.

Action: Gradually bend your knees to squat down, keeping both feet flat on the floor, counterbalanced by each other's weight and outstretched arms. Remain squatting for a couple of minutes. Hold your arms straight; bending your elbows will tire your biceps. Keep your feet flat or there'll be too much weight on the forefeet, which also makes you less stable. If your heels do not reach the floor, and for most people in our culture they won't, place a book under each heel. **Keep the weight on the outer borders of your feet,** lest the inner borders roll over and strain your knees and arches.

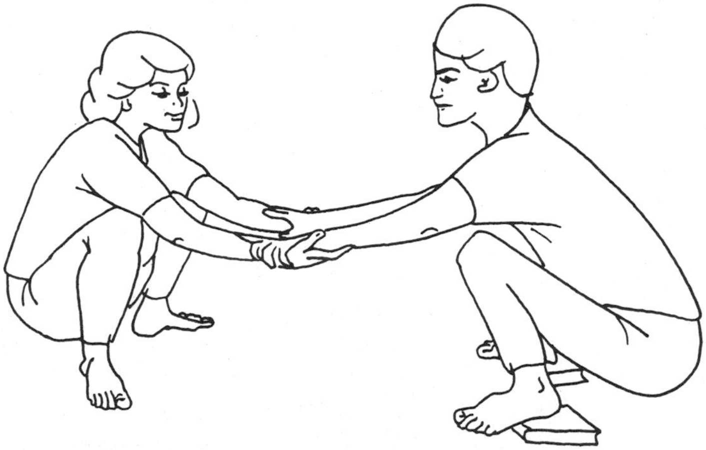

Figure 122. Squatting is easy with a partner for support.

Squatting is an excellent position for practicing pelvic floor exercises and for stretching your heel cords. It is also the easiest position for birth. At first because your legs may go to sleep before your circulation adjusts to the regular use of this position. If your legs become numb, stand up together using your thigh muscles (rising bottom-first is most inelegant), and squat down again.

Most adults in the United States are not used to squatting at all and find it difficult unless they do a lot of gardening. It is much easier—and always possible—with a partner. Begin slowly if you have stiff knees and ankles. Remember, children squat easily before school age, when they begin prolonged sitting in chairs that shortens their muscles. Adults need to re-learn the art of squatting for flexibility and proper body mechanics.

Exercise 3. Circling Stretch

Position: This is the same starting position for all the forward-facing stretches.

Both partners are seated on the floor with legs astride and soles of the feet together. Your knees must be straight and you should be sitting on your "sit-bones." If not, raise your pelvis by sitting on a large book. This will enable you to straighten your knees and back at the same time and to avoid slouching on to your sacrum. Most men have very tight hamstring muscles and need a thick book or telephone directory under their buttocks to achieve this starting position. If you experience any central tenderness between your pubic bones, keep your legs closer together, which may mean putting your feet against your partner's calves. Hold hands with arms outstretched in front.

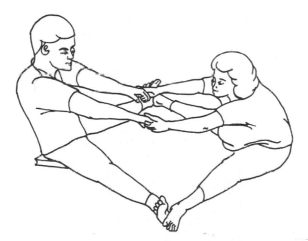

Figure 123. Circle around to loosen your legs and back.

Action: Move your arms and trunk slowly around in a complete circle, keeping your buttocks on the floor. Change direction. Remember to keep breathing throughout.

This limbering stretch loosens the trunk and legs, and prepares you for the stationary stretches that follow. The stretch should be felt in your inner thigh muscles and behind the knees more than in your lower back. If you feel the stretch primarily in your back, sit on a telephone directory.

Exercise 4. Side Bend Stretch
Position: As above, but partners hold right hands.

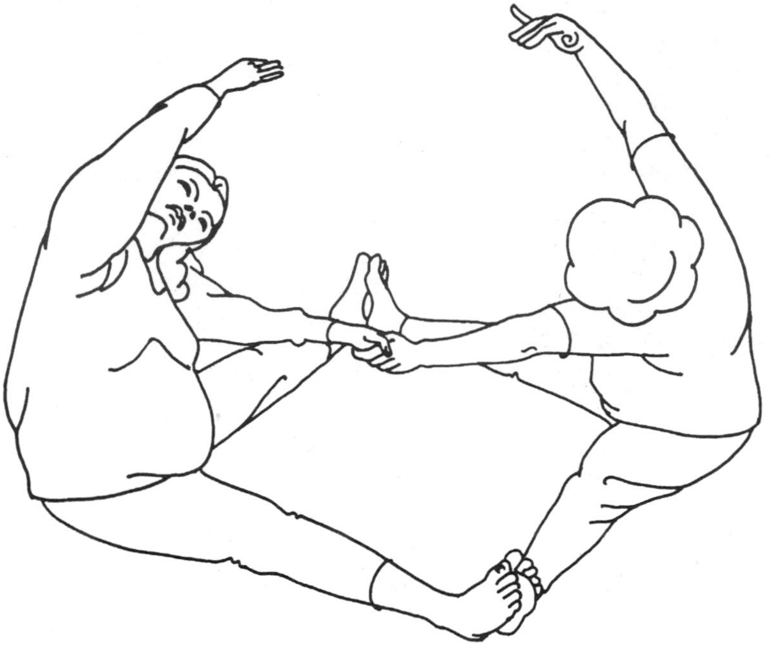

Figure 124. Open your chest as you bend from side to side.

Action: Both partners stretch toward the ceiling with the free arm, keeping it in a vertical line with the trunk. Next, each one bends to the opposite side with the elevated arm stretching over the head in the direction of the movement. For example, one partner is bending to the right while stretching the left arm, and the other partner is bending to the left while stretching the right arm.

Return to the central position, change hands and **stretch tall in the midline position before bending to the other side.**

This exercise continues to stretch your hamstrings as long as your knees remain straight. It also expands the side of your chest and trunk for easier breathing. Increased mobility of the shoulder and neck muscles is another benefit of this stretch.

Exercise 5. Surrender Stretch
Position: As above, both hands held.
Action: One partner leans back with outstretched arms, pulling the other member to his or her limit. As you are pulled forward, allow yourself to go to your "edge of pain," which you experience along your hamstrings and the inner

borders of your thighs. Keep your back straight. If you feel any pulling sensation in your lower back, elevate your buttocks on a book so that you feel the pull in your hamstrings instead. Hamstring muscles are usually tight and need a long, slow, consistent stretch.

Remember, the partner who is leaning back should keep the elbows straight, as bent arms tire the biceps. Leaning back provides **steady** traction to avoid injury. As the forward partner releases, the other partner providing the traction will lean a little farther back and take the stretch to a new limit. Thus the forward partner moves progressively in the direction of the stretch, each limit becoming more of a challenge.

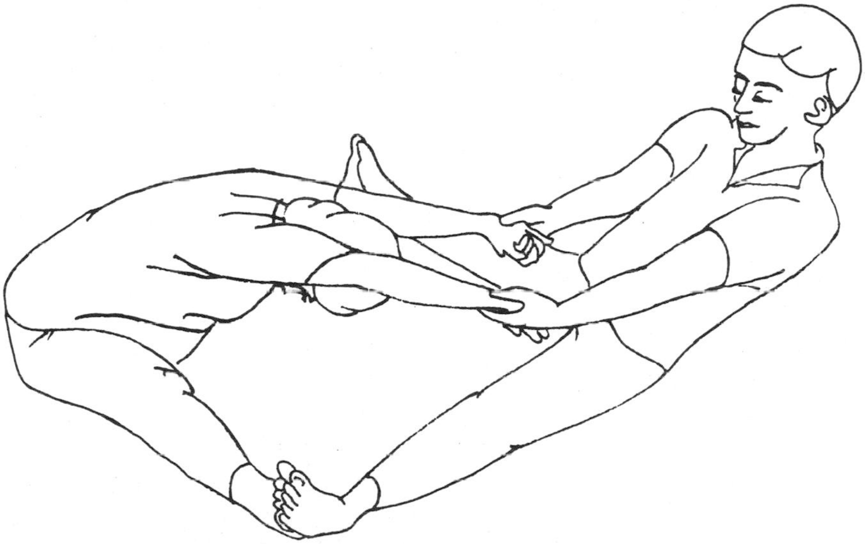

Figure 123. Explore your limits as you surrender on outward breath.

Simulated Contraction. Stay in the forward stretch for at least a minute, about the length of a contraction. Experience some simulated contractions for two minutes as well, to prepare you for contractions of longer duration.

This intense stretch is especially helpful for learning to surrender in labor while building your courage. The ability to feel the sensations (association rather than dissociation) without either pulling back or forcing forward takes practice. Allowing your body and mind to yield needs commitment to a whole different philosphy. Mothers who have participated in my programs over the years claim that these stretches are the most helpful of all the possible prenatal techniques[106] they can learn for coping with pain in labor. They also know that the sound helps surrender, too. Your partner will realize that opening up comes only from within, and that surrender is indeed difficult to learn. Partners who have practiced this stretch provide labor support with deeper understanding.

The key to surrender is releasing on the **outward** breath, which is the natural relaxation phase of the respiratory cycle. Moaning and groaning also help. Opening your mouth allows your pelvis to open. Bouncing or forcing is counterproductive; you actually stimulate the muscle to tighten against the direction of movement. You increase your flexibility by learning to let go, not by pulling yourself apart! It's not a goal to reach the floor, it is a **process of surrender.**

Back–to–Back Exercises

Starting Position: Both partners sit with their backs touching, knees bent and ankles crossed. An optional, more difficult, position is with the soles of your own two feet together (butterly position).

In the following exercises, you should maintain firm back–to–back contact from the buttocks to the head, which strengthens the muscles that extend the spine and thus posture improves. As it is difficult to strengthen back muscles in pregnancy (you can't readily lie on your front), these partner exercises are an effective and enjoyable substitute. Do them for the rest of your life to counteract all those times when you bend forward.

Figure 126. Twisting loosens the deepest muscles of your spine.

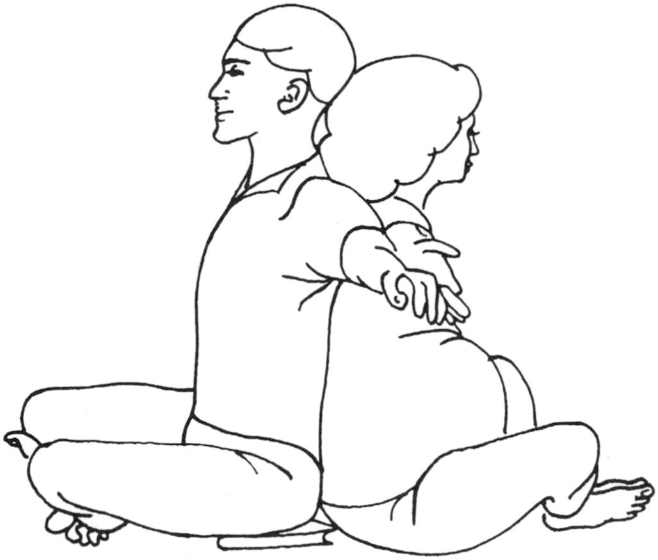

Exercise 6. Twisting
Action: Stretch out each arm sideways, **clasp** your partner's hands, and twist your trunk and arms from side to side. Turn your head and eyes, too, watching your hands. Keep firm contact between your backs. Twisting is excellent for spinal mobility and stretching the pectoral muscles of the chest. **Variation: Press backs of hands** together to work the muscles along the back of your arms and trunks.

Twisting relieves the middle and upper backache that is common in pregnancy and improves circulation to the deeper muscles of the spine.

Exercise 7. Side-Bending

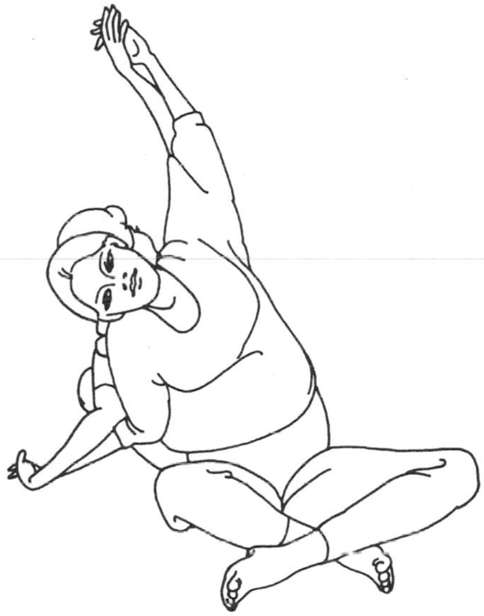

Figure 127. Press your arms and backs together as you stretch your ribcage.

Action: With both partners' arms outstretched and hands held, bend from side to side. Go over on to your elbow if each of you can keep both buttocks on the floor. Remember to maintain the pressure between your backs.

Variation: Press backs of hands together to work the muscles along the back of your arms and trunks.

Side-bending activities facilitate the expansion of the rib cage, which compensates for the reduced movement of the diaphragm in pregnancy.

Exercise 8. "Hold-Up" Press

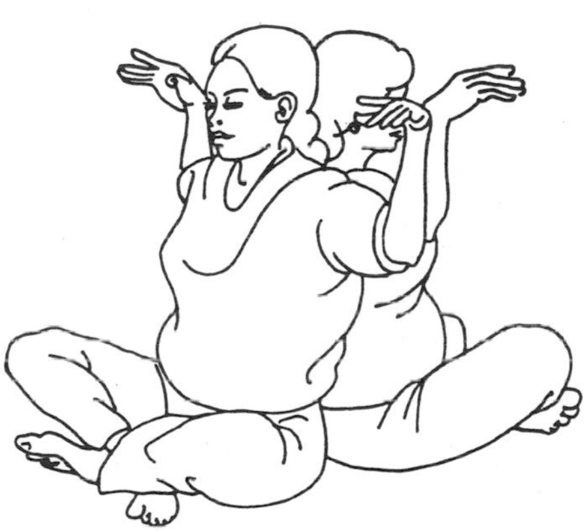

Figure 128. The hold-up position strengthens the muscles between your shoulder blades.

Position: Bend your shoulders and elbows at right angles and press them against the back of your partner's arms, also bent at right angles. Start with fingers touching.

Action: Hold the position and keep breathing. This requires a lot of effort from your neck and shoulder muscles. Then gradually straighten your elbows all surfaces of your arms pressing and moving together. Return to the starting position between attempts.

Progression: This time, drop your fingers forward and **press wrists together**. Now you really feel the muscles between your shoulder blades.

These partner presses build endurance in your back and neck muscles. This strength means better posture through your pregnancy, and prepares you for lifting and carrying your baby. Holding this position is hard work and the following exercise will stretch out any tension in your upper back.

Exercise 9. Trunk Twist and Forward Stretch

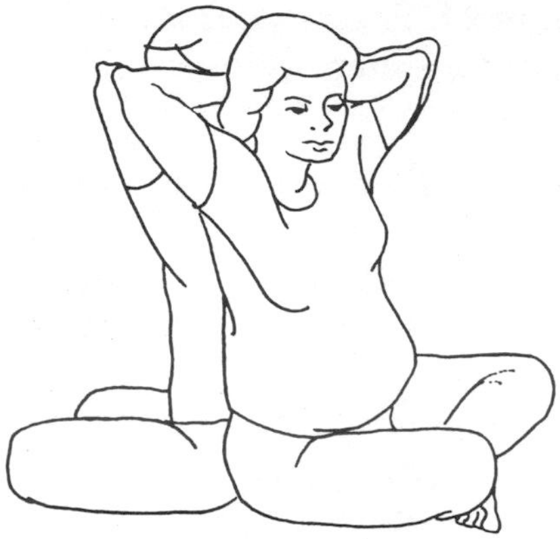

Figure 129. Stretch out your lower back as you strengthen your upper back. If you can press your elbows together, add a twist from side to side.

Position: Clasp hands behind your neck, both elbows touching your partner's elbows.

Action: Keep pressing your elbows together as you slowly twist. If the elbows lose contact, simply stay with the starting position.

After a few twists, each partner stretches forward away from the other. Keep your spine straight, so that you bend primarily from the waist. The buttocks must stay on the floor. Go to a 45 degree angle to strengthen your upper back. You will feel a stretch in the lower back now that your knees are bent, which makes your hamstrings slack.

The benefits of this movement include increasing mobility of your upper spine, stretching the hollow in the your lower back, and challenging your upper back muscles while you spread your "wings." The goal is not to reach the floor but to feel a general stretch in your lower back and experience the slow surrender of muscle resistance to help prepare you for labor.

Exercise 10. Trunk Twist and Diagonal Stretch

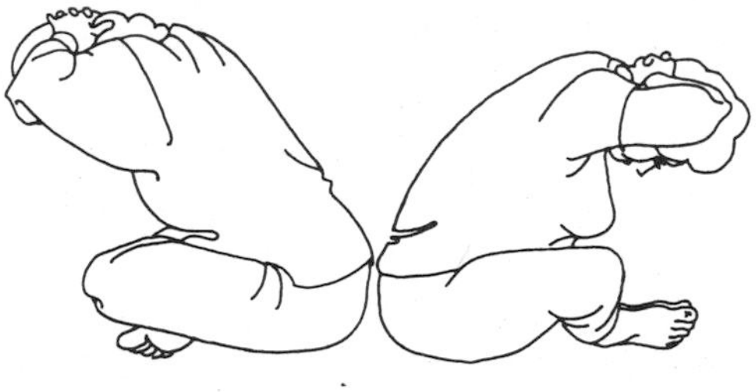

Figure 130. Bend to a 45 degree angle to stretch your lower back.

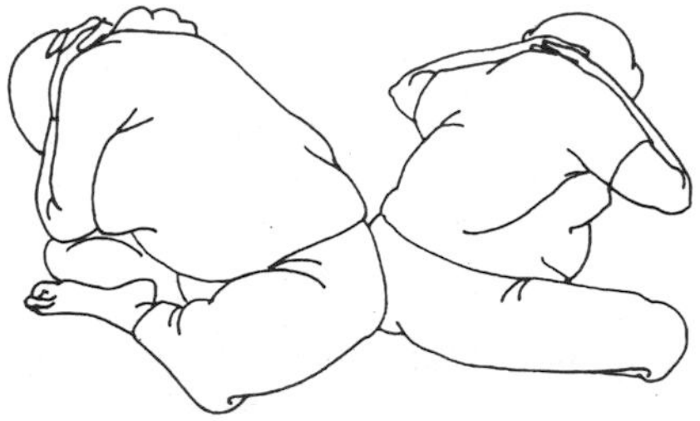

Figure 131. Let your shoulder blade glide across your ribs as you stretch one elbow toward the opposite knee.

Position: As above.

Action: Press elbows together and twist a couple of times. Then, turn your trunk as you bend forward so that your right elbow touches your left knee or reaches even beyond it to the floor. This movement provides a good stretch across the shoulder blade of the forward arm and relieves the common backache between and around the shoulder blades in pregnancy.

Between each diagonal movement, return to the starting position. Press against your partner's elbows again and turn your upper trunks in unison.

Repeat these two stretches with your ankles crossed the other way. You will then feel the stretch at the opposite hip as you go forward.

Exercise 11. Relaxation

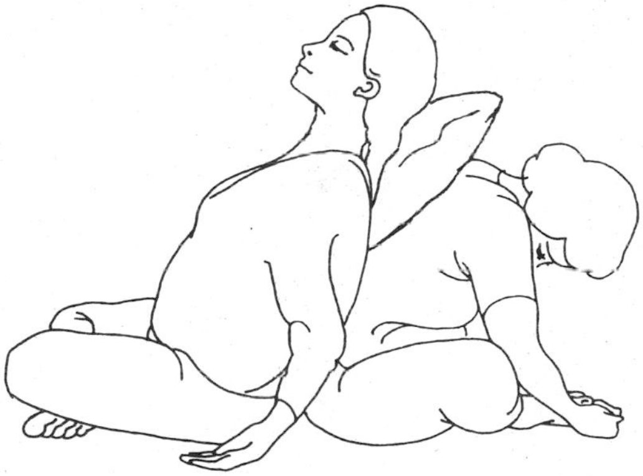

Figure 132. Use your partner's back for support during a relaxing stretch.

Action: One partner leans forward to support the other, who leans back, with head and shoulders supported. Arms are outstretched to the side to open the chest. Commonly, a pillow, sometimes folded for double thickness, is needed to align the neck with the spine.

This relaxation position facilitates diaphragmatic breathing. Spinal extension can be safely achieved in pregnancy because of the support of your partner's back from start to finish. Instead of working your elongated abdominals when lying back over your partner, you are raised to the vertical position when your partner becomes upright again.

Working with a partner enables you to get more leverage and distance than if you did these movements alone. I have taught partner exercises to many different groups: prenatal, postpartum, back class, mid-life women. Some of the exercises can be done against a wall, but a partner is much warmer, more comfortable and more conversational! Furthermore, you cannot twist against the wall. Make these exercises a regular practice for the rest of your life.

9

Cesarean Birth

Cesarean birth is the surgical delivery of the baby through the wall of the uterus and abdomen instead of the vagina. Since 1985 it has been the most frequently performed major surgery in the U.S. One third of Cesareans are elective repeat operations, and this has been the situation for the past 16 years.[107]

The Cesarean rate in the U.S. was less than 5 percent for a century. It began to rise in the Seventies. It peaked at almost 29 percent of births in 1989, and in 1992 it was 23 percent. In the Netherlands the rate remains around 6 percent, but in some South American capitals it is as high as 65 percent. The teaching hospitals of large urban centers in the U.S. often have 30 to 40 percent Cesarean deliveries, because they not only handle more complications but they also train residents. Regardless, rates above 10 percent are excessive.

Malpractice may play a role in defensive medical decisions that cause one quarter of U.S. women to undergo major surgery for the birth of their children. In less litigious societies, however, the rate can be even higher as noted above. Other influences on the final decision regarding the route of delivery include convenience, fear, misuse of technology and financial remuneration. Some women demand a C-section, too, for fear of labor or vaginal stretching.

Having a section is also having a baby.

Couples who genuinely need this type of delivery require information, understanding and support because the fact may be overlooked that having a section is also having a baby. The couple committed to natural childbirth is often sorely disappointed. Fortunately, many support groups have formed in response to the large number of Cesarean parents. Their purpose is to change the attitudes and policies of doctors and hospitals. Beginning with C/SEC (Cesareans/Support Education and Concern), which formed in Boston in the early Seventies, these groups have helped significantly to improve the Cesarean birth experience.

Today, many books, films and classes for planned Cesareans and vaginal birth after Cesarean (VBAC) are available. The International Cesarean Awareness Network (ICAN) began as the Cesarean Prevention Movement and has chapters in many states. A major part of their inspiration comes from the als of women who have successfully given birth vaginally, some even at home, and often a larger baby, following a Cesarean. A side effect of all this public information and education, however, is that the huge number of Cesarean deliveries is more easily accepted.

Indications

A planned Cesarean birth is termed *elective.* Although one third of the sections in this country are performed because of the presence of a uterine scar from an earlier Cesarean, the belief that "once a Cesarean, always a Cesarean" is outdated and not in accord with the latest recommendations of the American College of Obstetricians and Gynecologists. The College presently considers that 80 percent of women who gave birth by Cesarean could deliver vaginally the next time. Despite this, only about 25 percent actually do so.

In reality, some women may prefer a subsequent Cesarean. The ability to schedule the birth and the use of regional anesthesia as well as postpartum self-administered pain relief, is attractive to many women who fear that they may not be able to go through labor again.

In the Nineties, as in the Eighties, almost two thirds of all Cesareans are performed for the same two indications: prior Cesarean delivery and failure to progress.

Previous Cesarean Section

If a section is done because of a uterine abnormality, then that problem will continue in subsequent pregnancies. However, if the baby was breech, or the mother had an active herpes infection, it is unlikely that such events will recur.

Often a subsequent Cesarean birth may be anticipated by the physician but the mother is "allowed a trial of labor." The authoritarian terminology of *allowed* and *trial of labor* both represent a weak commitment with an attitude that undermines the power of women to create their own birth experience.

Cephalo-fetal Disproportion

A common reason given for abdominal rather than vaginal delivery is a disproportion between the size of the baby and the mother's pelvis. On rare occasions this may be the case, but often these same women go on to deliver larger babies the next time.[108]

General Disease

Sometimes the mother suffers from a disease, such as diabetes or pregnancy-induced hypertension (high blood pressure), which can lead to a medical decision to terminate a pregnancy before the due date for the sake of the mother, the baby or both. Cesarean delivery may be the only practical alternative.

Uterine Conditions

If the baby is in a transverse presentation (lying horizontally), the obstetrician may attempt to turn the baby to vertex (head-down). Regardless, some babies just seem to prefer certain positions and return to the undesirable presentation after being turned. Another, infrequent reason for a Cesarean is *placenta previa;* the placenta lies across the cervix, partially or totally blocking the baby's exit. In this case, the operation can be lifesaving.

Fetal Distress

During labor, emergencies can arise, such as fetal distress and/or the need to avoid a risky instrumental delivery. Separation of the placenta from the uterine wall with bleeding *(abruptio placenta),* or prolapse of the umbilical cord, also call for a section.

Failure to Progress

Failure of the uterine muscle to coordinate its action and dilate the cervix or push the baby through the bony pelvis (despite a prolonged period of time) accounts for many Cesareans. Terms such as *uterine inertia, dysfunctional labor* or *failure to progress* are used. As long as the vital signs are normal, and the baby is not becoming acidotic, slow labor is not a problem. However, obstetrician or maternal distress is common, especially when patience runs out.

Breech Presentation

Breech presentation (babies presenting with their feet or buttocks) accounts for 23 percent of Cesareans. Because about 4 percent of babies choose this presentation, ACOG has recommended that more obstetricians gain skills in vaginal breech birth. The poorer statistics for vaginal breech births relate more to the prematurity of the babies (as many premature babies are breech) than to the breech presentation. Dr. Sorger, my husband, has turned many babies into a head-down position. Often these women came from out of town or out of state for the procedure because their obstetricians were not comfortable performing external version.

Anesthesia

Most commonly, *spinal* or *epidural* anesthesia is provided to achieve numbness below the waist. In either case, the mother is fully conscious for the birth (although she does not observe the actual surgery, of course, as there is a screen in front or her face and she is lying flat.) However, she can see her baby as soon as it is lifted from her body.

General anesthesia is used when there is a need for speed, if there are contra-indications to the use of spinal anesthesia, or if mother or doctor prefer it. The fact is, the use of general anesthesia for a Cesarean is infrequent today.

The body's reflexes are eliminated under general anesthesia and there is a risk that the stomach contents may be regurgitated and enter the lungs. This is why, on admission to hospital, all mothers are questioned thoroughly with regard to what they have recently had to eat or drink. Women admitted for elective Cesareans must fast before surgery and drink antacids to neutralize the acid gastric juices. Food and fluids other than IVs and ice chips are generally denied or restricted for most women in labor. A tube will be placed in your windpipe during the operation if general anesthesia is required. Despite this, almost 4 million women a year in the United States are deprived of nourishment during labor, a time of great exertion.

Family-centered Cesarean Birth

It is now generally accepted that the mother has the right to have her partner present in the operating room. Her body is draped, and delivery of the baby takes just a few minutes. The presence of support person(s) is essential to the mother at this stressful time and the importance of early bonding between the baby and family members is now well-recognized. With regional anesthesia you are awake and can hold your baby right away (as long as the baby does not require the attention of a pediatrician or is routinely whisked away to the nursery).

Post-operative Recovery

Cesarean delivery is major surgery and as after other operations with abdominal incisions you may have the discomfort of various tubes for a while. The intravenous drip and catheter from your bladder may be retained for as long as 48 hours. Fever, pain and gas are common postoperative problems for which medication may be required. Cesarean mothers used to stay in hospital for two weeks, now they go home on the third day. This is when the milk comes in and mother and baby begin to learn the art of breastfeeding. Lots of help and support are needed because the mother is also recovering from the operation.

Rehabilitation

It is essential for your comfort that you bridge the gap between the operating table and what is known as *early ambulation* (walking as soon as possible). Otherwise you will be hauled to your feet the following day without the transition of gradual exercise or body movement to prepare you. Pain may make it hard for you to stand with good posture; apprehension will cause you to lean protectively forward over the incision. The following exercises are very simple and safe, and will condition you for other activities, such as going home on the third day. Such exercises have been routinely given to abdominal surgery patients for decades in other countries, yet Cesarean mothers rarely receive this form of postoperative care in the United States.

Muscles waste very rapidly without exercise, **especially after pregnancy and surgery.** I emphasize that these exercises will cause no damage to your incision, although for the first few days you may feel more secure if you support the area with your hands. Gentle muscular activity stimulates healing. If the area is allowed to stiffen and the circulation to stagnate, the ache becomes worse and later movement is even more painful. The stitches will not pull out unless the wound is infected or the suturing was very inadequate—and in these rare instances, it is much better to make this discovery as soon as possible. Correct isometric exercises encourage the edges of the incision to come together, whether the incision is vertical or more typically, horizontal. With each exercise, the muscles are shortened and pulled in **always on the outward breath**. Because it is difficult to inflict discomfort on yourself—even though you realize it is beneficial—you need encouragement.

Cesarean rehabilitation exercises are exactly the same exercises that should be done after any form of abdominal surgery. Remember this for the future and consider sharing this chapter with a friend who may be undergoing an operation. Dr. Sorger clearly recalls a dancer's recovery from Cesarean section more than twenty-five years ago. She exercised intensively and left in excellent condition after just three days, at a time when most women stayed in bed for over a week.

Exercise 1. Breathing and Huffing

Understandably, patients who have undergone abdominal surgery are reluctant to breathe deeply. However, breathing exercises will help to clear your body of the effects of the anesthetic and will tone the muscles of your abdominal wall. Although most Cesarean incisions do not go through the actual muscles—the doctor just pushes them aside—you will have pain and tenderness from the tissues that were cut.

The lungs require extra attention whether or not general anesthesia was used, as mucus may collect from shallow breathing. On coming out of the anesthetic or heavy sedation if epidural anesthesia was used, you must clear your lungs of any mucus; if it sinks to the lower lobes it will take more effort to loosen. Smokers often have problems with chest secretions after the operation.

Breathing must be done completely to ventilate all parts of each lung. Expand your chest in three ways, inhaling two breaths at each region to increase your capacity. Do this slowly to avoid dizziness. Pull **in** your abdominal muscles as you breathe **out**—doing this more strongly when the pain lessens.

- *Diaphragmatic breathing* (see page 150): Movement here may be diminished because of your abdominal wall's sensitivity. Expansion at this region is important for a complete breath.

- *Mid-chest expansion*: Placing hands over each side of your chest with gentle pressure will stimulate the sideways movement of your chest wall.
- *Upper chest expansion*: Place one hand beneath each collar bone, over your breastbone, and inflate your chest underneath.
- *Back-breathing*. Place hands on each side of your back and feel your ribs expand.

Coughing as it is generally understood is ineffective and uncomfortable for people in general, and for the postoperative patient in particular. A mother with an incision in her abdomen is naturally afraid that coughing will strain her stitches and at best she will just grunt feebly if asked to perform this painful effort. The brief closing of the throat causes a substantial increase of pressure within. Chronic coughing strains the abdominal wall and pelvic floor muscles, whereas huffing safeguards and actually benefits them.

A *huff* is a forced exhalation. Huffing is easier and more effective than coughing. It's also less painful. You use your abdominals and diaphragm to expel air from your lungs. **The key difference is that the abdominal wall is pulled in rather than pushed out.** Your diaphragm is moving up in the chest and your abdominal muscles are shortening (instead of just tensing). In this way, pressure is being decreased inside your abdominal cavity and your wound is safe from strain. Huffing must be done with sufficient speed and force to dislodge any mucus. It is like saying "ha" loudly and briskly, with a rapid, maximal contraction of your abdominal muscles. Open your mouth wide and allow your jaw to relax. (Have a tissue ready for any expectorate.) As a comfort measure, you may want to support the incision area with your hands or a pillow; however, be reassured again that the stitches will not pull out.

Huffing is also a good test to check if there are any secretions in your lungs. When a moist rattle is heard during this outburst of exhaled air, mucus is present and must be brought up. Huffing is more tiring than breathing; one or two huffs is all that is usually necessary. Do another round of breathing in the different chest regions between huffs to further loosen the chest secretions. When you huff and it sounds clear—then it is!

This sequence of breathing and huffing is the first line of chest care for anyone at any time when there is a productive cough. It is a great advantage to learn it now and you can teach your other family members and friends. With prolific secretions it may be necessary to have a physical therapist assist you with percussion on your chest and rib cage compression during huffing.

Abdominal tightening on outward breath automatically occurs with the above chest program. Shortening the muscles isometrically (without movements) also helps to shrink the skin and other tissues, avoiding a flabby belly later on, as long as you begin these exercises right after birth.

Muscles must always be shortened before they are strengthened.

Your partner can remind you to take a couple of deep breaths, to wiggle your toes and bend your feet up and down, and to tighten and relax your leg muscles frequently during the first few hours after surgery.

Exercise 2. Foot Movements (See page 145-146)
Ankle stretches and circles prevent thrombosis, particularly after anesthesia and if you are confined to bed. They can be discontinued when you walk again.
Position: Legs may be out straight or loosely bent over a pillow.
Action: Bend and stretch your feet at the ankles. Make circles with your feet at the ankles, together or separately.

Exercise 3. Leg Bracing

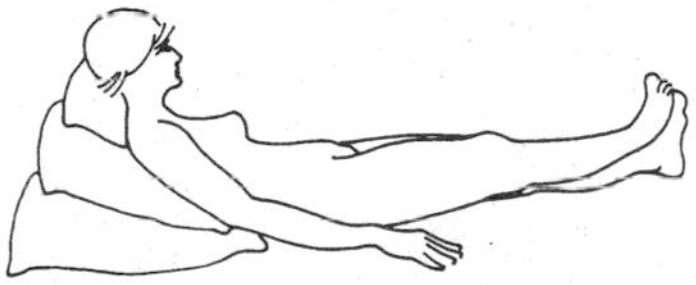

Figure 133. Ankles crossed, pull up the feet and brace the legs and buttocks.

Position: Legs out straight, ankles crossed.
Action: Tighten all the muscles in your legs, then press your knees down, tense your thigh muscles, and pull your buttocks hard together as if you were holding a coin between them. Point your heels to stretch your calves.

Exercise 4. Knee Bending and Straightening
Position: Lying on your back, one knee bent and the other straight.
Action: Slide the heel of the bent leg down the bed and back to the bent position again. Repeat with your other leg.
Progression: Bend one knee as you straighten the other so that you are working them together but in opposite directions.

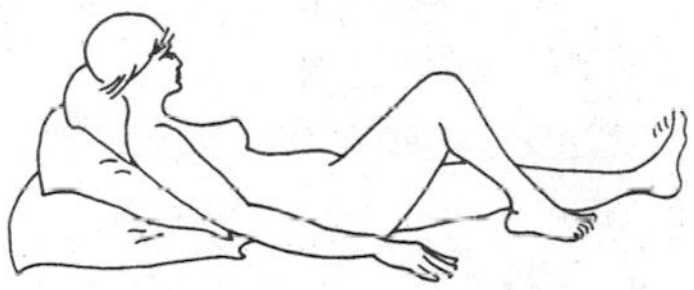

Figure 134. Bending and straightening alternate knees.

The exercises discussed so far hasten your recovery from the anesthetic and prepare you for the effort required in first getting out of bed and standing. The first time that you do this, make sure that you have someone standing by in case you become dizzy or faint. Ask for help with the intravenous tube and catheter.

Exercise 5. Bridge and Twist

This exercise will prevent gas pain if done at least twice a day for the first three days. Your intestines are passively moved which is a substitute for the normal intestinal movement that was interrupted by the surgery.

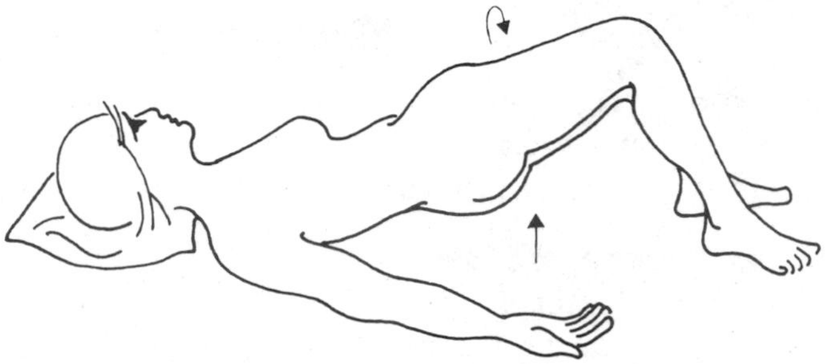

Figure 135. Bridge and twist the hips—first to the right, then to the left—and lower.

Position: Lie on your back with knees bent and feet as close as possible to your buttocks to use as much leverage as you can from your hamstrings. Place your arms alongside your body to press into the mattress for additional assistance.

Action: Contract your pelvic floor, buttocks and abdominal muscles, push through your feet and raise your hips a few inches off the bed, pressing with your arms as well. Maintain this elevated position as you drop one hip to the right and then to the left, which twists your pelvis from side to side. Lower your buttocks back to the bed and rest. Tighten both your abdominals and buttocks during these movements.

Exercise 6. Pelvic Rocking

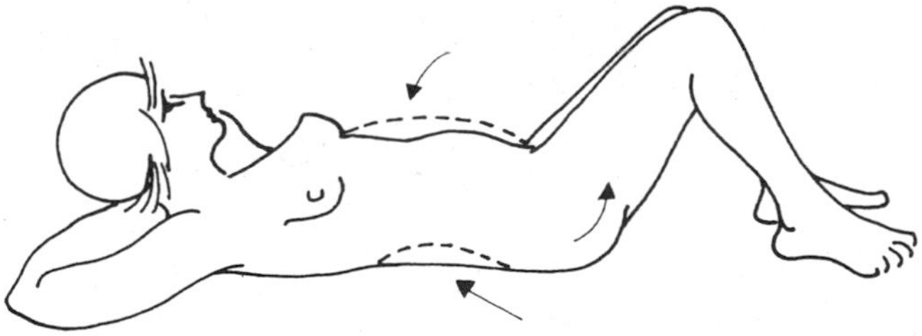

Figure 136. Rock your pelvis up and down.

Position: Lying on your back or side, with bent knees.

Action: This is similar to the pelvic tilting described on pages 95-96, but in this case it is done with the intent to stimulate sluggish intestinal activity rather than to strengthen the muscles that control the pelvic tilt.

Gently rock your pelvis from front to back, using your abdominal and buttock muscles. Breathe out simultaneously and pull in your abdominal muscles, all the while pressing your pelvis into the bed. The subsequent inhalation takes care of itself. Support the incision with your hands if you wish.

Getting Out of Bed

First, lower your bed, if possible, so that it is closer to the floor. Bend your knees and slowly slide each leg, one at a time, to the edge of the bed. Turn your shoulders to the same side and push yourself up with the arm closest to the edge of the bed. For comfort, support your incision with your other hand. Move closer to the edge of the bed so that your legs can drop over. Sit for a minute or two and move your feet up and down a few times. Brace your abdominal and buttock muscles as you gradually put the weight on your feet, breathing out. Lift your upper back and stand tall. By tightening your abdominal muscles, you support the area with a muscular "splint." This is also known as *stabilization,* which protects your pelvis and back when you lift. The early bed exercises prepare your natural corset—your abdominal muscles—for this exertion. New mothers who cannot do this yet can use their hands or a binder for support.

After a Cesarean, deep breathing and abdominal wall tightening, as already described, help relieve discomfort from air that may be trapped under the diaphragm causing shoulder pain. The bowel and bladder reflexes are always sluggish for a day or so postpartum and are further depressed by the effects of surgery. The greatest discomfort postpartum is gas within the intestines (known as *wind* in other English-speaking countries). The pain peaks around the second or third postoperative day, when the natural waves of intestinal movement *(peristalsis)* recur. The abdomen can become bloated and the movement of the gas within the intestines may be even visible. Exercises that provide gentle movement and compression of the abdominal wall helps prevent these problems. Some relief from these symptoms can be obtained by lying on your left side, with your knees bent, so that gravity encourages the natural progress of the gas through the intestines, and gently kneading the abdominal wall. Remember when you massage your abdomen that the colon goes up, across and then down so your hands must move in a **clockwise** direction.

Check Your Midline

On the third day, check your recti muscles (see pages 91–92) and then progress at your own pace with the exercises recommended for the normal postpartum mother. With advances in surgery and anesthesia today, Cesarean mothers recover so well that by the second week I am not able to pick them out in a postpartum exercise class. For this reason I have never developed a separate class for Cesarean recovery. Many women, regardless of whether they deliver vaginally or by Cesarean, have unresolved feelings and missing pieces from their expectations of birth. They process their disappointments, laughing and crying together, as they resume intensive abdominal and pelvic floor exercises in a postpartum exercise class. Cesarean mothers, while not giving birth vaginally, may nevertheless have experienced incontinence or developed pelvic floor weakness from the weight of the pregnancy. Therefore, they follow the same regimen for the pelvic floor.

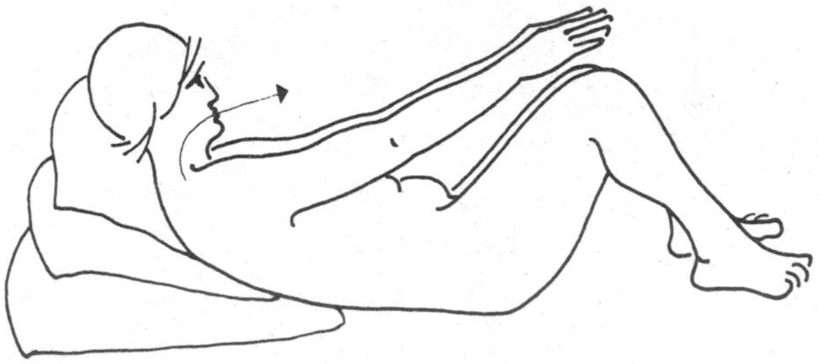

Figure 137. After surgery, start curl-ups on pillows

Comfort Measures

Ask for all the help you need to breastfeed with your abdominal discomfort. It boosts your self-esteem to nurse your baby after surgery and the experience will heal and unite you both. Mothers who feel disappointed that the birth ended with a Cesarean are overjoyed to breastfeed as nature intended, which the many mothers who give birth vaginally choose *not* to do.

When nursing, place a pillow between the baby and your incision, or lie on your side. You can also place your baby against you so that his or her head is at your breast, but the feet in the opposite direction, that is, under your arm and behind your shoulder in the so-called *football hold.*

Take it easy. This does not mean refrain from rehabilitation exercises, as they are the very ones that will hasten your recovery and ease your discomfort. But you will experience much fatigue since you have had not only a baby but surgery as well. Sometimes mothers are warned against climbing stairs or even driving a car for weeks after a Cesarean! Unfortunately, this well-intended advice prolongs your convalescence. Stairs are more tiring than regular walking, because they demand muscle work against gravity—thus they are an excellent exercise. You have no choice if your house has stairs! Exhale, keep your buttocks and belly tight and use your legs to propel your body upward. (See page 132 for the correct way to go up and down stairs.) For your comfort in the car, place a pillow or maxi-pad between you and the seatbelt while there is tenderness around the incision.

Your Incision

Your stitches may itch as they start to heal. Some doctors use dissolvable sutures whereas others use staples which have to be removed around the fifth day. Most incisions heal uneventfully, but some may develop thickened areas[109] and/or adhesions between the scar and underlying tissues that can cause discomfort months after the surgery. Massage can help. Castor oil or vitamin E is excellent for healing, although your fingers may be slippery for the precise friction massage that you need to do perpendicular to the scar. Rolling the skin and plucking it helps too.[110]

TENS (Transcutaneous Electrical Nerve Stimulation)

This physical therapy modality works on the same principle as scratching an itch. Another message gets to your brain before the pain, traveling over nerves with faster transmission speed. Electrodes are taped above and below your incision. These electrodes are then connected to a hand-held unit with adjustable controls. You can choose the type and speed of electrical current to meet your needs. Patients who use TENS after any kind of abdominal surgery require less or no pain medication, an important advantage to breastfeeding mothers. The stimulation also reduces the incidence of *paralytic ileus* (intestinal distention and symptoms of obstruction). I also believe it helps to prevent the formation of a *dead zone* around the scar. A *dead zone* occurs from pain, disuse, and the mother's reluctance to examine or palpate this area. The tissues are like dough, many women feel "cut off" from that part of the body, and nerves to the skin may indeed be injured and take many months to recover.

Sometimes knee and foot problems manifest after a Cesarean for which no cause can be found. In my experience this has to do with disturbances in the body's energy field. We know from Kirlian (laser) photography that all living things are surrounded by this field, also known as the aura. Some intuitive people can even see this. Photographs of a torn leaf, for example, show how the energy field is absent around the injury. I have found that polarity balancing for the entire body (see Appendix) resolves these obscure dysfunctions.

Emotional Processing

Some Cesareans are genuinely necessary, but most are not, considering the 5 percent rate for a century prior to 1970. Mothers may or may not be pleased with their doctor's decision and feel that they were in the category of a life saved. I support women wherever they are in their personal process. Those who are at peace with the outcome are at peace. Those who are not may be ambivalent or even angry—at themselves, their doctor, their partner, their baby, whomever. In my experience, reassurance is not helpful; in fact, it's a form of denial. Women who are integrating the Cesarean birth experience do not want to hear that the nurse had several Cesareans and she's just fine, or that a mother's feelings are irrelevant because she now has a wonderful, healthy baby. This has the effect of making her feel doubly sad and negating her feelings which are not only hers but to which she is entitled. Rather, women need to be listened to, to receive encouragement to finish their broken sentences and to let their emotions flow. Otherwise the repressed feelings will linger on, and in some women they don't emerge until the next pregnancy.

There are several excellent books that I recommend (see Further Reading) about Cesareans. Jane English's *A Different Doorway* describes the experience from the baby's point of view through adults' regression experiences. Nancy Cohen's *Silent Knife* will empower you to give birth vaginally next time. Bruce Flamm's book *Birth After Cesarean* gives you the medical perspective from an physician–activist working for fewer Cesareans.

10

Bed Rest

As I have suggested earlier, anxiety is the common denominator of illness and crisis. Nowhere is this clearer than in the case of a pregnant woman because two lives are at stake. Unfortunately, life is becoming ever-more stressful for most people. Even in middle-class and professional women, career commitments and financial obligations can cause major pressure. Economic and political uncertainties surround us as we journey through the Nineties. We have outgrown the old ways, but we have not yet evolved into the people we need to become. These diffuse concerns also contribute to anxiety during pregnancy and birth. Regrettably, most pregnant women today work too hard and too long into their pregnancies.

Obstetrical interventions, when pregnancy becomes complicated, do not address anxiety; on the contrary, they usually compound it. The term *high-risk* is but one example. Dr. Michel Odent always avoids classifying pregnant women into categories.[111] He believes that **being classified high-risk by itself is a cause for complications** (via a placebo effect that works in reverse). In his hospital outside Paris, women classified as high-risk by others could use the home-like birthing rooms with mats and pillows and enjoy the same degree of privacy and freedom as any other woman who came to his hospital in labor.

Women need the most validation when activity levels are restricted for obstetric reasons, rather than for maternal conditions like a broken leg.

Bed rest has been prescribed for:

- ✦ Pre-term labor contractions or "irritable" uterus.
- ✦ Bleeding at any stage of pregnancy.
- ✦ Hypertensive disorders of pregnancy.
- ✦ Placenta previa.
- ✦ Pre-term rupture of membranes (PROM).
- ✦ "Incompetent cervix" from diethylstilbestrol[112] (DES), cone biopsies, laceration and also for no obvious reasons.
- ✦ Multiple pregnancy, especially higher-order multiples.
- ✦ Trauma aftermath.
- ✦ Cardiac disease and other rare medical complications.

Pre-Term Labor

Preterm labor, as it is now called, refers to contractions that dilate the cervix prior to 37 weeks. It may result from "silent" infections with no noticeable symptoms. As a result, some obstetricians routinely prescribe antibiotics when preterm labor contractions occur. However, I feel the causes of preterm labor are multiple, and looking for a lone bacterial invader, despite increased incidence of sexually transmitted infections, is simplistic. The fact remains that the preterm birth rate has increased 15 percent in the last decade (varying from 6 to 10 percent, and up to 18 percent for African–Americans[113]) despite the use of tocolytic drugs to stop contractions and a variety of other means that supposedly guard women from this problem.

If a woman is also experiencing strong and frequent Braxton–Hicks contractions, it may be incorrectly assumed that she is in labor. As many as 80 percent of hospital admissions for supposed preterm labor turn out to be false labor, and after staying a few to 24 hours, the mothers are sent home.[114]

Excessive uterine activity, cervical effacement (thinning out of the cervix) or dilation (opening of the cervix) prior to 36 weeks increases the likelihood of preterm birth. If you can detect preterm contractions before your cervix has undergone significant changes and before the membranes have ruptured, sometimes they can be stopped with rest and increased fluid intake. Just as a marathon runner drinks frequently to prevent muscle cramps, so hydration must be adequate in pregnancy to prevent falling blood volume and the onset of preterm contractions. Often, just drinking several glasses of water and lying on your left side will take care of the contractions or, in the hospital, you may be put on intravenous fluids for hydration. Sometimes a glass of wine helps; in the past intravenous alcohol was administered to stop contractions.

Today when there is increased activity of the uterus accompanied by changes in the cervix, tocolytic drugs are usually prescribed despite controversy over whether they are useful for all patients. The side effects are most anxiety-provoking and include increased heart rate for mother and baby, palpitations, tremors and low blood pressure.

Hypnosis for Preterm Labor

David Cheek, a obstetrician retired from clinical work and a skillful hypnotherapist, considers that "preterm labor is a preventable disease—if you can talk to the mother." Before he learned to ask his expectant mothers about fear, he had a 6.5 percent prematurity rate in his practice. After he learned to help women in preterm labor to bring unresolved issues to their conscious minds, prematurity rate in his practice rapidly dropped to 2.3 percent.[115]

Dr. Cheek feels that preterm labor is often the result of fear put into the minds of women by their well-meaning but anxious obstetricians, or sometimes it has to do with anger experienced by the expectant mother toward her partner or some of her in-laws. This or some other problem in a woman's life may haunt her and cause her to build up a stress response. Preterm labor contractions develop when the mother dreams at a deep level that precludes recall, but she tunes in to the normal contractions of her uterus, which she suddenly experiences as painful.[116] She responds with anxiety and tension that increase her uterine sensations and the cycle begins that can eventually lead to preterm birth.

When a woman calls Dr. Cheek with preterm contractions, she is almost in a trance with fear. Over the phone, he sets ups a system of signals[117] and asks her to go back to the time when she is comfortable and nothing is going on and then to move forward to the event that disturbed her. Out of fear, the mother stops communicating with her baby, and the baby in turn feels alarmed that the telepathic communication has ceased. From regression hypnosis with adults who were born prematurely, Dr. Cheek has concluded that the baby does not feel safe and initiates labor.

Telepathic communication is just as important in humans as animals but it has been demoted in modern society. We have all seen how baby animals will scurry because of some silent message they received from their mother. Telepathic communication among Australian aborigines served them for centuries, for example, guiding them to row to a distant island for a funeral, because they "knew" of the death. Our personal origins of telepathic experience begin inside our mother, and pregnancy complications may arise when this goes awry. The well-known telepathic communication between twins is also established prenatally. Actual verbal communication is important, too; women with pregnancy complications **must** talk to their babies.

Dr. Cheek offers this service for free, a fact which I published in the Resources of the second edition of my book *Having Twins.* As a result, Dr. Cheek has enabled many expectant mothers (of both twins and singletons) in preterm labor to resolve the crisis and complete their pregnancies uneventfully. Pediatrician Marshall Klaus, social workers Phyllis Klaus and Gayle Peterson, among others, also offer telephone hypnosis for complications of pregnancy. (See Resources.)

Castor Oil Packs for Bleeding

Castor oil packs can be used successfully for a number of conditions, such as uterine bleeding, bruises, and injuries, although it is not known exactly how or why they work.[118] A compress for the abdominal wall is made of wool flannel saturated (but not dripping) with cold-pressed castor oil. Cover the pack with plastic wrap since castor oil is sticky and soaks into sheets and clothes. This is applied to your belly. Heat from a hot water bottle helps keep the oil warm longer and be absorbed better. (Bleeding may also cease with hypnosis.)

Hypertension (High blood pressure)

Studies are in process to determine whether exercise helps reduce hypertension in pregnancy as it does in essential hypertension. According to Dr. Odent, pregnancy-induced hypertension without protein in the urine is not a disease but an indicator of placental activity. In fact, the babies he followed did better than babies carried by women whose blood pressure did not elevate. Dr. Odent also found that blood pressure is lowered after a few minutes of immersion in water that is close to body temperature.

Placenta Previa, Cerclage

Women with placenta previa or a cerclage (sutured cervix) have often passed miserable pregnancies because of very restricted activity. I once knew a woman with a cerclage who was not allowed to drive during her pregnancy! Another woman, I recall, was admitted to hospital with placenta previa only to circumnavigate the maternity floor in her wheelchair for months. In contrast, Dr. Cheek describes one of his patients who spent the last six weeks of her pregnancy with her cervix dilated to 6 centimeters, but with hypnosis, and no restrictions on her activity level, carried to term.

Clearly, there are two opposing schools of thought: one that believes complications are physical and the other that looks for causes in the mind and emotions. When women with such conditions attend my exercise class, I simply advise them to skip exercises that intuitively don't feel right. For example, they may not want to squat or do curl-ups. However, encouraging physical movement raises a woman's confidence in her ability to carry her baby to term. In addition, my exercise classes offer psychological support in a safe environment for sharing anxiety.

Benefits of Bed Rest

I advocate plenty of rest for all pregnant women. Ideally, they should often rest in a semi-recumbent position or lie on one side, preferably the left. However, definitions of "bed rest" vary greatly, from sitting up in bed for a few days to lying down continuously for weeks, without even "bathroom privileges."

Increased rest for an *acute* crisis, such as threatened miscarriage, preterm labor, elevated blood pressure or bleeding, makes sense. Most women have experienced heavy menstrual flow at one time or another, when it felt right to lie down and rest. When we do too much, we often develop a cold, which forces us to take to our beds and give us the break that we need.

In pregnancy, short-term restricted activity gives you, your physician and your family a chance to acknowledge the circumstances and focus on the options. The rationale given for bed rest is that it takes the force of gravity off the cervix and the major blood vessels draining the legs and abdomen, and obviously it limits physical activity. However, what rests tends to rust, and other problems can arise.

Hazards of Bed Rest

Among the *diseases of recumbency*, there is loss of calcium from bones, loss of appetite, increased indigestion and constipation, muscle weakness and joint stiffness, the risk of thromboembolism, utter boredom and depression. While most people think of bed as a place of rest and refuge, when one is confined, the experience becomes stressful. Dependence on others, guilt, anger, sexual abstinence or being labeled *sick* contribute to the anxiety arising from prolonged bed rest. Common discomforts of pregnancy such as heartburn, constipation, swelling of the legs and backache are increased by inactivity.

Almost a century of studies have shown that these side effects tend to counteract any potential benefits. I consider that bed rest is a conservative approach taken when there is nothing more constructive to recommend.

Orthopedic surgeons have ordered bed rest, some of it prolonged, for patients with back or pubic pain, especially during pregnancy. Such patients should request physical therapy immediately. The nutrition of the discs between the vertebrae depends entirely on osmosis, and spinal movements are essential for circulation of fluids containing nutrients. Some patients respond well on bed rest and may become pain free but develop a significant loss of function, as in cases of severe constant low back pain (with or without *sciatica*), where symptoms are markedly worse during weight bearing, and when no movement or position can be found to reduce the pain. Immediate and ongoing assessment is required, and treatment must be instituted as early as possible. Restoring function and full rehabilitation is a priority. I have treated women who had been on bed rest for three to four months, and who came to me after birth because severe physical problems affected their ability to care for the new baby. Manual therapy and exercise could have alleviated such problems. (Remedies for back and pelvic pain can be found in the Appendix.)

With advances in medical research, critically ill patients who have suffered a stroke or a heart attack are no longer immobilized as they were in the past. On the contrary, today they are encouraged to assume progressively more challenging levels of fitness. It appears that in obstetrics the practice of bed rest remains where cardiovascular medicine was 20 years ago.

If you are ordered to go on prolonged bed rest, I advise you to seek a second opinion and to consider the services of Dr. Cheek and others who provide telephone hypnosis. They usually offer these services for free because they need to research this simple, non-interventionist approach. Certainly you have nothing to lose as you lie in bed! Also find a therapist[119] who can offer a good preventive exercise program to balance your restricted activity.

Physical Therapy is Much More than Just Exercise

Typically, a woman placed on bed rest feels isolated, inadequate and frustrated. Unless she can work from her bed, she probably must quit and the family may suffer economically from the loss of her income. If other children in the family make demands to which she cannot respond, these stresses understandably aggravate her anxiety.

The physical therapist is not the harbinger of ominous monitor readings nor the dispenser of unpleasant medication. The therapist offers a half to one hour's encouragement to the bed-ridden women. In my experience, hospital patients look forward with enthusiasm to this cheerful part of their day when they learn what they **can** do. The expectant mother, with spirits lifted and no longer feeling like a "failing incubator," can enjoy a program that stretches, strengthens, relaxes, and reassures. Exercises against the graded manual resistance of a physical therapist are ideal; massage and relaxation skills are also part of a bed rest program. The psychological benefits are just as significant as the physical activities.

If an individualized exercise program is not possible, you can perform the exercises described below to balance your level of restricted activity.

Recommended Exercises for Pregnant Women on Bed Rest

Bed mobility

The easiest way to get in and out of bed is to bend your knees (one at a time), keep them parallel and roll to the side of the bed where you plan to get out. Lower one leg at a time over the edge of the bed and use your arms to assist you into a sitting position. Reverse this process when you return to bed. (See page 201 for a full description.)

Using a Bedpan

If you may not leave your bed at all, you will be using a bed pan. Unpleasant as this is, lying down on your back makes it even worse. You need to have the back of your bed raised to vertical and both your knees bent, with your heels close to your buttocks. Grip the rails of your bed, or press on the mattress with your hands, as you **exhale** and push through your feet, lifting your buttocks into a bridge so that the bedpan can be slid underneath.

Joint Mobility for your Neck, Arms and Legs while you Sit

- ✦ Bend and stretch your ankles and toes, fingers and wrists to keep your blood moving (and you have fifty percent more of it).
- ✦ Circle your head to loosen your neck muscles.
- ✦ Bend your neck slowly forward and back. Keep your mouth closed as

you move your head backward for a nice stretch of your throat area.

- Bend your neck from side to side. Look straight ahead and keep your nose facing forward as you increase the distance between the ear and shoulder on that side. This will relieve tension in your neck and shoulders.
- Bend your knees, one at a time, and slide one heel along the bed until your knee is straight with your other knee bent.
- Bend and straighten your elbows.
- Fingers on shoulders, circle your elbows backward.
- Stretch open your arms and make backward circles. Imagine you have colored paint on your fingers and each circle is larger than the one before.

On your Side

- Raise and lower your top leg in a direction toward the back wall to strengthen your buttock muscles.
- Make circles with your outstretched leg, keeping your knee straight for a variation.
- Bend your knees and tilt your pelvis, sucking **in** your belly button and pelvic floor.
- Hold your uppermost leg so that your foot and hip are level, and hike your hip, moving your pelvis toward your shoulder. This exercises your side abdominal muscles.
- Cross over your top leg in front of the other, while your uppermost arm goes behind your trunk. On exhalation, bring your top leg over your other leg, all the way behind, as the arm from behind moves at the same time, all the way in front. Raise the legs high to give a good stretch. This cross-over exercise challenges your coordination.
- Bend your top leg and place the foot on the floor behind or in front of your other leg. Raise the lower leg to strengthen your inner thigh muscles.

These basic exercises will maintain the range of motion that you have in your arms and legs. You can use these movements to strengthen muscles with Theraband, which is like elastic and comes in different grades/colors. (See Resources.) This flexible tubing can be hooked around the foot or siderail of your bed, a door knob or a nearby chair to form a stirrup so you can work your hips, knees and feet against resistance.

Trunk Movements

These are controversial with U.S.-trained obstetricians who want to eliminate the effects of gravity and increases in intra-abdominal pressure if they fear pregnancy loss. Yet most women who are forced to stay in bed are given no advice on how to change position and often do so at the expense of increasing their intra-abdominal pressure. An example of what **not** to do is gripping an overhead bar, holding your breath and lifting your body from backlying to sitting. This exertion is much more strenuous than any of the safe and sane bed exercises that physical therapists recommend!

I frequently hear of physicians requesting a PT to "instruct the patient how to get in and out of bed without using her abdominal muscles." Not only is this impossible, but abdominal muscles must be used correctly (exhaling during exertion) to support the spine! All pregnant women, **especially those on bed rest,** should be taught correct, safe and efficient ways to maintain trunk muscle strength and flexibility, including how to transfer in and out of bed.

Abdominal Muscles

Your recti muscles should be checked and the appropriate modification or curl-ups commenced. The belly button moves toward the spine as your breath goes out, whether you are doing isometrics to tone your abdominal wall or actual movements to strengthen your muscles. Always stop before you are out of breath and **suck in your belly.** A bulging belly is proof that you are doing it wrongly because the pressure inside is increased like a balloon inflating.

Buttock Muscles

Bridging (page 143) is necessary to get on a bed pan as described above.
Bridge and Twist (page 200) is a good exercise to maintain adequate intestinal movement and prevent gas.

Pelvic Floor

These exercises can and should be done frequently through the day and in any position. Always exercise your pelvic floor while in the bridge position because then gravity assists.

General Precautions

The only exercises that may increase pressure on your uterus and cervix are squatting and incorrectly-performed abdominal exercises. When you exercise, listen to your body. If contractions, blood pressure, or bleeding increase, ease off. If not, then increase your activity level.

Modify abdominal exercises by simply doing frequent head raises on outward breath, supporting your abdominal muscles if necessary with your hands as described on page 91. Pelvic tilting on hands and knees is another alternative that will also give you a welcome change of position.

Generally the pregnant woman on bed rest will be using her arms and legs in some activities. However, the limbs will get progressively weaker from lack of use. Take the longest route to the bathroom and consider lifting weights.

Simple Adjustable Home-Made Weights

You can make weights out of strong, doubled plastic bags of sand or rice. For your legs, fill two bags, tie the ends together and put them on your ankle so that the bags hang down on each side. Wearing a weight like this, you can sit over the side of the bed and straighten one knee or lie down in bed and raise one leg while holding it straight. Start off with just enough weight to feel mild effort after a couple of repetitions. You should exhale easily throughout. Add more weight as you progress. Exhaling will prevent increases in pressure in your abdomen as well as fluctuations in circulation that occur with straining. I cannot sufficiently emphasize the importance of **proper breathing. Without exhaling during exertion, you may do more harm than good.**

Hydrotherapy (Water)

Suggest to your doctor that you be allowed to take frequent tub baths or, better still, swim gently in a pool to maintain mobility. A 1990 article in *Obstetrics and Gynecology* found immersion more effective than bed rest in treating *edema* of pregnancy as have other researchers.[120]

Dr. Michel Odent is the world's most experienced obstetrician with the use of water during labor and birth. It is common knowledge among those who assist at water births that the relaxing effects of immersion often slow down or stop contractions in early labor. Therefore, women are encouraged to get into the tub only when in active labor. By the same token, it make sense to use the special properties of water to reduce contractions and irritability of the uterus, and to induce relaxation and lower blood pressure.

Bed rest obviously limits your positions, and in most cases you will be encouraged to lie on your left side, predominantly, to improve blood flow back to your heart. Yet in water you can move as freely as a fish. Aquatic exercise reduces swelling, increases venous return and lowers blood pressure.

Making the Best of Bed Rest

If bed rest is unavoidable, you can take a few steps to lighten the sentence. Home visits by childbirth educators, physical therapists and mothers who underwent bed rest and experienced a good outcome are all valuable. Arrange regular massage for your circulation and relaxation. A foam wedge to support your belly when you rest on your side is very comfortable. Consider purchase-ing a bodyCushion™, see Appendix and Resources.

Take this time to educate yourself about birth and parenting. In the Resources is a list of organizations that specialize in educational materials for pregnancy, birth and postpartum. Join some of these groups and send for their literature and newsletters. They will help occupy your mind, because you don't want to put your brain to rest, too!

Some women are so diligent with bed rest that they don't even think to ask their doctor about going out for a quiet dinner with their partner, which in most cases would be a welcome boost to their morale.

Bed rest provides plenty of time for sharing with older siblings and communicating with your baby through touch, visualization and meditation. In this stressful situation you want to communicate your feelings to them, yes, even of frustration, impatience, anger or fear. Talk to your baby and explain what is happening. Daily singing is recommended because it is a joyful activity that will enhance your breathing. It also exposes your baby to a wide range of pitch, which is good for his or her learning skills. This will help to compensate for the lack of prenatal movement that your baby will experience.[121]

Social Support

The United States is not a society that affirms mothers and babies, in contrast to other industrial nations where prenatal care is free and maternity leave is at least as long as the pregnancy, or longer. Women's health issues in general have been on the back burner for too long. The National Center for Education and Maternal and Child Health at Georgetown University asked not to be listed in the Resources of this book, as according to the project librarian, there are no materials in their inventory addressing exercise for women! This organization does, however, provide "assistance and information to policymakers, state, and local health departments." I received a similar letter from the American College of Preventive Medicine!

Often complications of pregnancy occur among disadvantaged mothers, who have inadequate nutrition, housing and finances. It is much more cost-effective to take care of the basic prenatal requirements than to spend a fortune in the NICU for a preterm baby's life support systems. It was shown many years ago at the Montreal Diet Dispensary that supplementing the diet of poor pregnant women, in this case simply with oranges, eggs and milk, greatly improved the outcome of their pregnancies.[122]

Psychological Issues in Prenatal Complications

Ambivalence, at one time or another, is quite common during pregnancy. Discussion groups, exercise classes and childbirth education sessions all must acknowledge the differing personal realities of the individuals involved. While positive messages about pregnancy and motherhood are essential, time must be provided for women to express their anxieties. Once an issue is acknowledged and named, it loses some of its power to disrupt harmony and health, and appropriate remedial action can be taken.

Understanding causes is the most important and perhaps most difficult challenge in health care. It is completely different from "blaming the victim". As mind and body are one, our health problems generally have a symbolic role. This approach leads us to understand a symptom with greater insight—not simply to get rid of it. Holistic health care, in addition to providing relief from symptoms, asks why a person has certain symptoms at a specific point in time, and at a particular location in the body. Individuals may genuinely deny any factors that may be contributing to their medical condition, as our conscious mind is but a veneer of our true existence.

Like the proverbial iceberg, the greater part of our functioning—certainly in reproductive matters—goes on at deeper levels inaccessible to ordinary awareness. However, through hypnosis, dreams, art and guided imagery, it is possible to tap into old memories and make connections. Interpretations of disease and dysfunction, such as Louise Hay's *You Can Heal Your Body* and her suggested affirmations (positive statements), are well worth exploring. Journal writing, especially with your non-dominant hand, is explained in *Creating a Joyful Birth Experience*. (See Further Reading.)

While pregnancy is the literal and metaphorical embodiment of a woman's creative energy, her partner's support remains essential. Mothers who are teenagers, single, or whose partners abuse or abandon them, understandably have more complications during this vulnerable time. A woman's own pre- and perinatal experiences also affect her pregnancy and birth, just as those early experiences influence the care that her midwife or physician provides.

A crucial dimension of carrying a baby to term is a woman's belief in her ability to nurture her baby on all levels. We must foster the *concept of nurturing* through the months of development, both for mother and for her baby. This experience is not only physical, but sexual, emotional and spiritual as well. Ideally, when pregnant women move and stretch together, they also open up to these diverse dimensions of the mothering experience. For a woman whose own mother provided a suboptimal prenatal environment this can be a challenge. Other factors that interfere with the self-concept of a nurturer include sexual abuse in childhood, and loss of a twin. (Many twins vanish during pregnancy; at least 15% of pregnancies start out as multiple conceptions although only 1% of births involve twins.[123])

Sociologist Ann Evans[124] found that if a woman had experienced sexual abuse by a caretaker prior to the age of eighteen, she was twice as likely to deliver before thirty-four weeks of gestation and two and a half times more likely to have a newborn with a medical problem. This occurred regardless of the number of previous babies, education, race, alcohol or cigarette abuse, or history of other physical abuse in childhood. According to Lloyd deMause,[125] 60 percent of girls and 45 percent of boys experience some form of unwanted sexual encounter from a trusted caregiver.

Domestic violence is frequently the reason for a woman to seek medical care in an emergency room these days, and a recent article in the *New England Journal of Medicine*[126] lamented the fact that some pediatricians now treat more victims of violence than they do children with allergies and ear infections. Yet, when I ask both physicians and women who consult them if the question of abuse is ever raised, the answer is usually "no"! Many obstetricians request a psychological consultation only if the woman is in severe emotional distress. Even then, it is more likely that they will just order sedatives.

Bonding with Your Baby

Babies in the uterus are highly conscious beings. By the fifth month the ear is fully developed but even prior to that babies respond in many ways to their environment. The unborn baby is awash in the mother's hormones that pour out in response to her emotions. Talk to your baby, explain the circumstances.

An accumulating body of evidence demonstrates that adults can recall preverbal and prenatal experiences as far back as conception. Testimonies include my own book, *Primal Connections, The Application of Ideomotor Techniques in Hypnosis* by David Cheek, M.D., *Babies Remember Birth* by David Chamberlain, Ph.D., and the classic *The Secret Life of the Unborn Child*, by Thomas Verny, M.D. Members of the Association for Pre- and Perinatal Psychology and Health have produced various video and audio tapes and they offer specialized services for pregnant and postartum women experiencing problems (see Resources).

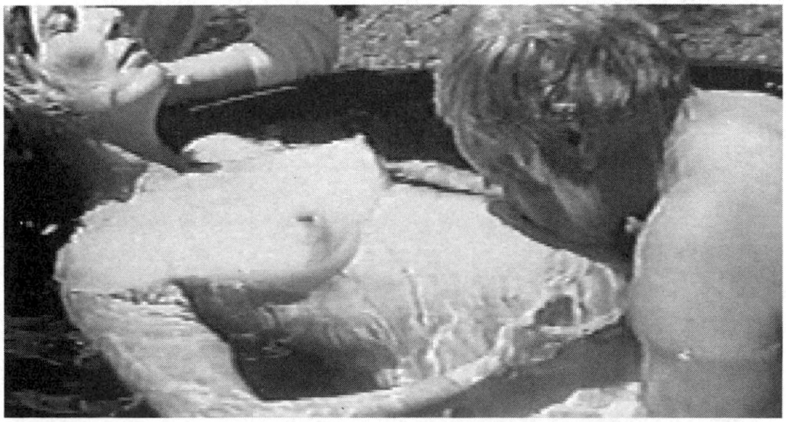

Figure 138. Always stay in touch with your baby.

Afterword

I was pleased, honored, and somewhat excited when Elizabeth Noble asked me to "look over" the manuscript for this, her latest book. My sense of excitement arose from the fact that several readers of my foreword to *Having Twins* had called or written with questions or comments—a circumstance that had never happened before with my medical readership.

These inquiries, along with the content of the manuscript, suggested two things: the first was that this book was truly written for the intended audience in a reader-friendly language chosen to make the point and, I might add, reinforce it. Indeed, as I read along I could hear Elizabeth's voice, exhorting and encouraging the reader in her clear tones and flawless diction. The words she has chosen are, by virtue of their numerous positive encouraging references, are not to be confused with the stern commands of a drill sergeant barking to a group of recruits. Rather, they sound more like the soft, kind advice of the Japanese "Senje" who taught the novice in the movie *Karate Kid*. The second point is that unlike medical texts, a goodly proportion of Elizabeth's works are read from start to finish.

Fortunately, I completed my editing of this book the morning I left for a two week visit to China. During my last conversation with Elizabeth, she asked me to inquire about the incidence of urinary incontinence among Chinese women. It was her recollection that this condition had been conspicuous by its absence when she visited there fourteen years before. I set about inquiring shortly after I arrived in Beijing. During my first and subsequent hospital visits, I received the same response, "very low." Elizabeth believed that this low rate, especially compared to the incidence in the United States and other developed countries, was due to the Asian everyday practice of squatting.

The Chinese squat frequently—to work and to rest. This position is the protective measure suggested by Elizabeth to prevent stress incontinence. Unlike North Americans, who usually can teeter for only a few moments on the balls of their feet, the Chinese can squat with both feet flat, maintaining their balance with the back coming forward like an airplane seat to stabilize their center of gravity.

Throughout the volume you have just read, there are numerous statements that exercise should be a part of everyone's life—not just during the pregnancy year—but for *the whole life.* This, in my opinion, is the most important message. Remember it, but do more than just remember it: Get on it! One of the few regrets I harbor about my childhood and young adult life is that physical exercise was not a part of it. Mental exercise came aplenty, but it was sedentary. The German term "sitzfleisch" best describes this—sitting on one's rear end. Russian novels, Greek drama, German grammar and masterpieces of English and French literature were all absorbed in a chair or on my bed. I had a bike and loved to cycle, but my bike was stolen one day and I was so mad that I gave up what I had loved, my sole opportunity to exercise.

Something tells me that my story is not unique. As I walked from three to six hours per day in China, the contrast between our cultures was never as vivid as it was with regard to physical activity. In a nutshell, the Chinese do not need to "exercise" with aerobics, yoga or any other type of classes because they, for the most part, live an active life. Before and after work, they can be observed practicing Tai Chi informally in the parks as well.

I encourage all readers, their partners and families, and anyone interested living more comfortably with their body to change their sedentary ways and become more active. Otherwise, you will soon find out that once the long muscles that support, move, twist, rotate or bend your body become shortened, it takes work—often painful work—to lengthen them again. The same may be said for ligaments, but only more so. Think of it: one does not start studying Chinese acrobatics at age sixty! For some people it's all they can do to get out of bed at that age.

So what's the answer? Here it is a case of "Don't think—Just do!" "Do" can mean many things: walk, run, climb, push, pull, lift, squeeze, squat, bend, twist, turn, jump, roll, skate, cycle, swim, throw, catch, kick, dance etc. Do something like walking to the store for a loaf of bread. Paint a room, but not during pregnancy. You know what I mean. As you read this book, make your plans, not only for your pregnancy year, but for the rest of your life.

Louis Keith, M.D.
Professor of Obstetrics and Gynecology
Northwestern University Medical School
Chicago, Illinois

Appendix

Pain Syndromes

The following suggestions are intended as safe self-help remedies. These useful techniques, however, are no substitute for a personal evaluation by a physical therapist or orthopedic specialist. Serious pathology, although uncommon, should be ruled out if your symptoms do not abate within two weeks.

General laxity that causes overall joint pain is rare, but disabling. Exercise makes the symptoms worse. The only successful treatment I know is a full-body polarity balancing session. (See American Polarity Therapy Association in Resources.)

Pubic Symphysis (PS)

The connective tissue uniting both pubic bones becomes softer during pregnancy and the increased mobility at this joint may become painful. No muscles span this joint, therefore no specific exercise can be done to protect it. In fact, exercise usually makes the condition worse, especially moving one leg. Keep your thighs parallel during exercises and rolling in and out of bed.

A diagnostic test is to get on your hands and knees and raise one leg off the floor. If this does not aggravate the PS symptoms at the **center** of your vulnerable midline, you may have *adductor tendinitis* or *round ligament spasm*, the discomfort of which is felt on one side.

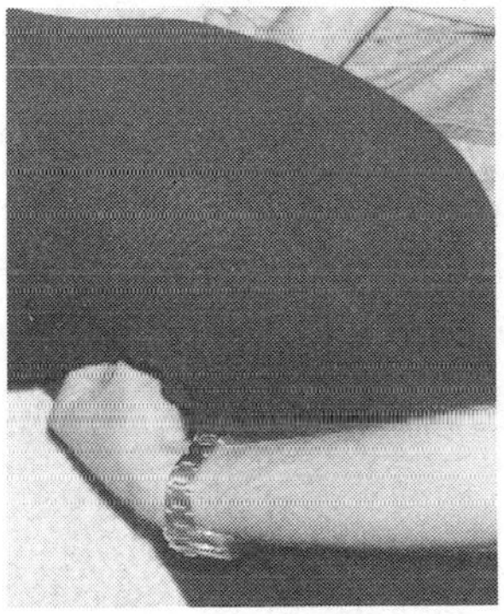

Treatment: Local polarity therapy.

Position: Lying on your side, a partner places all five finger tips firmly at the union of your pubic bones, and the other hand rests flat on your sacrum. The hands should remain still on these two points until warmth, tingling, vibration, pulsing or other evidence of your body's electric field can be felt equally in your partner's both hands. Usually only one to two treatments is necessary. I have successfully used polarity balancing to treat painful PS laxity for fifteen years.

Figure 139. Hands on for pain relief.

Round Ligament Spasm

This knife-like sensation in one groin may come after prolonged standing or with sudden changes of position.

Treatment: Avoid the factors listed above which aggravate it, and when it occurs, go on hands and knees to perform pelvic tilting exercises. The **V**-stretch helps too, but do it only for a few minutes because of the extra blood volume flowing to your head.

Adductor Tendinitis

This tendon inflammation results from stretches done with the legs astride and forceful bouncing. This produces a tender area on one pubic bone, usually about an inch away from the midline.

Treatment: Friction massage.

Massage, with firm pressure, perpendicular to the direction of the tendon. You can feel this tendon as a ridge if you squeeze something between your knees and place your fingers to the side of your PS. Friction massage is painful initially, but if done for about three to five minutes the area will become numb. If you persevere to the point of numbness, only a couple of treatments should be necessary.

Sacro–Iliac Joint Pain

This is characteristically felt in the upper quadrant of one buttock. You can experience pain at this location that is referred from your lumbar spine which makes this a much more difficult area to diagnose. Although it is an **L**-shaped joint and too deep to palpate, the Australian technique below has worked for my patients in over 90 percent of cases. (I have also used it successfully on many physical therapists who have taken my courses!) It takes less than ten minutes. To ensure that the adjustment holds, follow with polarity balancing.

A diagnostic test is to lie flat on your back with the soles of your feet together. Rotate your pelvis around like a clock. This movement will aggravate a problematic SI joint.

Treatment: Local traction and polarity.

There are many manual therapy techniques for SI treatment. A simple one that you can try at home is to lie with the leg on the painful side supported on a chair . Both your hip and knee should be bent at a 90 degree angle. Your relaxed weight provides the traction that relieves the discomfort in the SI joint. If rest in this position doesn't achieve this, you will need help.

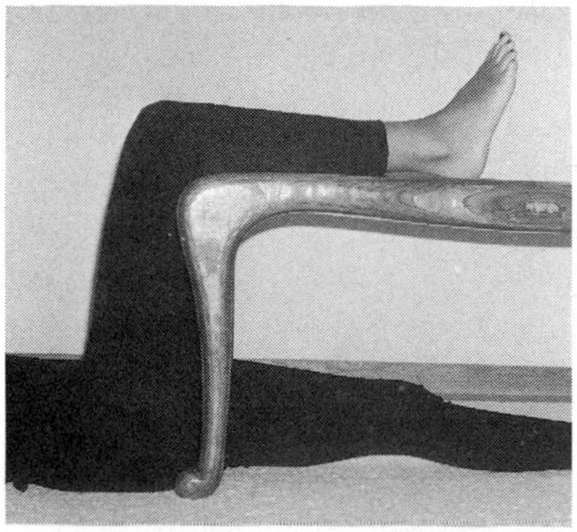

Figure 140. Sacro-iliac joint pain is relieved by positioning.

You partner removes the chair and holds your thigh between two hands. Your calf rests on his shoulder. Compression, that is, pressing directly down to the floor, aggravates SI joint pain. Pulling the leg up toward the ceiling will relieve it. It is important to take up the slack in the joint (buttock stays on the floor) and give some gentle jiggles at the limit.

Your partner must check after each traction by compressing the joint again. Pain should be substantially reduced each time. When zero pain is experienced, usually within five minutes, you should receive a polarity session.

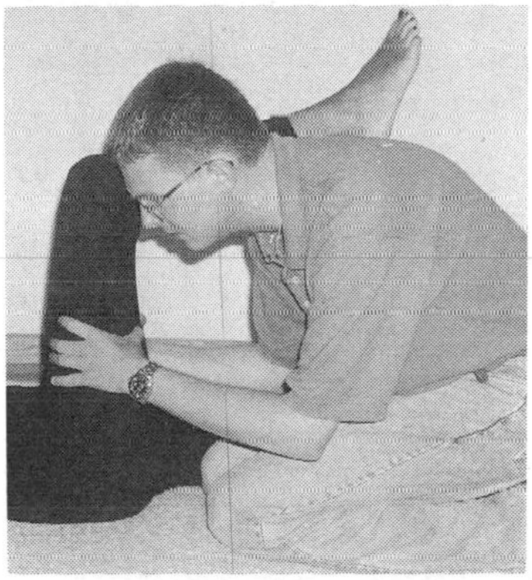

Figure 141. A partner can provide gentle traction.

The finger tips of your partner's one hand press on the dimple of your buttock, and fingertips of the other hand on the front of your pelvic crest (anterior and posterior superior iliac spines). The hands should remain still on these two points until warmth, tingling, vibration, pulsing or other evidence of your body's electric field can be felt equally in both of your partner's hands.

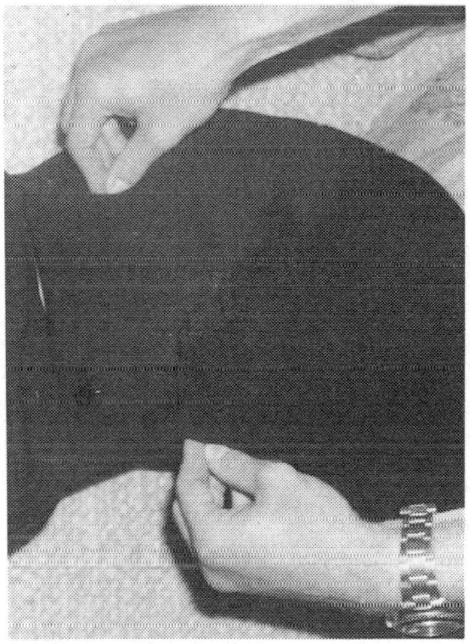

Figure 142. Polarity energy balancing stabilizes an adjustment.

In this area it may take 10 to 15 minutes depending on how much pain you have felt. Usually only one to two treatments is necessary.

If this remedy doesn't help, then you may have a spinal problem referring pain to your buttock or localized buttock pain. Seek a complete physical evaluation.

Back Pain

Approximately 90 percent of the U.S. population suffers from back pain at some stage of their lives. Most back pain results from a sedentary lifestyle and inappropriate body mechanics, whether lifting, shoveling snow or exercising. Bed rest is appropriate for a couple of days when the pain is acute, but movements and positions must be found that reduce and resolve the pain. The pain has to first go out of the leg or arm and centralize at the spine. Avoiding painful movements will allow the disc to heal and then you can gradually resume those same movements.

A regular exercise class often takes care of diffuse central aches *(the postural syndrome)* that do not radiate to the limbs. Choose a class with emphasis on stretching and relaxation, such as yoga or a Back School class, if you cannot find a specialized prenatal or postpartum exercise class.

Lumbar Pain

Spinal pain may be localized to the central lower back, or it may radiate down the leg, usually one side. Sitting is usually the worst position because it increases the pressure on the spinal discs. If you hurt your back by bending forward and lifting, it is helpful to reverse that movement.
Treatment: Positioning, Stretching, Traction.

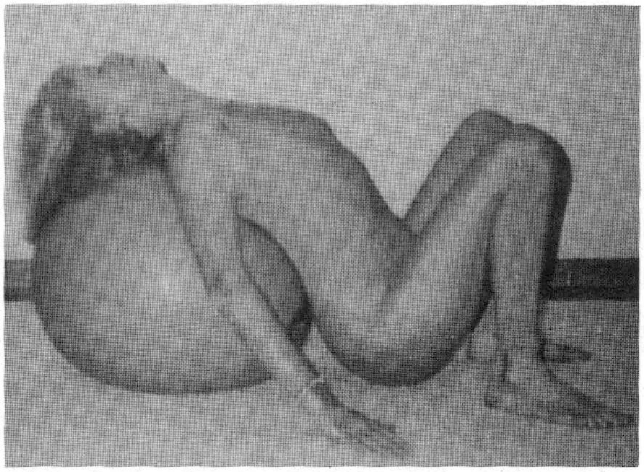

Figure 143. Resting backward over a large gymnastic ball for a few minutes several times a day relieves backache.

Sciatica may be helped if you stretch your hamstring muscles with a stirrup around your foot. Tie two neck ties together, or join two belts. Rest on your back and hook the strap round your foot. Slowly pull your leg high, exhaling, until you reach your limit. Stay there and keep breathing until you can raise the leg a little more.

Symptoms that you feel below the knee, such as tingling in your toes, indicate nerve compression. Traction is my first choice to relieve such pain, but in pregnancy this can be difficult. I have a *Backswing*, an inversion device wherein the ankles are fixed and the whole frame tilts at varying angles. This provides traction without needing a belt around the abdomen. (See Resources.) A gymnastic ball decompresses your spine and massages the muscles as you slowly rock back and forth from a squatting position.

If these techniques do not resolve your pain in a few days, find a physical therapist who can provide manual therapy. (See Resources for the American Physical Therapy Association, or call your local state chapter.)

Thoracic Pain

Pain in the "area of the bra strap" comes on during early pregnancy with the increased weight of the breasts. Resting backward over a gymnastic ball provides relief.

Sometimes pain is experienced in the area of one of the ribs, often from the baby's foot. A castor oil pack (see Resources) may help any local inflammation of the cartilage or friction massage can be tried. If the pain is referred from the thoracic spine you will need manual therapy.

Positioning for Comfort, Massage and Manual Therapy

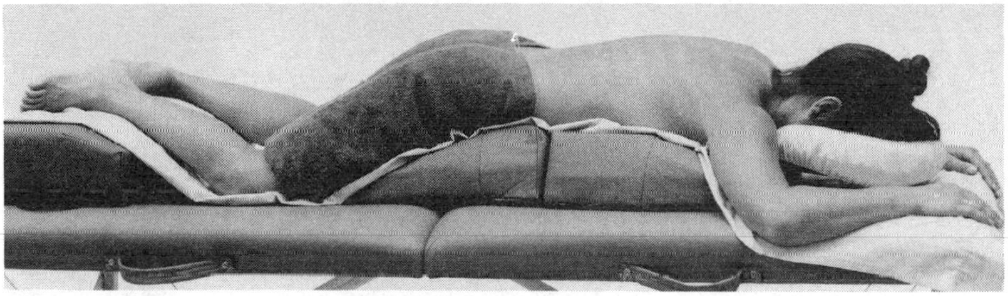

Figure 144. The bodyCushion™ accommodates prone lying through the end of pregnancy because the body is suspended on its bony frame.

The bodyCushion™, a combination of contoured cushions with a central concavity, allows you to lie on your front during pregnancy. Additional concavities accommodate the breasts. This support system is also ideal after birth and Cesarean section. It is highly recommended for women on prolonged bed rest, if affordable.

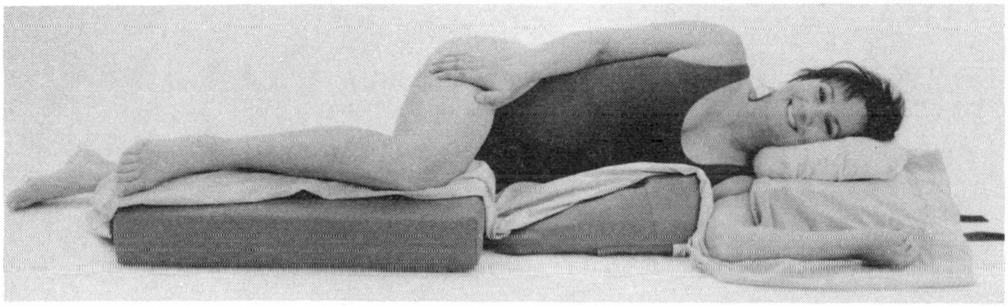

Figure 145. The bodyCushion™ can also position you optimally on your side.

Figure 148.

Posture Checklist

Incorrect Posture

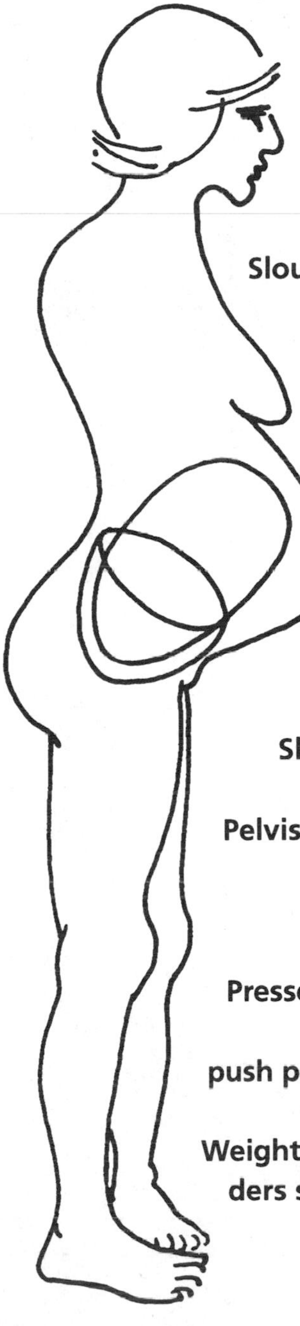

If neck sags, chin pokes forward, and whole body slumps.

Slouching cramps the rib cage and makes breathing difficult. Shoulders turn forward, arms roll in.

Slack muscles = hollow back. Pelvis tilts forward.

Pressed back knees strain joints, push pelvis forward.

Weight on inner borders strains arches.

To correct posture

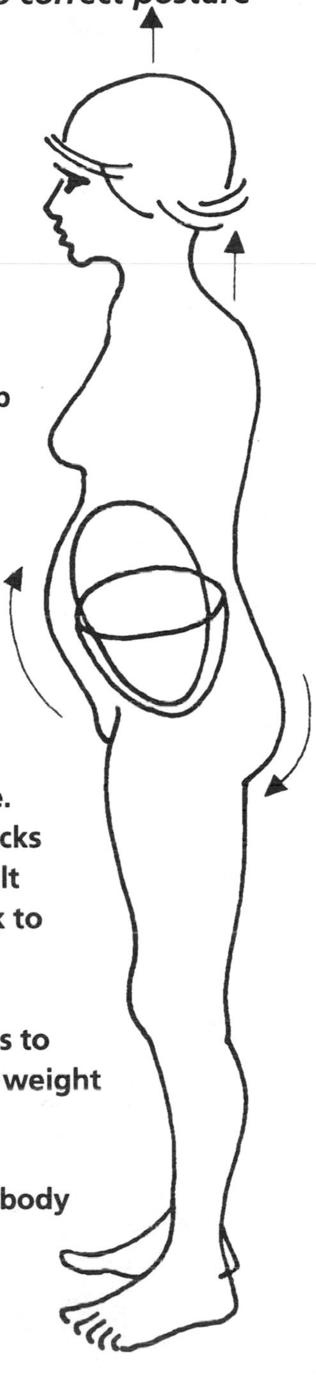

Straighten neck, tuck chin in so ear lines up with shoulder.

Lift up through rib cage and lower shoulders. Roll arms out.

Contract abdominal muscles to align spine. Tuck buttocks under to tilt pelvis back to neutral.

Bend knees to ease body weight over feet.

Distribute body weight through center of each foot.

Summary of Essential Prenatal Exercises

Do each exercise twice at first, progressing at your own pace to 5 times. The sequence can be repeated in reverse order. Rest and breathe deeply between each exercise.

1. Abdominal Wall Tightening on Outward Breath (page 94)

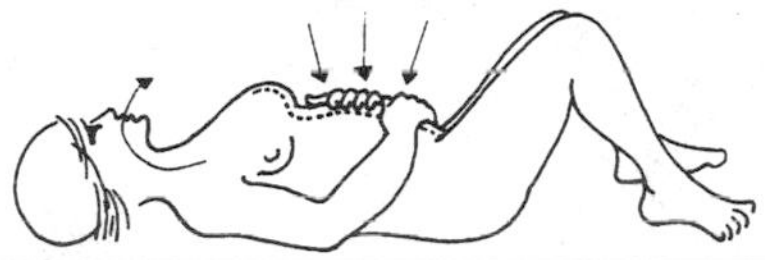

2. Pelvic Floor (See pages 75-80 for a full description.)

3. Stretch Out the Kinks on the bed, against the wall (page 142)

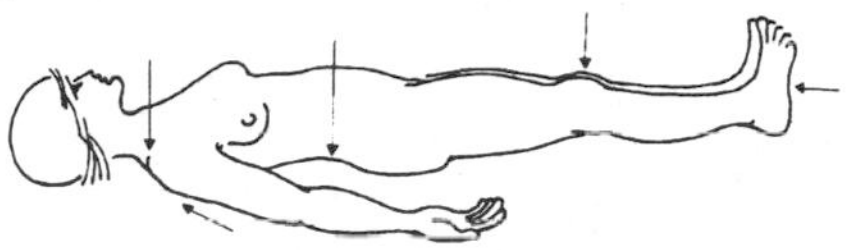

4. Pelvic Tilting in various positions (page 70)

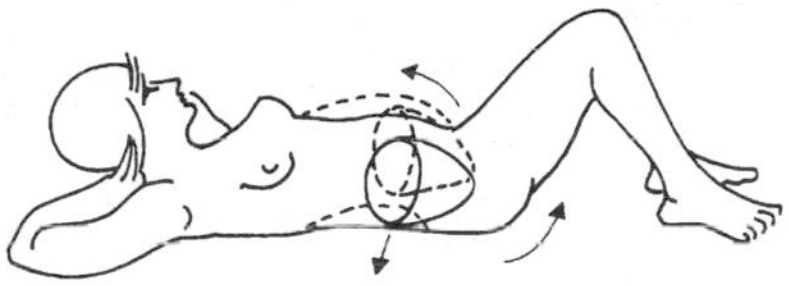

5. Heel-sliding (page 77)

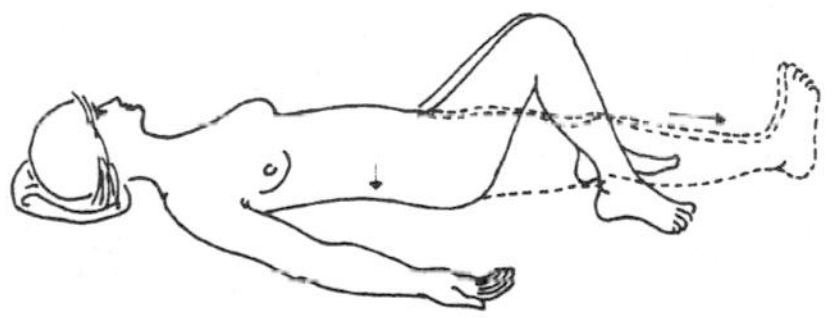

6. Bridging (page 118)

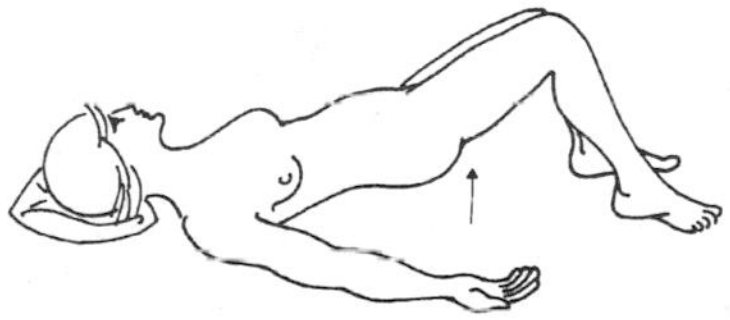

7. Straight Curl-up (page 78)

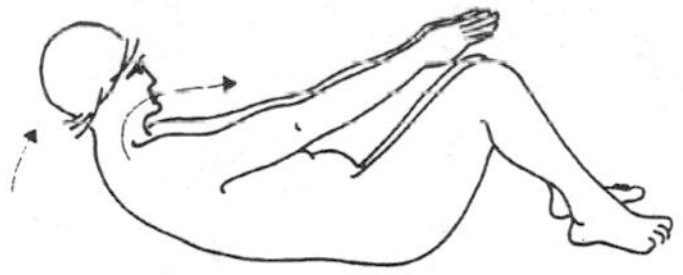

8. Diagonal Curl-up (page 79)

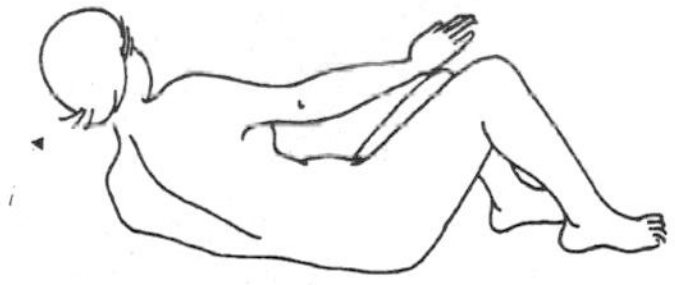

9. Squatting (page 129)

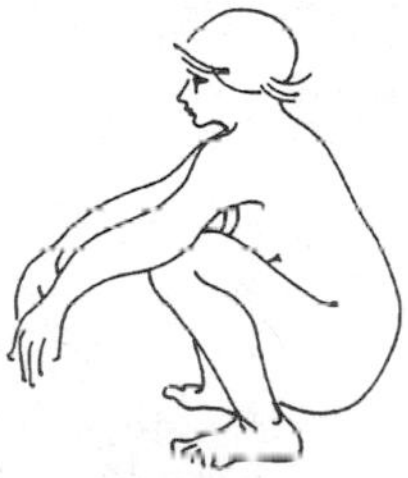

When **standing up**, roll over onto your knees and push off with your arms. When rising from the bed or floor, go on to one knee and straighten your legs to stand.

Posture Check (page 225)
Relaxation Session: Twenty minutes' complete tension release in any comfortable position twice daily.

Summary of Essential Postpartum Exercises

Commence within 24 hours; repeat each exercise twice to start, progressing at your own pace through the phases. Rest between each exercise and continue with normal breathing. The sequence can be repeated in reverse order for variety.

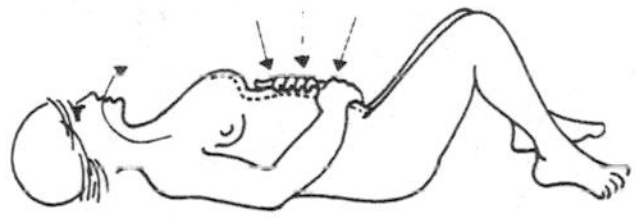

1. Deep Breathing with Abdominal Wall Tightening on outward breath (page 94)

2. Pelvic Floor Contractions (page 75)

Posture Check (page 225)
Before standing: Sit with legs over bed for a few minutes and swing your feet. Brace abdominals, buttocks, and pelvic floor when upright and walking around.

Relaxation: Lying on the front. (page 121-122) Half an hour, twice daily.

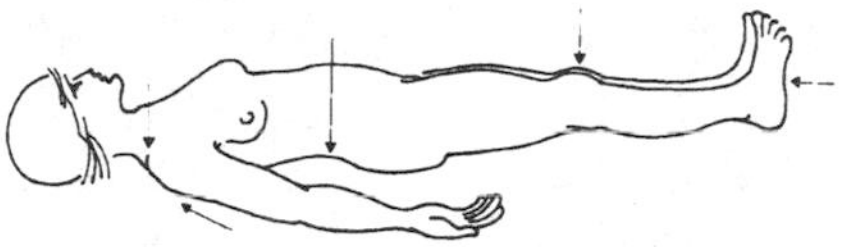

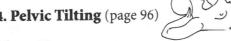

3. Stretch Out the Kinks (page 142)

4. Pelvic Tilting (page 96)

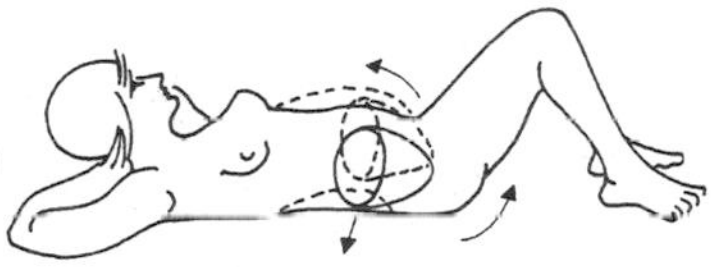

Phase II

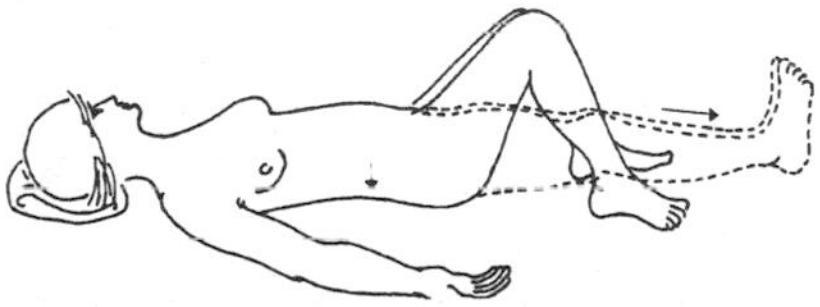

5. Heel Sliding (page 96)

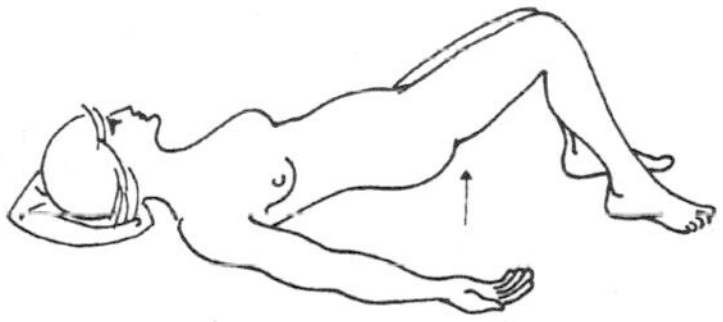

6. Bridging (page 143-44)

Phase III
Check your recti muscles after the third day (page 91). Check stopping and starting your urine flow (page 78).

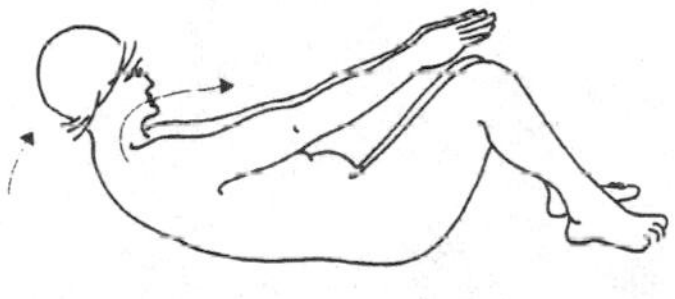

7. Straight Curl-up (page 78)

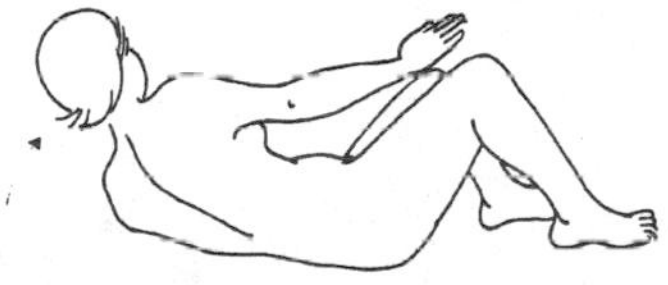

8. Diagonal Curl-up (page 79)

Phase IV
Progressive abdominal exercises (pages 103-105)

Summary of Post-Cesarean Essential Exercises

Commence as soon as you recover from the anesthetic. Do each exercise twice to start, progressing at your own pace through the phases. Relax and breathe deeply between each exercise. The sequence can be repeated in reverse order.

1. Breathing Exercises: Upper chest, mid-chest, diaphragmatic with abdominal wall-tightening (pages 94, 150).

2. Huffing (page 163). These two are very important if general anesthesia was used.

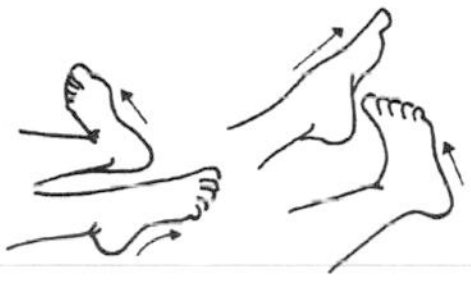

3. Foot Exercises (page 145)

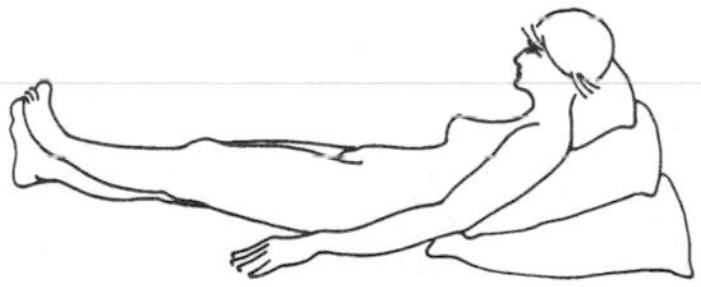

4. Leg Bracing (page 199)

Continue Exercises 3,4,5, for as long as you are confined to bed.

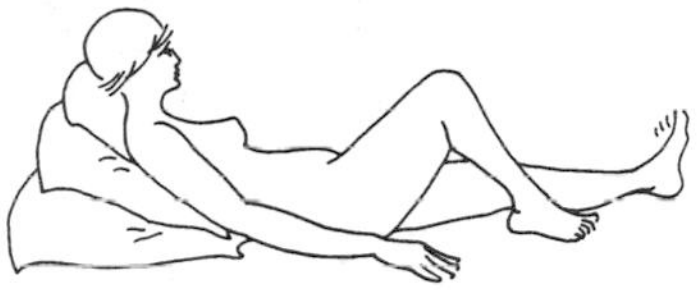

5. Bending and Straightening Alternate Knee (page 199)

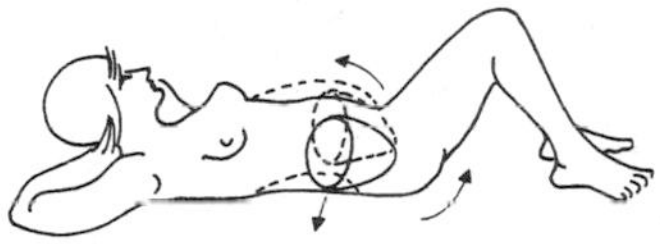

6. Pelvic Rocking (page 96)
Combine with pelvic floor contractions.

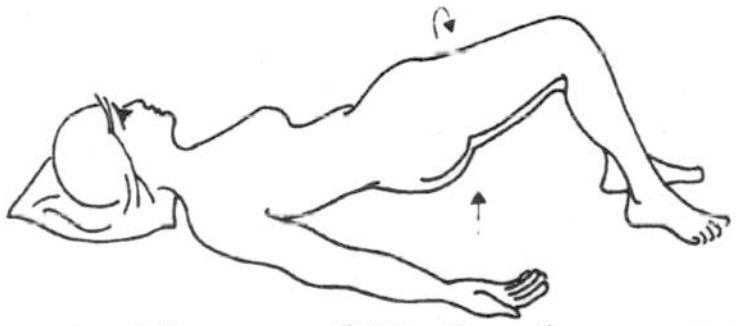

7. Bridge and Twist (page 200)

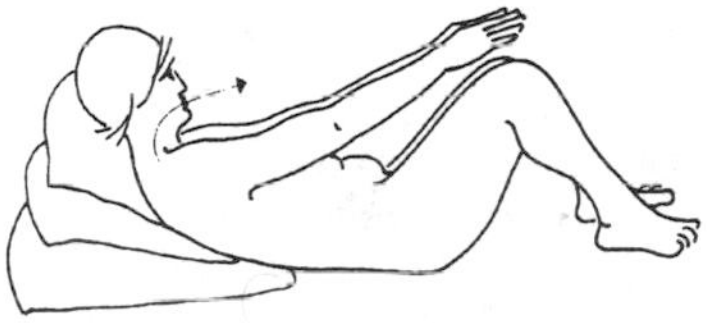

8. Straight Curl-up (page 102)

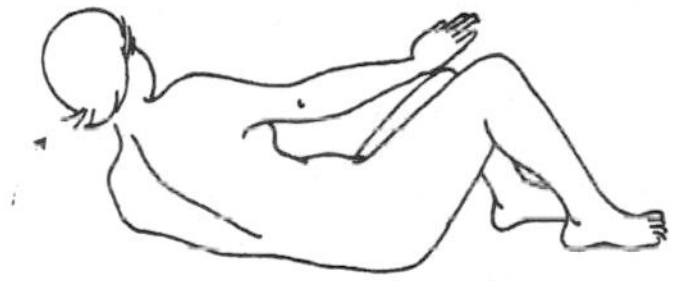

9. Diagonal Curl-up (page 102)

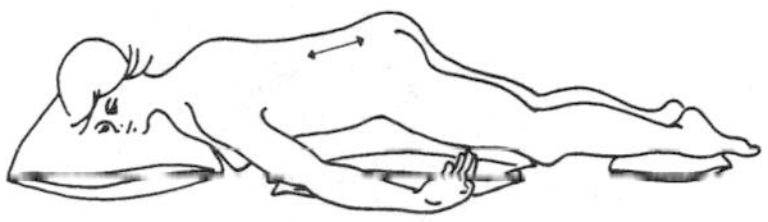

Relaxation on front when comfort permits (page 121-122)

Posture Check (page 225): Before standing, bend knees and use arms to turn toward edge of bed. Sit first and swing feet a few times. Brace abdominal muscles as you stand upright.

Phase II Check recti muscles after day 3 (page 91)
Stop and start urine flow (page 78)
Phase III **Progressive abdominal exercises** (pages 103-105)

List of Illustrations

Footnotes

Introduction

1 *Vaginal Birth After Cesarean.* For many decades it was a standard policy in the United States that "once a Cesarean, always a Cesarean."

2 The childbearing year officially consists of 9 prenatal and 3 postpartum months.

3 This weekend, which couples often find more convenient than a series of evening lectures, is described in my book, *Primal Connections,* New York: Simon and Schuster, 1993.

4 Balaskas, Janet. *Active Birth,* Boston: Harvard Common Press, 1992.

5 Bing, Elisabeth and Colman, Libby. "Better than Ever: Build your energy with our easy-to-follow diet and exercise plan." Lamaze Baby, 1994.

6 *After Baby Comes,* Woman's Hospital, Baton Rouge, LA.

7 Veldman, Frans. *L'Haptonomie,* Paris: Presses Universitaires de France, 1989.

Chapter 1

8 Kraus, Hans, MD. *Backache, Stress and Tension: Their Cause, Prevention and Treatment.* New York: Pocket Books, 1984.

9 The pelvic floor is also known as the perineum, perineal area, levator/es ani, pubococcygeus/ci, Kegel muscle, pelvic or urogenital diaphragm.

10 Premenstrual syndrome and dysmenorrhea are greatly helped by regular exercise.

11 Some physicians advise their patients to wait until the second trimester to start exercising for fear of spontaneous abortion (miscarriage.) Approximately one-quarter of conceptions fail (and at least one in eight persons is an unknowing surviving twin) Such loss is related usually to hormonal or chromosomal problems. If exercise caused miscarriage, women seeking abortions could go instead to aerobics classes, and we know that this is not true. The argument cannot be used in the reverse.

Chapter 2

12 Adapted from Peterson, James, *Strength Training for Women,* Champaign, IL: Human Kinetics, 1995.

13 Choprak, Deepak. *Magical Mind, Magical Body.* (Audiocassette tapes) 1993. Nightingale-Conant. See Resources.

14 Sometimes you may hear warnings about hyperflexion, too. However, hyperflexion is not a problem because when you bend elbows, knees, thighs or fingers, your soft tissues meet; thus you do not stretch your ligaments into any danger zone.

15 Adapted from *After Baby Comes,* Woman's Hospital, Baton Rouge, LA.

16 Adapted from unknown source.

17 An air bubble can enter the bloodstream via the unhealed placental site on the uterus and can result in sudden death. This completely passive position, when the vagina is still wide after birth, encourages a negative vacuum for air entry.

[18] The theory is that if you are upside down, your baby is now head-down, instead of presenting bottom first. It is hoped that s/he prefers the normal position and will turn; also the compression is less because gravity is assisting Baby to move.

[19] In Fonda's first pregnancy workout tape many exercises were repeated over 100 times!

[20] The American College of Obstetricians and Gynecologists (ACOG) considers the following conditions to be contraindications to vigorous exercise in pregnancy: history of three or more miscarriages, ruptured membranes, premature labor, incompetent cervix, bleeding or diagnosis of placenta previa, diagnosed heart disease, and multiple gestation. However, as a physical therapist who has worked with high-risk mothers in hospital, I believe in appropriate exercise; muscle atrophy must be avoided, especially in twin pregnancies, because the mother has so much extra physical work afterward.

[21] Never diet to lose weight during pregnancy. In fact, obese women are often malnourished and need careful dietary analysis. If they are morbidly obese, (body mass index—height/weight ratio—over 35) weight gain is typically limited to 15 pounds.

[22] Clapp, JF et al. "Exercise in Pregnancy—Good, Bad, or Indifferent?" Available from James F. Clapp, MD, Dept of OB-GYN, MetroHealth Medical Center, 2500 MetroHealth Drive, Cleveland, OH 44109.

_____"Exercise in Pregnancy." *Med Sci Sports Exercise,* 1992: 24 (suppl): S294—300.

_____"Exercise and Fetal Health." *J. Dev Physiol,* 1991 15:9-14.

_____"The course and outcome of labor following endurance exercise during pregnancy." *Am J Obstet Gynecol* 1990: 163 (6): 1799-1805.

[23] Bailey, Covert. *Smart Exercise.* Boston: Houghton Mifflin, 1994.

[24] *Marie Osmond's Exercises for Mothers-to-Be* is available only from New Life Images. See Resources and Order Form.

Chapter 3

[25] I developed a presentation called *Pelvic Integrity: Psychophysical Challenges in a Woman's Lifetime,* exploring both the inevitable and the preventable life events that we experience in this part of our body.

[26] A diagnostic exercise for SI pain is the *pelvic clock,* lying flat on your back. Bend your knees and place the soles of your feet together. Now circle your pelvis around like a belly dancer. If an SI joint is the problem, this movement will cause pain on one side.

[27] While there is no evidence that therapeutic ultrasound is harmful when given in pregnancy, and indeed it is given in many countries abroad, this modality is rarely used on pregnant women in the litigious United States because the effects are not known.

[28] Pronounced *pewbo-coxeegeeus.*

[29] Kegel, Arnold. "Stress incontinence of urine in women: physiologic treatment". *J Int. Coll Surgeons* 1956 (25)487-99.

______*The Pathological Physiology of the Pubococcygeus Muscle in Women.* (Film) Hollywood, CA: Morgan Camera Shop, 1953.

[30] Pessaries are mechanical devices of various shapes that are inserted into the vagina to provide support for the bladder or uterus.

[31] Even if you do not experience regular monthly bleeding after birth, it is possible to get pregnant from one unprotected intercourse because ovulation precedes menstruation.

[32] See the warning about postpartum air embolism on page 42.

[33] Bø Kari, et al. "Prevalence of stress urinary incontinence among physically active and sedentary female students." *Scand. J. Sports Sci* 1989 11(3):113-116.

[34] These may vary with gender. For example, little boys may play peeing games to direct their stream at objects. Boys and men typically find more convenient places to urinate than girls who are taught from an early age to hold it. Grown women frequently ignore the desire to void longer than men do.

[35] Paciornik, Claudio and Moyses. "Implications of the birth in the squatting position for the mother-child relationship," "Iatrogenicity of delivery in dorsal decubitus positon," "A comparsion between EEGs of Indians born through squatting position and Indians and civilized people born through dorsal decutibus delivery." Available from CCP Pesquisas, Rue Baltazar, Carrasco do Reis, 2245, Curitiba, Brazil, 80,000.

Paciornik, Moyses, Aprenda a Viver Com Os Indios. Rio De Janiero, Brasil: Editora Espaço e Tempo Ltda.

[36] Zaccharin, R.F. "A Chinese anatomy—the pelvis supports of the Chinese and occidentals compared and contrasted." Australian and New Zealand Journal of Obstetrics and Gynaecology February 1977 17(1): 1-11.

[37] *Urge incontinence* is experienced as an overwhelming need to void, simultaneously with the loss of urine. It is not provoked by mechanical stress like sneezing or jumping. In fact, it can happen lying in bed at night. There is a reciprocal relationship between your voluntary PF and the involuntary muscle of the bladder, although they are composed of different types of muscle fibers. Pelvic floor exercises help this condition by coordinating your voiding functions better and raising your confidence that if you *do* get the urge, then you have the external sphincter strength to control it long enough to find a toilet. Urge incontinence also has many other contributing factors, especially psychological ones, and may also be provoked by sudden increases in abdominal pressure, too.

[38] Benson, Ralph. *Handbook of Obstetrics and Gynecology.* New York: McGraw Hill, 1994.

[39] Episiotomy is our culture's vestige of genital mutilation, a problem of enormous proportions in Africa and the Middle East. North Americans are becoming aware of these barbaric practices because refugees from these countries have sought asylum, or arrests have been made for the hemorrhage or death of young girls in the United States, Canada, Australia and Europe. In its worst form, the procedure removes the inner and outer lips surrounding the vagina, and the clitoris, usually with a razor blade or a sharpened shell. The raw edges of the wound are sewn together leaving

just a matchstick-sized opening for both urine and menstrual flow. The girls often die of shock, bleeding, infection, or kidney failure because fluids are restricted and the legs are bound together for several weeks. Further cuts are necessary to prepare the "virgin" for first intercourse and again for childbirth, which otherwise would result in obstructed labor and death of mother and child. It has been estimated that there are between 40,000 and 60,000 women in the United States who have suffered genital mutilation or who are in danger of being "scraped clean." While North Americans are disgusted by these customs, this continent has the world's highest rate of non-ritualized circumcision of newborn males. This surgery is also done without the consent of the usually unanesthetized victim, and is also a form of sexual amputation. The adult circumcised male has lost 12 square inches of specialized erogenous tissue. See Resources and Further Reading for information on how to honor the integrity of the male infant body and just say "NO" to circumcision.

40 Some women suffer permanent damage from their episiotomies. As I write this I was consulted about an infected episiotomy in another state. Sadly, the therapist reported back to me that the mother died, in 1995!

41 If you have had anesthesia, you will be told what to do.

42 Occasionally one reads instructions to differentiate between anal and vaginal contractions. But they share the same nerve supply and it is only a matter of emphasis.

43 Single or lesbian women have used a dildo or vibrator, available from Eve's Garden or Good Vibrations. (See Resources.)

44 While I have emphasized strengthening in this chapter, it is just as important that a muscle be able to relax. Some women, especially those who have been sexually abused, may experience painful chronic tension in the PF. These muscles also are usually weak as the muscle never fully works or rests.

Chapter 4

45 Because the birth occurred outdoors, our next-door neighbors heard my primal sounds and thought we were using a chain-saw! A woman wrote to me after seeing my birth video, *Channel for a New Life* (see Resources). She remarked: "I just loved your birth. It seemed so self-indulgent—how wonderful!"

46 One of the first births I saw as a student was a young woman with paraplegia. I was impressed with the power of the uterus. In my own two births, however, I used my abdominal muscles very strongly.

47 Experienced birth attendants are not at all concerned by urine and/or feces around the time of birth. When they next see you, they will only be interested in the state of your health and your baby.

48 Learn to bear down with exhalation (as if for the second stage) and intermittently. Relax your legs with your feet on a stool and correct your diet to avoid constipation. Constipation refers to hard stool; frequency varies widely among people

49 If all fails, then there is always a "tummy tuck" done as outpatient surgery.

[54] You cannot do a pelvic tilt in squatting, because your pelvis is as far back as it will go. This makes squatting an ideal birth position, one less movement you need to do.

[51] In late pregnancy, however, the weight of the uterus compresses the major blood vessels in this position, so if you experience discomfort or feel faint, practise this in one of the other recommended positions.

[52] Raising both legs at any time overpowers your abdominal strength: the belly will bulge. Anyone can raise and lower their legs, but very few do the movement correctly without strain or injury. Occasionally, a woman can control her pelvic tilt only with single heel sliding. All exercises must be individualized—modification is as important as progression.

[53] Gymnastic balls in several sizes can be ordered from ***New Life Images.*** See order form at the of the book.

[54] Pelvic movements are practically impossible with the knees locked.

[55] I don't believe I have ever given anybody, man or woman, a thoracic flexion (rounding) exercise! On the contrary, we need to extend the thoracic spine (move backward instead of forward). Exercises that achieve this include back-to-back partner exercises, and stretching backward over a large gymnastic ball.

[56] Adapted from Simons, Jane. *Pregnant and in Perfect Shape.* Melbourne, Australia, Thomas Nelson, 1987.

[57] Adapted from Polden, Margie and Barbara Whiteford. *Postpartum Exercises.* London, UK: Century Hutchinson, 1984.

[58] It is easy enough to check **just once,** by curling-up half way, and then moving into a full sit-up. You'll feel when your muscles "change gear." In future, stop **before** that point when your hip flexors take over from your abdominals. Do curl-ups staying in low gear only!

[59] Your diagonal abdominal muscles work as soon as your shoulders leave the floor, even in a straight direction. They work more when you curl-up bringing one shoulder to the opposite knee.

[60] Avoid pulling on your neck.

[61] In contrast, double-leg-raising **begins** at the point of maximum difficulty and exertion. You will not know if you cannot hold your back flat until it **has** arched, as you strain to lift both legs off the ground simultaneously.

Chapter 5

[62] Even if a mother is comfortable breastfeeding in public, sometimes people around her avert their gaze as if she were doing something inherently wrong. New York State recently passed a law that it is legal to breastfeed in public and mothers, the few who dare cannot be stopped from doing this! African women who breastfeed anywhere are amazed that there is even a book on breastfeeding (such a normal body function) and of course, there are **many** books on the subject!

[63] The *anterior superior iliac spine.*

[64] Most commonly, pelvic tilt correction to neutral involves a backward movement of your wrists in this position. However, sexologists, among others, may refer to this as a forward pelvic tilt, because the pubic bone and genital area is raised.

[65] See Resources and Order Form for the videotape I made with Marie Osmond demonstrating palming.

[66] Some doctors even say that the rapidity with which a woman combs her hair or applies makeup (if she uses it) is a sure sign of recovery from delivery or surgery!

[67] Adapted by Vivienne White from the *Journal of the American Osteopathic Association,* August 1990, 90 (8) 686-703.

[68] Refer to the book *The Family Bed* by Tine Thevenin, for reassurance about sexual activity (It's simple: wait till the child is asleep.) and other concerns you may have.

[69] Even slight auto collisions may trigger preterm labor. If you should be this unlucky, be sure to report to your doctor or hospital for monitoring and perhaps 24 hours of observation.

[70] See page 99 for advice on back labor.

[71] Dunn, P. "Obstetric Delivery Today: For Better or For Worse?" *Lancet,* April 1976;1:7963.

Ehrstrom, Chr. "Forlossingstolar." Reprint from Recip Relex 13, 72 (1973) cited in Kirchoff, H. "The Woman's Posture During Childbirth." Organorama 14:1. 9 Organanon, Oss, The Netherlands.)

Fisher, Chloe. "The Management of Labour: A Midwife's View." In *Episiotomy: Physical and Emotional Aspects,* ed. Sheila Kitzinger, London: National Childbirth Trust, 9 Queensborough Terrace, London W.2 England, 1981.

Flynn, A.M., J. Kelly, F. Hollins. P.F. Lynch. "Ambulation in Labour," *British Medical Journal,* August 26, 1978: 591-93

[72] Cyriax, James, *Textbook of Orthopaedic Medicine,* Part 1. London, Balliere Tindall, 1978.

[73] This is part of a sequence of asanas that form the Salutation to the Sun in yoga. I recommend this daily routine for all women when the childbearing year is completed.

[74] A bra offers support but may compromise your lymph circulation. A 1995 book, *Dressed to Kill,* by Sydney Ross Signer and Soma Grismaijer makes a persuasive argument that wearing tight bras more than 12 hours a day can create a risk factor for breast cancer. Make sure that you take off your bra when you get home. If you have habitually worn tight, wired bras to push up your breasts, or sleep in your bra, I advise you to read this book. Women in traditional cultures are as astonished at the purpose of a bra as they are that a book would exist on such a basic function as breast-feeding!

[75] Ligaments are normally composed of connective tissue. However, the round ligaments grow out from the smooth or involuntary muscle of the uterus, becoming fibrous where they insert into a ligament in your groin on each side. Thus, this is the only ligament in the body that has some muscular components that go into spasm.

Chapter 6

[76] Gandevia, S.C., "Does the diaphragm fatigue during parturition?" Lancet Feb 6, 1993;341:347

[77] There is always residual air in your lungs which can be forcefully exhaled. This is a good abdominal exercise. The amount of air replaced is spontaneously regulated, making the need for conscious inhalation unnecessary

[78] Lamaze, Fernand. *Painless Childbirth: The Lamaze Method.* New York: Pocket, 1972.

[79] Psychoprophylaxis means "mind prevention." It is the basis of the Lamaze method which in the United States is promoted by the American Society for Psychoprophylaxis in Obstetrics.

[80] The Valsalva maneuver is named after the seventeenth century physician who recommended this technique to expel pus from the ear.

[81] Caldeyo-Barcia, R. "The influence of maternal position on labor," and "The influence of maternal bearing-down efforts in second stage of labor on fetal well-being." *Kaleidoscope of Childbearing: Preparation, Birth and Nurturing.* Simkin, Penny and Reinke, Carla. Eds. Seattle: the pennypress, 1978.

"Physiological and psychological bases for the modern and humanized management of normal labor," presented at the International Year of the Child, Commemorative International Congress, FIGO, Tokyo, October 21-22, 1979.

[82] Beynon, Constance. "The Normal Second Stage of Labour." *Journal of Obsterics and Gynaecology of the British Empire* December 1957; 64: 815-20

[83] Some people envisage the diaphragm pushing the baby out like a piston, or popping a cork out of a bottle!

Chapter 7

[84] I created, with a musician, a tape for guided recall of your experiences before and during birth. *Inside Experiences* is available for those born head-first, breech and also by Cesarean section. Most people find the tape very relaxing, and a way to connect more deeply with the growing baby inside. Some individuals connect with a prenatal incident or an event at the time of birth which is helpful in releasing misconceptions or negative judgments. Play this tape as often as you need to, and although it is never too late, begin as early as you can in the pregnancy. (See Resources.)

[85] Simonton, O. Carl, and Stephanie Matthews-Simonton, and James L. Creighton. *Getting Well Again.* New York: Bantam, 1978.

[86] Siegel, Bernie. *Peace, Love and Healing: Bodymind Communication and the Path of Self-Healing.* New York: Harper and Row 1990.

[87] Prenatal exercise classes that also facilitate discussion offer an opportunity for pregnant women to share their fears and expectations. In some cases, women have deep anxiety stemming from former reproductive experiences and need individual counseling in addition, which I call *personal reality therapy.*

[88] The uterus in labor is an exception. It contracts and retracts, that is, the muscle fibers never fully return to the prior length. Therefore, because the uterine cavity becomes increasingly smaller, the baby is squeezed out.

[89] Mitchell, Laura. *Simple Relaxation.* New York: Athaneum, 1979.

[90] Vellay, Pierre. *Childbirth without Pain.* London: Allen and Unwin, 1959.

[91] Huxley, Aldous. *The Art of Seeing.* London: Flamingo, 1994.

[92] Op cit. 78.

[93] Dick-Read, Grantly. *Childbirth without Fear.* New York: Harper and Row, 1979.

[94] Bradley, Robert. *Husband-Coached Childbirth.* New York: Harper and Row, 1974.

[95] Paciornik, Moyses. *Birth in the Squatting Position,* Boston: Polymorph Films, 1991.

[96] Remember to watch for curling toes during labor—a classic indicator of tension.

[97] You can make a deeper connection with your partner by "extending yourself into his or her hand, elbow, shoulder and ultimately the whole body," just as a person with visual impairment uses a cane to prolong his or her sense of touch all the way to the tip of that cane.

[98] This type of massage is known as *effleurage.*

[99] This angle is formed by the axes of the maternal and fetal spines, and is ideally between 60 and 80 degrees to guide the baby's head toward the back of the pelvis. In the supine position, this angle is diminished. In cases of severe *diastasis recti,* it is increased and may prevent engagement.

[100] Another very useful preparation for both expectant parents is to write a *Birth Story.* Describe the birth from start to finish in the past tense. Then compare stories with your partner. This is a process of deep personalization for the expectant father.

[101] Sosa, Roberto, John Kennell, Marshal Klaus, Steven Robertson and Juan Urrutia, "The effect of a supportive companion on perinatal problems, length of labor and maternal and infant attachment. *New England Journal of Medicine,* September 11, 1980; 303(11):597-600.

[102] In my book, *Primal Connections: How experiences from conception to birth affect our emotions, behavior and health,* I describe how people can relive their experiences of birth. For most adult Americans today, this invariably means reliving the effects of drugs and anesthetics. Adults commonly recall "being in a fog," passing out, as well as frightening moments of being unable to breathe. I have actually smelled anesthetic gas on their breath as their bodies recall and release the experience.

[103] Rigard, Lennart and Kittie Franz. *Delivery Self-Attachment.* See Resources.

[104] I am fully aware of the cardioprotective effect of these agents, and their effect on bone metabolism although I prefer a natural lifestyle and alternative remedies.

Chapter 8

[105] Inverted postures put you at risk of air embolism until all bleeding has ceased.

[106] Other attempts to simulate a contraction include your partner squeezing above your knee, or twisting the skin in opposite directions on your arm. The partner exercises

involve you both, provide for rest intervals as you alternate, and have the added benefit of stretching tight muscles. Most importantly, they allow you to learn surrender and to see your progress as you move forward to ever more challenging limits that you thought were beyond your ability.

[107] "Focus on Cesarean and VBAC." *International Journal of Childbirth Education,* November, 1994; 9(4) (The entire issue.)

[108] National Center for Health Statistics, 1992.

[109] Wound induration, a thickening of the skin and underlying tissues, is normally present for up to eight to twelve weeks, depending on the individual patient.

[110] Therapeutic ultrasound, as given for muscle injuries, relieves the pain and swelling of episiotomies and hemorrhoids. Unlike the different type of ultrasound used in medical diagnosis, it should not be given over your scar because of possible harm to your ovaries and uterus.

Chapter 10

[111] Personal communication.

[112] A drug given to women a generation ago to prevent miscarriage.

[113] National Center for Health Statistics, 1992

[114] Mothers are seldom kept in the hospital for more than a few days in the United States because of the cost.

[115] Since that year (1956) Dr. Cheek's practice had no more breech presentations or erythroblastosis (Rh incompatibility), two more conditions which he believes are associated with maternal anxiety.

[116] Dr. John Braxton-Hicks, after whom the uterine contractions of pregnancy are named, wrote in 1871 that women did not notice these contractions unless they were worried about something. These contractions begin in the third month, and an outsider can also feel the uterus tightening (which lasts from a few seconds to up to a half-hour) by resting a hand on the uterus.

[117] Ideomotor signals are an established component of hypnosis. The client chooses a "yes" finger, a "no" finger and an "I don't want to answer" finger. (There is never an "I don't know" finger.) Just as during conversation we nod or shake our heads unconsciously and repetitively, we can use the muscles of our fingers to tell us about unconscious feelings and memories. After setting up these ideomotor signals, the woman can scan her night's sleep on awakening for any events or emotions in her dreams that need to be brought to conscious awareness.

[118] Gladys McGarey, M.D., cites a case of a baby whom she delivered with a fine scar instead of a harelip and cleft palate. The condition was allegedly healed in the uterus when the castor oil pack was applied for bleeding. Further details on castor oil packs, and the materials, can be obtained from Dr. McGarey, the ARE Medical Clinic in Phoenix, Arizona, Women–to–Women in Yarmouth, Maine, and Home Health Products in Virginia Beach. (See Resources.)

[119] Since I founded the *Section on Women's Health* of the American Physical Therapy Association, we have gained over fifteen hundred members. Large hospitals have physical therapy departments but smaller units do not. You may need to search for a therapist. (See Resources.)

[120] Katz, VL. Et al. "A comparison of bed rest and immersion for treating the edema of pregnancy." *Obstetrics and Gynecology,* February, 1990, 75 (2):147-51. Franchio, M and A. Markell, "Immersion: alternative to bed rest for pregnancy-related edema." *Advance for PTs* 1994, 5 (41): 5.

[121] My mother was on bed rest when she carried me; I became a pioneer in prenatal exercise in general, and for mothers restricted to bed in particular!

[122] The work of dietician Agnes Higgins, cited in Brewer, Gail Sforza and Tom Brewer. *What Every Pregnant Woman Should Know: The Truth about Diet and Drugs in Pregnancy.* Rev. Ed. New York: Viking: Penguin, 1985.

[123] I have counseled expectant mothers whose spouse, mother, twin or child died during pregnancy, and these experiences can shake the very foundations of the new life. I speak from personal experience, as my sister died when my mother was six months' pregnant with me. She was on bed rest for spotting and I have recalled the loss of my twin as well.

[124] Evans, A. "Childhood sexual abuse, prematurity and neonatal medical problems." presented at the *Pre- and Perinatal Psychology Association of North America Congress* in Amherst, MA, 1989.

[125] L. DeMause, "The Universality of Incest," *J Psychohistory,* Fall 1991;19(2):123-164.

[126] Hutson, H. Range, Anglin, Deidre and Pratts, Michael. "Adolescents and Children Injured or Killed by Drive-by Shootings in Los Angeles. *New England Journal of Medicine,* 3/29/95;330 (5):324

References and Further Reading

Aivanhov, Master Omraam Mikhael. *Education Begins Before Birth*. Los Angeles: Editions Prosveta, 1982.

Anderson, Bob. *Stretching*. Bolinas, CA: Shelter Publications, 1980.

Arms, Suzanne. *Immaculate Deception II: A Fresh Look at Childbirth*. Berkeley: Celestial Arts, 1994.

_____*Seasons of Change: Growing through Pregnancy and Birth*. Durango, CO: Kivaki Press, 1995 (970) 385-1767.

Baker, Jeannine Parvati. *Conscious Conception: Elemental Journey Through the Labyrinth of Sexuality*. Monroe, UT: Freestone, 1986.

_____*Hygieia: A Woman's Herbal*. Monroe, UT: Freestone, 1978.

_____*Prenatal Yoga and Natural Birth*. Monroe, UT: Freestone, 1986.

Bailey, Covert, and L. Bishop. *The Fit or Fat Woman*. Boston, MA: Houghton Mifflin, 1989.

_____*Smart Exercise*. Boston, MA: Houghton Mifflin, 1994.

Bean, Constance. *Methods of Childbirth*, revised edition, New York: William Morrow, 1990.

Benson, Herbert, MD. *The Relaxation Response*. Avenal, NJ: Outlet Book Co. 1993.

Benson, Ralph. *Handbook of Obstetrics and Gynecology*. 11th ed., New York: McGraw Hill, 1994.

Bing, Elisabeth, and Libby Colman. *Making Love During Pregnancy*. New York: Bantam Books, 1994.

Boston Women's Health Book Collective. *The New Our Bodies, Ourselves*. New York: Simon & Schuster, 1992.

Brewer, Gail Sforza. rev. ed. *What Every Pregnant Woman Should Know: The Truth about Diet and Drugs in Pregnancy*. New York: Penguin, 1985.

Bright, Susie. *Susie Bright's Sexual Reality: A Virtual Sex World Reader*. Pittsburgh: Cleis, 1992.

Capacchione, Lucia, and Bardsley, Sandra. *Creating a Joyful Birth Experience*. New York: Simon and Schuster, 1995.

Chamberlain, David. *Babies Remember Birth*. L.A: Tarcher, 1988.

Cheek, David B. *Hypnosis: The Application of Ideomotor Techniques*. Boston: Allyn and Bacon, 1994.

Childs-Gowell, Elaine. *Good Grief Rituals: Tools for Healing*. Barrytown, NY: Station Hill Press, 1992.

Chopra, Deepak. *Quantum Healing: Exploring the Frontiers of Body, Mind and Medicine.* New York: Bantam, 1990.

Cohen, Nancy, and Lois Estner. *Silent Knife: Cesarean Birth and Vaginal Birth after Cesarean*. Westport CT: Bergin and Garvey, 1983.

_____*Open Season: Survival Guide for Natural Childbirth and VBAC in the 90s*. Westport CT: Bergin & Garvey, 1992.

Colbin, Annemarie. *Food and Healing*. New York: Ballantine, 1986.

Creager, Caroline Corning. *Therapeutic Exercises Using the Swiss Ball.* Minneapolis, MN: Executive, 1994.

Davis-Floyd, Robbie. *Birth as an American Rite of Passage*. Berkeley, CA: U. Cal. Press, 1992.

Dunham, Carol, and the Body Shop Team. *Mamatoto: A Celebration of Birth*. New York: Penguin 1991.

English, Jane. *Different Doorway: Adventures of a Caesarean Born*. Point Reyes Station, CA: Earth Hart, 1985.

Enkin, Murray, Marc J., N.C. Kierse, Mary Renfrew, and James Nielson. *A Guide to Effective Care In Pregnancy and Childbirth*. New York: Oxford University Press, 1995.

Faludi, Susan. *Backlash: The Undeclared War Against American Women*. New York: Crown, 1992.

Federation of Feminist Women's Health Centers. *A New View of a Woman's Body*. Feminist Health Press: West Hollywood, CA, 1991.

Frantz, Kittie. *Breastfeeding Product Guide*. Sunland, CA: Geddes Productions, 1994.

Gaskin, Ina May. *Babies, Breastfeeding and Bonding*. Westport, CT: Bergin and Garvey 1987.

_____*Spiritual Midwifery*. 3rd edition. Summertown, TN: Book Publishing Company, 1990.

Goer, Henci. *Obstetric Myths Versus Research Realities*. Westport, CT: Bergin and Garvey, 1995.

Hodson, Geoffrey. *The Miracle of Birth: A Clairvoyant Study of a Human Embryo*. Wheaton, IL: Theosophical Publishing House, 1981.

Johnson, Sonia. *Going Out of Our Minds: The Metaphysics of Liberation*. Freedom, CA: Crossing Press, 1987.

_____*Wildfire/Igniting the Shevolution*. Albuquerque, NM: Wildfire Books, 1989.

Jordan, Sandra. *Yoga During Pregnancy*. Honolulu: Sun Moon, 1987.

Kendall, Florence, and Dorothy Wadsworth. *Muscles: Testing and Function*. 4th edition. Baltimore: Williams and Wilkins, 1993.

Keith, L.G. and Keith, D., Papiernik-Berhauer, E., and Luke, B., eds. Multiple *Pregnancy: Epidemiology, Gestation, and Perinatal Outcome.* New York: Parthenon, 1995.

Kitzinger, Sheila. *The Experience of Childbirth*. New York: Viking Penguin, 1990.

Kitzinger, Sheila, and Penny Simkin, eds. *Episiotomy and the Second Stage of Labor*. Seattle: The pennypress, 1984 (Available from Birth and Life Bookstore and ICEA, see Resources.)

Kraus, Hans, MD. *Backache, Stress and Tension: Their Cause, Prevention and Treatment*. New York: Pocket Books, 1984.

Ladas, Alice, and Beverley Whipple. *The G-Spot and Other Recent Discoveries About Human Sexuality*. New York: Holt, Rinehart and Winston, 1982.

Lasater, Judith H. *Relax and Renew: Restful Yoga for Stressful Times*. Berkeley, CA: Rodmell Press, 1995.

Leboyer, Frederick. *Birth Without Violence*. New York: Knopf, 1975.

Levine, Stephen. *Who Dies?: An Investigation of Conscious Living and Conscious Dying*. New York: Doubleday, 1982.

Lichy, Roger, and E. Herzberg. *The Waterbirth Handbook*. Gateway Books, UK: Atrium, 1992.

Liedloff, Jean. *The Continuum Concept.* Reading, MA: Addison Wesley, 1985.

Lowen, Alexander, MD. *Bioenergetics*. New York: Penguin, 1976.

Miller, Alice. *For Your Own Good: Hidden Cruelty in Child-Rearing and the Roots of Violence*. New York: Farrar, Straus, Giroux, 1984.

Mitford, Jessica. *The American Way of Birth*. New York: Penguin, 1992.

Montagu, Ashley. *Touching: The Human Significance of the Skin*. New York: Harper & Row, Perennial Library, 1978.

Nathanielsz. Peter. *Life Before Birth and A Time to Be Born*. Ithaca, NY: Prometheus, 1992.

Nilsson, Lennart. *A Child is Born*. New York: Delacorte, 1990.

Noble, Elizabeth. *Childbirth with Insight*. Boston: Houghton Mifflin, 1983. Available from *New Life Images.*

_____*Primal Connections: How Our Experiences From Conception Through Birth Influence Our Emotions, Behavior and Health*. New York: Simon & Schuster, 1993. Available from *New Life Images.*

_____*Having Twins*. Boston: Houghton Mifflin, 1988.

Noble, Elizabeth. *Marie Osmond's Exercises for Mothers and Babies*. New York: New American Library, 1985. Available from *New Life Images*.

Northrup, Christiane. *Women's Bodies, Women's Wisdom*. New York: Bantam, 1994.

Odent, Michel. *The Nature of Birth and Breastfeeding*. Westport, CT: Bergin and Garvey, 1992.

Olkin, Sylvia Klein. *Positive Pregnancy Fitness*. New York: Avery, 1988.

_____*Positive Parenting Fitness*. New York: Avery, 1992.

Panuthos, Claudia. *Transformation through Birth.* Westport, CT: Bergin and Garvey.

Pearce, Joseph Chilton. *Magical Child.* New York: Bantam, 1981.

_____ *Magical Child Matures*. New York: Bantam, 1986.

Poole, Catherine, and Elizabeth Parr. *Choosing a Nurse-Midwife*. New York:Wiley, 1994.

Peterson, Gayle. *An Easier Childbirth*. Los Angeles: Tarcher, 1992.

Reich, Wilhelm. *The Function of the Orgasm*. Trans. Vincent R. Carfagno. New York: Simon and Schuster, 1973.

Renfrew, Mary, Chloe Fisher and Suzanne Arms. *Breastfeeding: Getting Breastfeeding Right for You*. Berkeley, CA: Celestial Arts, 1990.

Ritter, Thomas J. *Say No to Circumcision!* Aptos, CA: Hourglass, 1992.

Robertson, Laurel, Flinders, Carol and Godfrey, Bronwen. *Laurel's Kitchen: A Handbook for Vegetarian Cookery and Nutrition*. New York: Bantam Books, 1982.

Rothman, Barbara K. ed. *Encyclopedia of Childbearing: Critical Perspectives*. Washington, DC: Oryx Press, 1993.

________*Recreating Motherhood: Ideology and Technology in a Patriarchal Society.* New York: Norton, 1989.

Schwartz, Leni. *Bonding Before Birth*. Salem, MA: Sigo, 1991.

Shealy, C. Norman, and Caroline M. Myss. *The Creation of Health: Merging Traditional Medicine with Intuitive Diagnosis*. Walpole, NH: Stillpoint, 1988.

Siegel, Bernie. Peace, *Love and Healing: Body Mind Communication and the Path of Self-Healing*. New York: Harper and Row, 1990.

Signer, Sydney Ross, and Soma Grismaijer. *Dressed to Kill*. Garden City, NY: Avery, 1995.

Simonton, O. Carl, Matthews-Simonton, Stephanie, and Creighton, James L. *Getting Well Again*. New York: Bantam, 1978.

Solter, Aletha. *The Aware Baby*. Goleta, CA: Shining Star Press, 1984.

Stone, Randolph. *Polarity Therapy: Complete Works*. Vol. 1, 1986, Vol. II, 1987. Sebastopol, CA: CRCS Publishers.

Thevenin, Tine. *The Family Bed*. Wayne, NJ: Avery, 1987.

Verny, Thomas, M.D., with John Kelly. *The Secret Life of the Unborn Child.* New York: Summit, 1981.

Verny, Thomas, and Pamela Weintraub. *Nurturing the Unborn Child: A Nine-Month Program for Soothing, Stimulating and Communicating with Your Baby.* New York: Bantam, 1991.

Wagner, Marsden. *Pursuing the Birth Machine*. Camperdown, NSW, Australia: Ace Graphics, 1995.

Watts, Alan. *The Wisdom of Insecurity*. New York: Random House, 1951.

White, Gregory. *Emergency Childbirth*. Marble Hill, MO: NAPSAC Reproductions. 13th edition, 1994. (Available from Birth and Life Bookstore and ICEA. See Resources.)

Wolfe, Honora Lee. *How to Have a Healthy Pregnancy, Healthy Birth According to Traditional Chinese Medicine*. Boulder, CO: Blue Poppy Press (800) 487-9296) 1993.

Resources

Maternity Comfort Items

BabyHugger, Trennaventions, 131 Hill Street, Derry, PA 15627, (412) 694-5283 (abdominal support)

Backswing, Hammacher Schlemmer, 9180 Le Saint Drive, Fairfield, OH 45014, (800) 543-3366

Bailey Manufacturing, PO Box 130, Lodi, OH 44254, (800) 345-3371 (positioning wedges)

Bodycare, 315 Gilmer Ferry Road, Ball Ground, GA 30107, (800) 858-9888, (Posture-Curve Lumbar Cushion)

Body Support Systems, Inc., PO Box 337, Ashland, OR 97520, (800) 448-2400, (503) 488-1172 (bodyCushion™)

Carpal Care® Rehabilitation Program for Carpal Tunnel Syndrome, Repetitive Motion Trauma Corporation, 820 Arlington Heights Road, Itasca, IL 60143, (800) 860-RMTC, (708) 285-8900, Fax: (708) 773-0358

CMO Inc, PO Box 147, Barbeeton, OH 44203, (216) 745-9679, (800) 344-0011 (mother-to-be abdominal lift pad)

ComfyBack/ComfyWedge, PO Box 988, Venice, CA 90294 (seating wedge with removable coccyx insert)

Contour Form Products, PO Box 328, Greenville, PA 16125, (800) 223-8808, (412) 588- 4452, Fax: (412) 588-864 (moldable hot or cold gel packs that can be inserted into a custom-made maternity support)

D-Med, Inc.,/AOL), PO Box 700, Highland Park, IL 60035-0700, (800) USA D-MED, (708) 433-1021, Fax: (708) 433-1565, (customizable foot orthotics, (arch supports), call for referrals to clinicians in your area)

Embracing Concepts Inc, 76 Woodside Drive, Penfield, NY 14526, (716) 381-9229 Fax: (716) 458-0593, (*Isch-Dish* for coccyx and "sit-bone" pain and *Spinalign*)

Gottfried Medical, PO Box 8996, Toledo, OH 43623, (800) 537-1968, (419) 328-5216, (corset)

IEM Orthopedics, PO Box 592, Ravenna, OH 44266, (800) 992-6594, (216) 297-7652, Fax: (216) 297-6568, (maternity lumbo-pelvic support).

Jerome Medical, 102 Gaither Drive, Mt. Laurel, NJ 08054, (800) 257-8440. (Tummy grip)

Jobst, PO Box 471048, Charlotte, NC 28247-1048, (800) 537-1063, Fax: (704) 551-8581(support wear, leg health products, skin care)

Living Arts, PO Box 2939, Venice, CA 90291-2939, (800) 2-LIVING, (relaxation and yoga items)

Loving Lift™ and Action Lift™ Moore products, PO Box 647, Rewood, CA 94002-0647, (800) 457-1567, Ph/Fax: (415) 592-8174, (corset)

Medela Inc, PO Box 660, McHenry, IL 60051-0660, (800) 435-8316, Fax: (815) 363-1246, (maternity lumbo-pelvic support)

Medi Support Hose, 76 W. Seegers Road, Arlington Heights, IL 60005, (800) 633-6334

Natural Energy Works, PO Box 364, El Cerrito, CA 94530, Phone/Fax: (510) 526-5978, (products offering protecting from environmental hazards and related health and social issues)

Psychological Corporation, PO Box 839954, San Antonio, TX 78283-3954, (800) 228-0752, Fax: (800) 232-1223, (video: *Swiss Ball Exercises for Chronic Pain Patients)*

Tecnol, 6625 Industrial Park Boulevard, Fort Worth TX 76180, (800)523-3660, (817) 577-6426., (*Warm 'n Form*, moldable insert for lumbar support)

Quickmed Supplies, 3421 San Fernando Road, Los Angeles, CA 90065, (800) 966-1111, (213) 259-1000, Fax: (213) 259-0401, (Theraband®, posture pillows, wedges)

Scott Specialities, Inc., PO Box 508, Belleville, KS 66935, (913) 527-5627 (800) 255-7136, Fax: (800) 531-9826, (abdominal support)

Self Care Catalog, 5850 Shellmound Street, Emeryville, CA 94608-1901, (800) 345-3371, (Orthopod Inversion Machine, a type of backswing with weight taken on the upper thighs and lower abdomen suitable for postpartum)

Suits Me Swimwear, 2377 Deltona Boulevard, Spring Hill, FL 33526, (904) 666-1485, (adjustable for pregnancy or women with disabilities)

Visual Health Information, PO Box 44646, Tacoma, WA 98444, (800) 356-0709, (ball exercises on cards)

Telephone Hypnosis

Birth Resources, Gayle Peterson, Ph.D., 1749 Vine Street, Berkeley, CA 94703, (510) 526-5951

Cheek, David. B. M.D., 1140 Bel Air Drive, Santa Barbara, CA 93105 (805) 569-7161

Klaus, Marshall, M.D., and Phyllis Klaus, M.S.W., 657 Creston Road, Berkeley, CA 94708, (415) 528-4458

Organizations

Aerobics and Fitness Association of America, (AFAA), 15250 Ventura Boulevard, Suite 310, Sherman Oaks, CA 91403(818) 905-0040

Alliance of Genetic Support Groups, 35 Wisconsin Circle Suite 440, Chevy Chase, MD 20815, (800) 336-4363, Fax: (301) 654-0171

American Academy of Husband-Coached Childbirth, (AAHCC), PO Box 5244, Sherman Oaks, CA 91413, (818) 788-6662, (800) 423-2397 California: (800) 42-BIRTH

American Academy of Medical Hypnosis Analysts, (AAMH), 710 East Ogden, Suite 208, Naperville, IL 60563, (800) 34-HYPNO

American Association for Pre- and Peri-natal Psychology and Health, (APPPAH), 5999 Stevenson Avenue, Alexandria, VA 22304-3300 (703) 823-9800 extension 246, Fax: (703) 823-0252

American Board of Preventive Medicine, 9950 W. Lawrence Avenue, #106, Schiller Park, IL 60176, (708) 671-1750

American College of Home Obstetrics, PO Box 508, Oak Park, IL 60303 (708) 383-1461

American College of Nurse-Midwives, 818 Connecticut Avenue, Suite 900, Washington, DC 20006, (202) 728-9860, Fax: (202) 728-9897

American College of Obstetricians and Gynecologists, (ACOG), 409 12th Street SW, Washington, DC 20024-2188, (800) 762-ACOG, (202) 638-5577

American College of Osteopathic Obstetricians and Gynecologists, (ACOOG), 900 Auburn Road, Pontiac, MI 48342-3365, (800) 875-6360, (810) 332-6360, Fax: (810) 332-4607

American College of Sports Medicine, PO Box 1440, Indianapolis, IN 46206-1440, (317) 637-9200

American Council on Exercise, (ACE), 5820 Oberlin Drive, #102, San Diego, CA 92121, (800) 529-8227, Fax: (619) 535-1778

American Foundation for Maternal and Child Health, 439 E. 51st Street, New York, NY 10022, (212) 759-5510

American Holistic Medical Association, 4101 Lake Boone Trail, Suite 201, Raleigh, NC 27607, (919) 787-0116

American Holistic Nurses Association, 4101 Lake Boone Trail, Suite 201, Raleigh, NC 27607, (919) 787-5181, Fax: (919) 787-4916

American Institute of Preventive Medicine, 30445 NW Highway, Suite 350, Farmington Hills, MI 48334, (810) 539-1800

American Gentle Birthing Association, 1804 SW Oak Knoll Court, Lake Oswego, OR 97034, (503) 636-7823

American Nurses Association, 600 Maryland Avenue, SW Suite 100, Washington, DC 20024, (202) 554-4444

American Physical Therapy Association, 333 North Fairfax Street, Suite 400, Alexandria, VA 22314, (800) 999-APTA, (extension 3237 for *Section on Women's Health)*

American Polarity Therapy Association, 2888 Bluff Street, Suite 149, Boulder, CO 80301, (800) 878-3373, (303) 545-2080, Fax: (303) 545-2161

American Society for Psychoprophylaxis in Obstetrics, (ASPO), 110 Connecticut Avenue NW, Washington, DC 20036, (800) 368-4404, (Lamaze method)
American Society for Psychosocial Obstetrics and Gynecology, 409 12th Street SW, Suite 700, Washington, DC 20024-2188, (202) 863-1648, Fax: (202) 554-0453
American Society of Clinical Hypnosis, 2200 E. Devon Ave., Suite 291, Des Plaines, IL 60018, (708) 297-3317, Fax: (708) 297-7309
American Society of Dowsers, Inc., Danville, VT 05828, (802) 684-3417, Fax: (802) 684-2565, (for information not available through the conscious mind)
Association for Childbirth at Home International, (ACHI), PO Box 430, Glendale, CA 91209, (818) 545-7128, Fax: (818) 409-1728
Association of Labor Assistants and Childbirth Educators, (ALACE), 174 Cushing Street, Cambridge, MA 02138, (617) 441-2500
Association of Women's Health, Obstetric and Neonatal Nurses, 700 14th Street NW, Suite 600, Washington, DC 20025, (800) 673-8499, (202) 662-1600, Fax: (202) 737-0575
Association for Research and Enlightenment, (ARE), PO Box 595, Virginia Beach, VA 23451, (800) 333-4499, (based on the work of Edgar Cayce)
Association for Research and Enlightenment, (ARE) Medical Clinic, 4018 N. 41st Street, Phoenix, AZ 85018, (602) 955-0551, (information on castor oil packs and Edgar Cayce remedies)
Association for Treatment and Training in the Attachment of Children, (ATTACh), 2775 Villa Creek, Suite 240, Dallas, TX 75234, (214) 247-2329
Athena Institute for Women's Wellness, 30 Coopertown Road, Haverford, PA 19041, (610) 642-3073, Fax: (610) 642-5497., (After 1996, location will be Chester Springs, PA)
Be Healthy Inc/Positive Pregnancy and Parenting Fitness, RR#1 Box 172, Waitsfield, VT 05673, (800) 433-5523
Biofeedback Training Associates, 255 W. 98th Street, New York, NY 10025, (212) 222-5665
Birth Resources, 1749 Vine Street, Berkeley, CA 94703, (510) 526-5951
Boston Women's Health Book Collective, 240A Elm Street, Somerville, MA 02144, (617) 625-0271
C/SEC Inc, 22 Forest Street, Framingham, MA 01701, (508) 877-8266
Center for Dance Medicine, 41 E 42nd St., NY, NY 10017, (212) 661-8401
Center for Humane Options in Childbirth Experiences, (CHOICE), 3474 N. High Street, Columbus, OH 43214
Center for Women's Policy Studies, 2000 P. Street NW, Suite 508, Washington, DC 20036, (202) 872-1770

Childbirth Education Foundation, (CEF), PO Box 5, Richboro, PA 18954, (215) 357-2792

Childbirth Without Pain Education Association, (CWPEA), 20134 Snowden Avenue, Detroit, MI 48235-11170, (313) 341-3816

Circumcision Resource Center, PO Box 232, Boston, MA 02133, (617) 523-0088

Confinement Line, PO Box 1609, Springfield, VA 22151, (703) 941-7183, (for mothers on bed rest)

Dancing Thru Pregnancy, Inc. Pre/Postnatal Health and Fitness Programs, PO Box 3083, Stony Creek, CT 06405-1683, (800) 442-9034, (203) 481-2200
eMail: images@yalevm.ycc.yale.edu
homepage: http://www.dataimages.com/dtp/
(Also consulting for adolescent mothers' programs)

Doulas of North America, (DONA), 1100 23rd Avenue East, Seattle, WA 98112, (800) 448-DONA, Fax: (206) 325-0472, (resources for labor support)

Families USA, 1334 G. St. NW, 3rd Floor, Washington, DC 20005, (202) 628-3030, Fax: (202) 347-2417, eMail: HNO156@HANDSNET.ORG

Global Maternal/Child Health Association, Inc., PO Box 1400, Wilsonville, OR 97070, (503) 682-3600, (800) 641-BABY, Fax: (503) 682-3434, (resources for waterbirth)

Healthy Mothers, Healthy Babies, (HMHB), 409 12th Street SW, Room 309, Washington, DC 20024, (202) 863-2458

Home Health Products, 949 Seehawk Circle, Virginia Beach, VA 23452, (800) 284-9123

IDEA Inc, 6190 Cornerstone Court East Suite 204, San Diego, CA 92121-3773, (800) 999-IDEA, (aerobics)

National Association of Childbirth Assistants, 936-B 7th Street #301, Novato, CA 94945, (408) 225-9169

National Women's Health Network, 1325 G. Street NW, Lower Level B, Washington, DC 20005, (202) 347-1140

OB-GYN Courses, 448 Pleasant Lake Avenue, Harwich, MA 02645, (508) 432-8040, Fax: (508) 432-9685

Pacific Women's Health Services, 533 Castro Street, San Francisco, CA 94114, (415) 861-3558, (lesbian health care)

Parent Care International Inc, 9041 Colgate Street, Indianapolis, IN 46268, (317) 872-9913

Parent-to Parent, 50 North Medical Drive, Rm 2553, University of Utah Hospital, Salt Lake City, UT 84132, (801) 581-2098, (preterm and high-risk infants)

Pocket Ranch/STAR Foundation, 3960 West Sausal Lane, Healdsburg, CA 95448, (707) 431-1516, (crisis and therapy center)

Pregnancy and Infant Loss Center, 1421 E. Wayzata Blvd #30, Wayzata, MN 55391, Phone/Fax: (612) 473-9372

President's Council on Physical Fitness and Sports, Department of Health and Human Services, Washington, DC 20002

Read Natural Childbirth Foundation, PO Box 150956, San Rafael, CA 94915-0956, (415) 456-8462 or 456 3143

Sidelines National Support Network, PO Box 1808, Laguna Beach, CA 92652. Referrals and Patient Information: (714) 497 2265, magazine and educational materials, (714) 651 8673, Fax: (714) 497 5598, (complications of pregnancy)

Twin Services Inc., PO Box 1066, Berkeley, CA 94709, (510) 524 0863, Fax: (510) 524 0894

Twinless Twin Support Group International. 11220 St. Joe Road, Ft. Wayne, IN 46835, (219) 627-5414

Women to Women, 1 Pleasant Street, Yarmouth ME 04096, (207) 846-6163

Bookstores and Mail Order Items

Artemis/ Harriette Hartigan, 3337 McComb Sreet, Ann Arbor, MI 48108, (313) 677-0519, Fax: (313) 677-6606, (birth images on slides, laser disc, greeting cards, art prints)

Association for Research and Enlightenment, (ARE) Bookstore, PO Box 656 Virginia Beach VA 23451-0656, (804) 428-3588

ASPO/ Lamaze National Bookstore, 2931 S. Sepulveda Blvd., Suite F, Los Angeles, CA 90064, (800) 650-0818

Ball Dynamics, Interntional, 1616 Glenarm Place, Suite 1900, Denver, CO 80202, (800) 752-2255, Fax: (303) 893-0524

BeHealthy Inc, RR1 Box 172, Waitesfield, VT 05673, (800) 433-5523, (expectant and new parents' catalog)

Birth and Life Bookstore, 141 Commercial St. NE, Salem, OR 97301, (800) 443-9942, (503) 371-4445, (birth and health books and supplies)

Blue Poppy Press, 1775 Linden Ave, Boulder, CO 80304, (800) 487-9296, (Chinese medicine for women's health).

Cascade Health Care Products, 141 Commercial St. NE, Salem, OR 97301, (503) 371-4445, (birth and health books and supplies).

The Childbearing Years, PO Box 245, Rochester, MN 55903, (507) 289-1088, Fax: (507) 281-9597

Childbirth Graphics, PO Box 21207, Waco, TX 76702-1207, (800) 299-3366, Fax: (817) 751-0221

Down-to-Earth Books, 72 Philip Street, Albany, NY 12202, (518) 432-1578, Fax: (508) 462-6836

Echo Communications Group, 97 Perry Street, Suite 13, New York, NY 10014, (212) 255-3839, (on-line computer network on alternative birth children)

Elginex, 270 Eisenhower Lane North, Unit 4-A, Lombard, IL 60148-5403, (800) 279-5955, (weights, Theraband® etc.)

Home Health Products, 949 Seahawk Circle, Virginia Beach, VA 23452. (800) 284-9123

ICEA Bookcenter, PO Box 20004, Minneapolis, MN 55420, Fax: (800) 624-4934

March of Dimes, *Catalog of Public Health Education Materials,* PO Box 1657, Wilkes-Barre, PA 18703-1657, (800) 367-6630, Fax: (717) 825-1987

Moonflower Birthing and Herbal Supply/Natural Baby Care Products Catalog, 141 Commerical St. NE, Salem, OR 97301, (503) 371-4445, (800) 443-9942

Mother Press, RR #2, Chesley, Ontario, N0G 1L0, CANADA, (519) 363-3378

Mystic Trader, 1334 Pacific Avenue, Forest Grove, OR 97116, (800) 634-9057, Fax: (503) 457-1669, (Chinese balls)

New Atlantean Press, PO Box 9638, Santa Fe, NM 87504 Fax: (505) 183-1856

New Directions in Sound and Sight, Box 327, Botsford, CT 06404, (800) 788-6543, Fax: (203) 268-1796, (music)

New Words: A Women's Bookstore, 186 Hampshire St., Cambridge, MA 02139, (617) 876 5310, Fax: (617) 354 9066

Northeast Homeopathic Products, 563 Mass Ave Route 111, Acton, MA 01720-2903, (800) 551-3611, (508) 264-4341, Fax: (508) 263-2305

Hygieia College/Prenatal Yoga, PO Box 398, Monroe, UT 84754, (801) 527-3738

Price-Pottenger Nutrition Foundation, PO Box 2614, La Mesa, CA **Self-Self-Health Systems/** Norman Shealy, MD, Route 1, Box 216, Fair Grove, MO 65648, (417) 467-2900

Audiovisual Resources

Awakenings: Creating a Joyful Birth Experience, Sandra Bardsley, Co-Creations, PO Box 3204, Ashland, OR 97520

The Miracle of Life, Lennart Nilsson, Boston: WGBH Educational Foundation, 1983

BabyJoy: Exercises and Activities for Parents and Newborns, Elizabeth Noble, P.T. and Leo Sorger, M.D., *New Life Images*, 448 Pleasant Lake Avenue, Harwich, MA 02645, (508) 432-8040, Fax: (508) 432-9685, (video)

Back Care in Pregnancy, Rebecca Gourley Stephenson, P.T., 335 Main Street, Medfield, MA 02052, (508) 359-7835, Fax: (506) 359-6310, (video)

Channel for a New Life, (Underwater birth with Elizabeth Noble, P.T., and Leo Sorger, M.D., and a 7 year-old sister present), *New Life Images*, 448 Pleasant Lake Avenue, Harwich, MA 02645, (508) 432-8040, Fax: (508) 432-9685, (video)

Children at Birth, Academy Communications, Box 5244, Sherman Oaks, CA 91413-5222, (800) 336-4363, (301) 625-553, Fax: (301) 654-0171, (video)

Churchill Media, 6901 Woodley Avenue, Van Nuys, CA 91406-4844, (800) 334-7830, (videos)

Gentle Birth Choices, PO Box 1400, Wilsonville, OR 97070, (503) 682-3600, (800) 641-BABY, Fax: (503) 682-3434

Heartland Music, 605 South Douglas Street, Box 1034, El Segundo, CA 90245, (800) 755-2400

Injoy Videos, 3970 Broadway, Suite B4, Boulder, CO 80304, (800) 326-2082, (303) 447-2082, Fax: (303) 449-8788

Marie Osmond's Exercises for Mothers to Be, Elizabeth Noble, P.T. *New Life Images*, 448 Pleasant Lake Avenue, Harwich, MA 02645, (508) 432-8040, Fax: (508) 432-9685, (video)

Nightingale-Conant, 7300 N. LeHigh Avenue, Niles, IL 60714, (800) 572-2770, Fax: (708) 647-7145, (audiocassettes and videos)

OB Back School: P.T. Department, Woman's Hospital, PO Box 95009, Baton Rouge, LA 70895-9009, (504) 924-8450, Fax: (504) 924-8647, (slides and text for back care in pregnancy and other patient education programs for the childbearing year)

Parenting Pictures, 121 NW Crystal Street, Crystal River, FL 32629, (904) 795-2156, Fax: (904) 795-6144

Parenting Video Resource Center Catalog, Consumer Vision Inc., 149 Fifth Ave. 8th Floor, New York, NY 10010, (800) 756-8792, Fax: (212) 677-7030

Polymorph Films, 118 South Street, Boston, MA 02111, (617) 542-2004, Fax: (617) 542-4957

Sahrmann, Shirley. Exercise Series 1. Videoscope, Inc., 7701 Forsyth Blvd, Suite 900, St. Louis, MO 63105-1813, (314) 854-0340

Soothing Sounds, 6600 Silacci Way, Gilroy, CA 95020, (800) 944-2250, (audiotapes)

Swing into Shape, Lutheran Hospital, 1910 A. Avenue, WI 54601, (608) 785-0530, (video of low intensity exercises)

Spirit Music, PO Box 2240, Boulder, CO 80306, (303) 443-8181, (audiotapes)

Vida Health Communications, 6 Bigelow Streeet, Cambridge, MA 02139, (617) 864-4334, Fax: (617) 864-7862

Pelvic Floor Resources

AquaFlex® Pelvic Floor Cones, DePuy® Healthcare, Millshaw House, Manor Lane, Leeds, LS11 8LQ England, (44) 113-270-6000, (44), (800) 526-177, (free phone), Fax: (44) 113-270-9490, (two different diameter cones with insertable weights)

Dacomed Corporation, 1701 East 79th Street, Minneapolis, MN 55425, (612) 854-7522, (Set of 5 Femina™ Cones)

Essential Control Systems, 4181 Lively Lane, Dallas, TX 75220, (800) 537-3779, Fax: (214) 350-1878, (rental and sales of EMG home trainers)

Eve's Garden, 119 West 57th Street, Suite 420, NY, NY 10019, (800) 848- 3837, (212) 757-8651, (212) 977-4306, (mail order for females and their partners)

Good Vibrations, 938 Howard Street, Suite 101, San Francisco, CA 94103, (800) 289-8423, (415) 974-8990, Fax: (415) 974-8989, eMail: goodvibe@well.com

Help for Incontinent People, (HIP), PO Box 8310, Spartanburg, SC 29305-8310, (800) BLADDER

Milex, 5915 NW Highway, Chicago, IL 60631(800) 621-1278, (Kegel-type perineometer)

Perry Institute and **Perrymeter Systems**, 362 Sunset Drive, Key West, FL 33040, (305) 294-3779, Fax: (305) 294-5115, (Perrymeter™ Certification Course, equipmental sales and support)

PFX: North American Distributors, 17300 17th Street, Suite J-134, Tustin, CA 92680, (800) 995-0510, Fax: (714) 836-8551, (Pelvic floor exerciser and book *Women's Waterworks* by Pauline Chiarelli)

Sex Over Forty, PO Box 1600, Chapel Hill, NC 27515

The Simon Foundation, Box 81, Wilmette, IL 60091

Family Health Media, PO Box 1842, Charlottesville, VA 22903, (800) 366-3641, Fax: (814) 296-2289, (video: *Treating Urinary Incontinence: A Guide to Behavioral Methods*)

Society of Urologic Nurses and Associates, (SUNA), PO Box 56, Pitman, NJ 08071-0056, (609) 256-2335, Fax: (609) 589-7463

U.S .Department of Health and Human Services, Agency for Health Care Policy and Research: Urinary Incontinence in Adults. AHCPR Clearinghouse, PO Box 8547, Silver Springs, MD 20907, (800) 358-9295

The Vulvar Pain Foundation, PO Drawer 177, Graham, NC 27253, (919) 226-0704, Fax: (919) 226-8518

Womankind, PO Box 1775, Sebastopol, CA 95473, (707) 829-2744, (Menstrual Health Foundation, Lifecycle)

Journals and Newsletters

Pregnancy, Childbirth and Parenting

Birth, Blackwell Science Inc., 238 Main Street, Cambridge, MA 02142

Birth Gazette, 42 The Farm, Summertown, TN 38483, (615) 964-3895

Childbirth Instructor, PO Box 15612, N. Hollywood, CA 91615-5612, (818) 760-8983

Clarion/International Cesarean Awareness Network, (ICAN), Box 276, Clark's Summit, PA 18411-0276, (310) 530-5545

Compleat Mother, PO Box 209, Minot, ND 58702, (701) 852-2822

Doula Magazine, PO Box 7l, Santa Cruz, CA 95063-0071

Growing Child, PO Box 620, Lafayette, IN 47902-0620, (800) 927-7289, Fax: (317) 423-4495

International Journal of Childbirth Education, PO Box 20004, Minneapolis, MN 55420-0048, Fax: (612) 854-8772

International Journal of Prenatal and Perinatal Psychology and Medicine, Mattes Verlag GmbH, Postfach 103866, 69028 Heidelberg, Germany, Fax: (4) 62 21 45-9322

Journal of Family Life, 72 Philip Street, Albany, NY 12202

Journal of Nurse-Midwifery, Elsevier Science Inc, 655 Avenue of the Americas, New York, NY 10010, (212) 989-5800, Fax: (212) 633-3990

Journal of Perinatal Education, ASPO/Lamaze, 409 12th Street SW, Suite 700, Washington, DC 20024-2188, (202) 863-1648, Fax: (202) 554-0453

Lamaze Parents' Magazine, 372 Danbury Road, Wilton, CT 06897-2523, (203) 834-2711, Fax: (203) 761-8696.

Midwifery Today, PO Box 2672, Eugene, OR 97402, (800) 743-0974, (503) 344-7438 Fax: (503) 344-1422, eMail: Midwifery@aol.com

Mothering Magazine, PO Box 1690, Santa Fe, NM 87504, (800) 984-8116, (505) 984-8116, Fax: (505) 986-8335

General Health

Action on Smoking and Health, (ASH), 2013 H Street NW, Washington, DC 20006, (202) 659-4310

Consumer Reports on Health, 101 Truman Avenue, Yonkers, NY 10703-1067

Covert Bailey Newsletter, PO Box 230877, Tigard, OR 97281

Environmental Nutrition, PO Box 420501, Palm Coast, FL 32142-0451

Family Connections, PO Box 782, Radford, VA 24141

Gender and Society/Department of Sociology, University of California, Santa Barbara, CA 93106

Harvard Women's Health Watch, 25 Shattuck Street, Boston, MA 02115
Health, PO Box 56878, Boulder, CO 80321-6878
Health News Naturally Inc, PO Box 876, New Canaan, CT 06840-0876, (800) 858-7014, (203) 972-3991
Health and Longevity. Robert D. Willix Jr., M.D., PO Box 17477, Baltimore, MD 21298
Health Wisdom for Women. Christiane Northrup MD, 7811 Montrose Road, Potomac, MD 20854, (301) 424-3700
Journal of Holistic Nursing, Sage Publications Inc., PO Box 5084, Thousand Oaks, CA 91359, (805) 499-0721.
Journal of Psychohistory, 140 Riverside Drive, Suite 14H, New York, NY 10024, (212) 799-2294
3 Henriette Street, London, WC2E 8LU, England, (071) 140-0856
Melpomene Institute, 1010 University Avenue, St Paul, MN 55104 Fax: (612) 642-1871, eMail: Melpomene@webaspan.com. (women's health research)
Primal Renaissance: The Journal of Primal Psychology, Sonoma Grove/44 Varda, Rohnert Park, CA 94928, (707) 792-9851, eMail: djdp2prodigy.com
Pure Water Gazette, PO Box 2783, Denton, TX 76202, (817) 382-3814
Second Opinion, PO Box 467939, Atlanta, GA 31146-7939, (800) 728-2288
WIN-NEWS, (Women's International Network), 187 Grant Street, Lexington, MA 02173, (617)862-9431
Women's Health Advocate Newsletter, Box 420235, Palm Coast, FL 32142-0235
Women's Health Letter, PO Box 467939, Atlanta, GA 31146-7939, (800) 728-2288
Violence Against Women, Sage Publications Inc., PO Box 5084, Thousand Oaks, CA 91359, (805) 499-0721

Index

W

Y

Z

Reader Response Card

State Zip

From

New Life Images

448 Pleasant Lake Avenue
Harwich, MA 02645

Reader Response Card

From

State Zip

New Life Images

448 Pleasant Lake Avenue
Harwich, MA 02645

448 Pleasant Lake Avenue
Harwich, MA 02645

New Life Images

Tel: (508) 432-8040
Fax: (508) 432-9685

Qty		Titles by Elizabeth Noble	Price	Total
	BOOKS	Essential Exercises for the Childbearing Year, 4th edition	16.95	
		Having Twins, 2nd edition	15.95	
		Primal Connections: How Our Experiences from Conception to Birth Influence Our Emotions, Behavior and Health.	12.00	
		Childbirth with Insight	16.95	
		Marie Osmond's Exercises for Mothers and Babies	12.95	
		Having Your Baby by Donor Insemination	15.95	
		The Joy of Being a Boy, with Leo Sorger, M.D.	4.95	
	VIDEOS	Channel for a New Life (underwater birth)	35.00	
		BabyJoy: Exercises & Activities for Parents & Newborns	25.00	
		Marie Osmond's Exercises for Mothers-to-Be	30.00	
		Flo® Tube Exercises	20.00	
	AUDIO	Inside Experiences: Guided Recall for Birth and Before ***Side A*** Vaginal /***B*** Breech ***or*** ***Side A*** Vaginal /***B*** Cesarean	15.00	
	EQUIPMENT	Orange Gymnastic Ball 53 cm. diameter	20.00	
		Green Gymnastic Ball 65 cm. diameter	25.00	
		Blue Gymnastic Ball 85 cm. diameter	36.00	
		Flo® Tubes ***State your height***	30.00	
	PAYMENT	**Number of items ordered**	**Subtotal**	
		Deduct 10% for 3 or more items ordered		
			Subtotal	
		Postage: $4 for first item, $2 each extra item, gymnastic balls $6		
			TOTAL	

Name

Address

City State Zip

Mastercard/VISA

Expiration Date Signature

448 Pleasant Lake Avenue
Harwich, MA 02645

New Life Images

Tel: (508) 432-8040
Fax: (508) 432-9685

Qty		Titles by Elizabeth Noble	Price	Total
	BOOKS	Essential Exercises for the Childbearing Year, 4th edition	16.95	
		Having Twins, 2nd edition	15.95	
		Primal Connections: How Our Experiences from Conception to Birth Influence Our Emotions, Behavior and Health.	12.00	
		Childbirth with Insight	16.95	
		Marie Osmond's Exercises for Mothers and Babies	12.95	
		Having Your Baby by Donor Insemination	15.95	
		The Joy of Being a Boy, with Leo Sorger, M.D.	4.95	
	VIDEOS	Channel for a New Life (underwater birth)	35.00	
		BabyJoy: Exercises & Activities for Parents & Newborns	25.00	
		Marie Osmond's Exercises for Mothers-to-Be	30.00	
		Flo® Tube Exercises	20.00	
	AUDIO	Inside Experiences: Guided Recall for Birth and Before ***Side A*** Vaginal /***B*** Breech ***or*** ***Side A*** Vaginal /***B*** Cesarean	15.00	
	EQUIPMENT	Orange Gymnastic Ball 53 cm. diameter	20.00	
		Green Gymnastic Ball 65 cm. diameter	25.00	
		Blue Gymnastic Ball 85 cm. diameter	36.00	
		Flo® Tubes ***State your height***	30.00	
	PAYMENT	**Number of items ordered**	**Subtotal**	
			Deduct 10% for 3 or more items ordered	
			Subtotal	
		Postage: $4 for first item, $2 each extra item, gymnastic balls $6		
			TOTAL	

Name

Address

City State Zip

Mastercard/VISA

Expiration Date Signature